Günther Kern
With Collaboration of Erika Kern-Bontke

Preinvasive Carcinoma of the Cervix

Theory and Practice

Translated by Ralph M. Wynn

With 118 Figures

Springer-Verlag
Berlin Heidelberg GmbH 1968

Privatdozent Dr. GÜNTHER KERN, Oberarzt an der Universitäts-Frauenklinik Köln

Dr. ERIKA KERN-BONTKE, Universitäts-Frauenklinik Köln

RALPH M. WYNN, M. D., Associate Professor, Department of Obstetrics and Gynecology, State University of New York, Downstate Medical Center, Brooklyn, New York

Title of the Original German Edition: Carcinoma in situ, Vorstadium des Gebärmutterhalskrebses, Grundlagen und Praxis

DOI 10.1007/978-3-662-25149-2

Originally published by Springer-Verlag Berlin Heidelberg New York in 1968

MyCopy version of the original edition 1968

 Title No. 1451

www.springer.com/mycopy

Preface

It is a well known fact that the earlier the illness is recognized and treatment initiated, the better are the results of cancer therapy. The demand for earliest possible treatment generated the necessity for development of methods for the diagnosis of the earliest forms of cancer. A search for the smallest cancer thus started, leading to the recognition of epithelial changes that were undoubtedly abnormal, although their malignant nature was dubious. The long interval before a true malignant tumor develops, according to observations made by various groups of investigators all over the globe, rendered the malignant nature of the primary epithelial change unlikely. In the search for the smallest cancer, its precursor was found. It thus became possible to interrupt the chain of changes leading to cancer, through less extensive surgical intervention, before the development of the typical destructive form.

Nowhere is this sequence of events more obvious than in cancer of the uterine cervix. The easy access to these tumors made the applications of the systematically developed ingenious methods of search especially successful. Only classical histologic examination, however, can form the basis for the correct evaluation of these methods.

A great number of early changes associated with cervical cancer were discovered in recent years in Cologne through the clever application of methods for early detection. These cases represent the basis of the work of the Köln-Bonn team with regard to the morphology and classification of carcinoma in situ. In the present volume, Dr. KERN has correlated and interpreted his experiences in the recognition of the early stages with the histologic knowledge of carcinoma in situ. We have been endeavoring, especially at the Women's Clinic of Cologne University, to achieve real correlation between histopathology, clinical examination and methods of early cancer detection, which together form the only possible basis of a synopsis like this.

We wish the book and its readers the greatest success, which will be achieved when these problems are more thoroughly understood, and many patients therefore spared the fate of cervical cancer.

July 1964

H. HAMPERL, Bonn
C. KAUFMANN, Köln

Introduction

Early detection of carcinoma of the cervix is being pursued in many parts of the world with great intensity. Special methods have been developed with increasing success, so that cancer of the cervix uteri may now be regarded as a "preventable disease." The success of early detection is the more significant in view of the incidence of the disease of 2 per cent.

There are, in addition to the literature accumulated over the decades, monographs on this subject in many languages, frequently describing only certain aspects of the problems involved. There are, for instance, magnificent atlases that deal with cytologic cancer detection and frequently exceed the realm of gynecology. Well-illustrated textbooks of colposcopy present all the basic concepts of this method, and the histopathological characteristics of early forms of carcinoma of the cervix have also been described often.

This book attempts to present a survey of the entire complex of the problems of the early detection of carcinoma of the cervix. The reader is given information about the basic nature of so-called carcinoma in situ, its symptomatology, and the available diagnostic and therapeutic procedures. In addition, detailed advice is given about clinical and laboratory methods, since they enhance the chances of successful cancer detection.

The following pages reflect the experiences gained in this field at the Women's Clinic of Cologne University. Only brief mention is made of those methods and problems not encompassed by our own experience.

The early diagnosis of carcinoma of the cervix has been greatly aided by the collaboration with Professor H. K. ZINSER, who was in charge of our cytological laboratory from 1955 to 1956.

The observations concerning the physiologic epithelial changes in the cervix uteri, as well as the technique developed in the histological laboratory of our clinic for the preparation of whole cervices and uteri, represent a great contribution to this book. Early detection and histopathology at the same clinic, but in different hands, complemented each other most favorably. The histologic examinations were conducted in collaboration with Professors H. HAMPERL, C. KAUFMANN, and K. G. OBER.

A study of the literature reveals the great interest in the early detection of carcinoma of the cervix. The abundance of relevant publications required restriction of citations to significant and historically important papers only; it was not easy to make a fair selection.

The following pages present the opinions and results of the Women's Clinic of Cologne University concerning the morphology, symptomatology, diagnosis, and therapy of carcinoma in situ. Each chapter is incomplete without the others, just as successful early detection of cervical carcinoma is possible only through close cooperation between clinician and histopathologist.

The mastery of such extensive material is not within the capability of one person. I should like at this point to thank my colleagues, H. P. Bötzelen, E. Hinderfeld, E. Rissmann, and G. Stadler, and the technical assistants, H. Gräfin zu Eulenburg, U. Kownatzki, I. Lange, M. Pletten, R. Sayffaerth and K. Wahlhäuser for their cooperation and help.

I thank the Kultusministerium des Landes Nordrhein-Westfalen for generous financial support of the work on the problems of early cancer detection.

Köln, July 1964 Günther Kern

Table of Contents

Early Stages of Carcinoma of the Cervix

Historical Introduction

The first description and illustration of a cancer that grew only on the surface of the cervix uteri is that of Sir J. WILLIAMS (1886). He emphasized that the change had been found incidentally and had remained symptomless. He noticed also that the change had remained for a long time on the surface. The histologic drawing showed a carcinoma in situ growing into cervical glands. There followed similar descriptions of the earliest phases of cervical carcinoma growing on the surface, by CULLEN (1900, 1921), SCHOTTLÄNDER (1907), SCHAUENSTEIN (1908), PRONAI (1909) and RUBIN (1910). The terms "surface carcinoma" or "early carcinoma" were coined in a monograph by SCHOTTLÄNDER and KERMAUNER (1912). Thereafter, interest in superficial cancer of the cervix seemed to subside temporarily.

The number of superficial cancers detected increased considerably in the German-speaking countries after the introduction of colposcopy by HINSELMANN (1925), and interest in problems of the "smallest cancer" reappeared. In 1927, SCHILLER tried to find clinical methods for the early recognition of these epithelial changes, which up to that time had been found only in operative specimens. SCHILLER called the surface carcinoma "preinvasive" and v. FRANQUÉ "precancerous" (1927). The designation "cancer" was at first rejected during the twenties, because infiltrating growth, as postulated by VIRCHOW, was absent. ROBERT MEYER, however, did not insist on this requirement and classified the malignant epithelium according to its structure and degree of maturity (1923).

BRODERS, in 1932, first used the term "carcinoma in situ", which has since been accepted internationally.

It was generally assumed that the superficial change, if untreated, progressed to an invasive stage and that radical removal or destruction through hysterectomy or irradiation was indicated. This assumption was corroborated by numerous publications, in which superficial carcinomas persisted after the diagnosis of invasive carcinomas had been made in previously performed biopsies. HINSELMANN was the first to demonstrate, in 1933, a case of this kind.

The diagnosis of the earliest stages of cervical carcinoma received new impetus through the introduction by PAPANICOLAOU of the cytologic method. It found wide acceptance in America at the beginning of the forties, while the second world war delayed its acceptance in Europe by several years.

Translator's Note. In preparing the English edition of this text I have attempted to make the translation as literal as possible, within the bounds of idiomatic American usage. The statements and concepts, however, are strictly those of the author.

R. M. W.

The more carcinomas in situ were detected, the more frequently it was observed that the change could remain stationary for a long period. It was slowly recognized that carcinoma in situ required less radical therapy than clinical carcinoma.

Gynecologists and pathologists have been and still are equally interested in the problems of carcinoma in situ of the cervix uteri.

Histologic Features of Early Stages of Cervical Carcinoma

Carcinoma of the cervix exhibits, in its clinical course, all the signs of malignancy. The tumor infiltrates and destroys neighboring organs; it metastasizes and kills the host within a predictable time. These characteristics mark a tumor as a cancer.

All therapeutic efforts to cure carcinoma of the cervix are directed toward the total removal or destruction of the cancerous tissue. The results, however, are not satisfactory because the tumor frequently has already followed its fateful tendency to metastasize when therapy is begun. If the cure rate of the most frequent female genital carcinoma is to be improved, it can be only by treatment at an early stage, when the malignant epithelium has not yet acquired all the potentialities of cancerous growth, especially metastasis. Through the use of certain diagnostic methods, many of these early stages have been detected during the past three or four decades, although their terminology, interpretation, and mode of treatment were far from uniform.

Nomenclature of the Early Stages of Carcinoma of the Cervix

In accordance with the historical development, the observed change was at first called a "surface carcinoma" because of the belief that it was a cancer that grew only on the surface of the cervix. The term "carcinoma in situ" originated in America; it was based on the impression that cancerous tissue was growing in situ, that is, in the location of normal epithelium. This term has been accepted internationally and will, therefore, be used here. The expression is, however, not entirely satisfactory, because it contains the ominous word "carcinoma". The term "markedly atypical epithelium" is more appropriate because it comprises in a short expression the morphologic feature of the change. Even in American literature the expression "markedly atypical epithelium" is used. In France, the term "intraepithelial epithelioma" (Funck-Brentano, 1960) is preferred. An international committee (Blaikley, Kottmeier, Martius and Meigs) in 1958 decided to call the preinvasive stages of carcinoma of the cervix Stage 0 without including this stage in the clinical classification I—IV, since it was doubtful that carcinoma in situ invariably represented a premalignant lesion.

The terms mentioned are, therefore, synonyms for the same epithelial change. In addition to this terminology, there are many other names. Held as far back as 1953 collected no fewer than 19 synonyms.

What Does "Carcinoma in Situ of the Cervix" Mean?

Carcinoma in situ is a disease of the squamous epithelium in the area of the cervix uteri. The epithelium shows a transformation with all the histologic signs of malignancy, without extending beyond the limits of the squamous epithelium. Thus, one of the most essential characteristics of malignant growth, invasion, is absent.

During the last decades, many cases of carcinoma in situ have been observed so that further statements may be made about their malignant potential: carcinoma in situ does not metastasize. The change has three very precise characteristics: histologic signs of malignancy in the epithelium, absence of infiltration and no metastases. These observations mean, furthermore, that carcinoma in situ is not a cancer, or, more precisely, not yet a cancer in the classical sense. This statement is extremely important, because the treatment of carcinoma in situ need not, or rather must not, be radical cancer therapy.

There are important reasons for considering carcinoma in situ a precursor of cervical carcinoma. The lesion must therefore be removed in order to save the patient from an invasive cancer of the cervix.

Histologic Characteristics of Carcinoma in Situ

The normal squamous epithelium of the portio is characterized by a distinct stratification.

Carcinoma in situ lacks the intraepithelial architecture of the normal squamous epithelium. There is either no stratification at all in the diseased epithelium or barely perceptible traces of it on the surface (Fig. 1). Usually, the so-called basal layer with very tightly packed rows of cells is not clearly defined. No differentiation occurs above this layer. The epithelium seems filled with tightly packed cells from the basal layer to the surface. Only on the surface may flattened cells with dark nuclei be found. The intraepithelial structure of carcinoma in situ is, however, not uniform in individual cases. Different degrees of maturation may be observed even within a single specimen. On examining the epithelium with a magnifying glass carcinoma in situ is recognized by its dark appearance, resulting from the increase in nuclear density. Its nuclei are round or oval with a coarse chromatin pattern. Variation in size is frequent, and the nuclear-cytoplasmic ratio is increased.

Hillemanns and Rha (1961 I, II) were able to confirm this impression by measuring nuclear and cytoplasmic volumes. In comparison with normal epithelium and with forms in transition to dysplasia, carcinoma in situ exhibits a minimum of cytoplasm and a maximum of nuclear volume. Infiltrating cancers do not exhibit these features.

Intercellular bridges are not usually visible in markedly atypical epithelium. The cells are so tightly packed that their individual outlines are obscured. Calculation of cellular density per unit of surface, likewise, indicated maximal values for carcinoma in situ (Foraker and Reagan, 1959; Hillemanns and Rha, 1961).

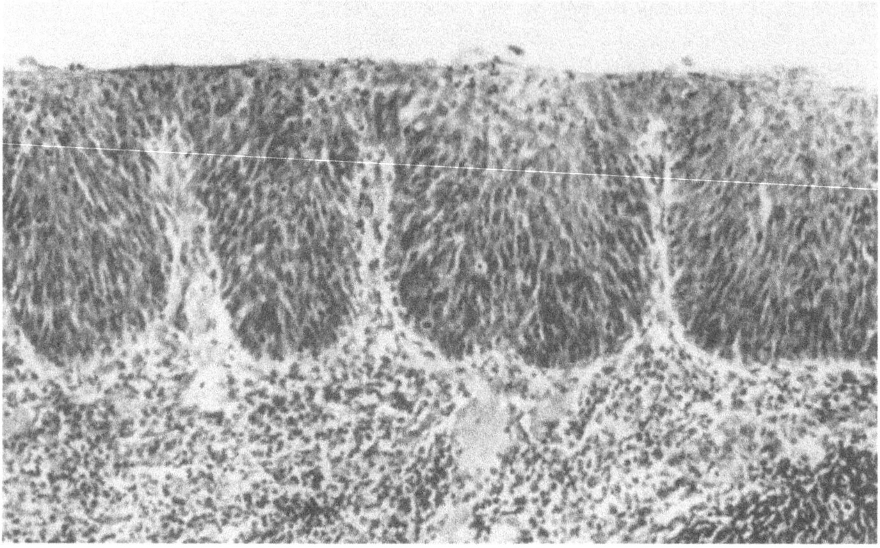

Fig. 1. Carcinoma in situ. The epithelium is characterized by the closely packed nuclei. The subepithelial leucocytic and lymphocytic infiltration is distinct

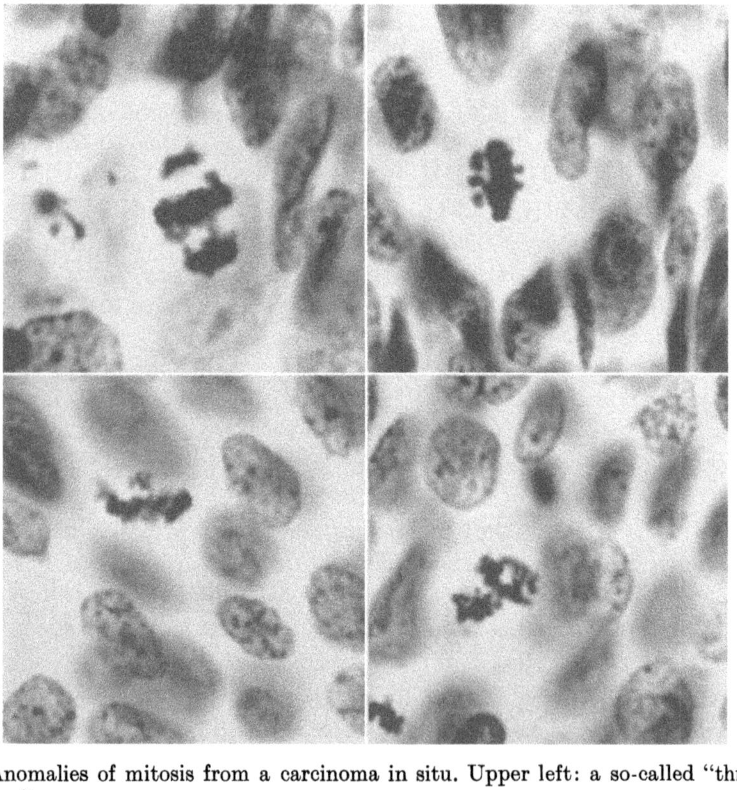

Fig. 2. Anomalies of mitosis from a carcinoma in situ. Upper left: a so-called "three-group metaphase"

The capacity to store glycogen has been lost in most cases. The markedly atypical epithelium contains virtually no glycogen. This property is utilized in one method of clinical examination (see Iodine test, p. 149).

The marked proliferation of the epithelium is reflected by numerous mitoses that are not limited to the basal layer but may be seen throughout the entire epithelium. Carcinoma in situ very often exhibits atypical mitoses that were

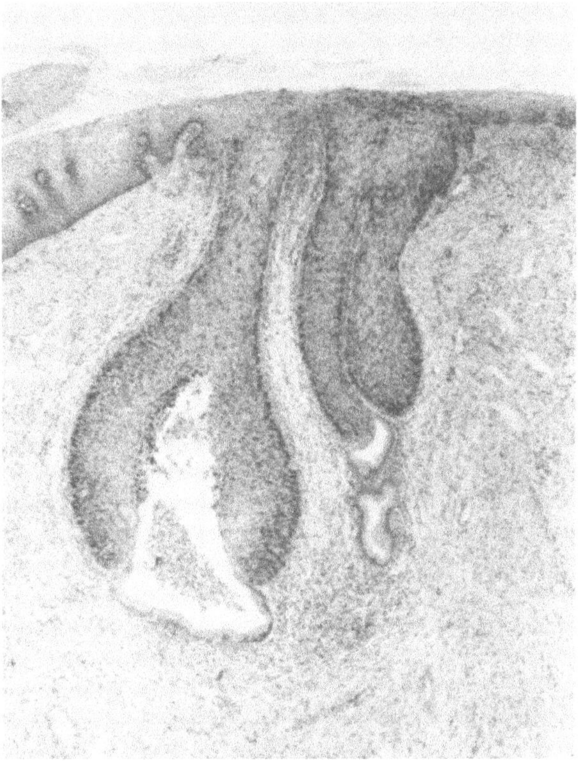

Fig. 3. Invasion of markedly atypical epithelium into cervical glands. In the left upper corner, normal squamous epithelium

described as "three-group metaphases" by DUSTIN and PARMENTIER (1953) (Fig. 2). These are mitoses in which the chromosomes are arranged at the equatorial plate, while some smaller groups of chromosomes appear at the poles; as a result, three groups of chromosomes appear during the division of the nucleus. There are, furthermore, many more varieties of atypical mitoses in carcinoma in situ.

The lateral boundary of a carcinoma in situ is usually the normal squamous epithelium of the part of the vaginal membrane that covers the surface of the portio distally, and the columnar epithelium of the cervical canal proximally (BAJARDI, 1962).

The transition from carcinoma in situ to normal squamous epithelium differs from case to case. The boundary is frequently so well defined that the separation of the two kinds of epithelium can be made from two adjacent cells. The line of separation often runs diagonally through the epithelium, causing the diseased portion to push against the normal like a plowshare (Fig. 6). It is difficult to tell whether its growth proceeds in this way.

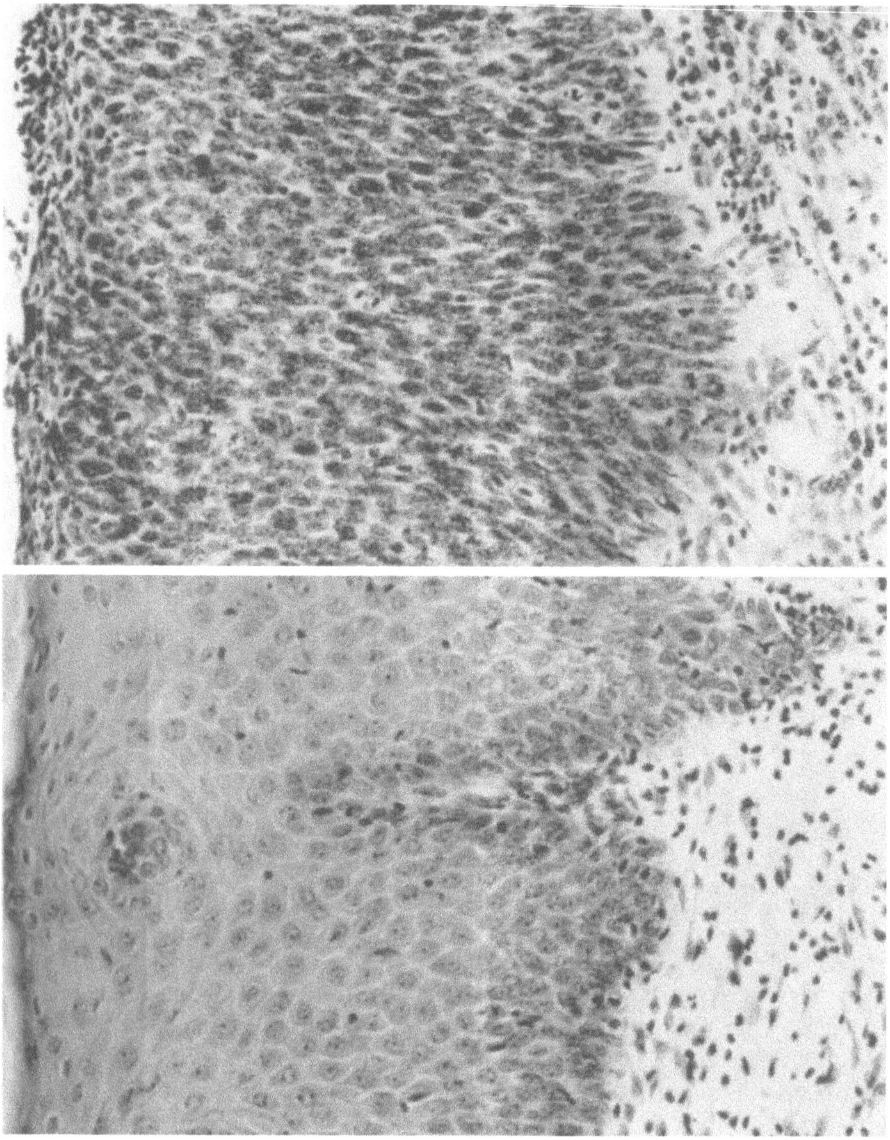

Fig. 4. Comparison of normal squamous epithelium (left) with markedly atypical epithelium (right)

In other cases, the separation is not well defined; the carcinoma in situ changes into a more dysplastic epithelium, which is followed by an epithelium exhibiting many mitoses and basal cell hyperactivity. There are many variations of this pattern.

The growth of carcinoma in situ towards the columnar epithelium resembles that of normal squamous epithelium. It may be immediately adjacent to the columnar epithelium without any reaction, but it may, on the other hand, lift it off its base by narrow tongues of epithelium. The impression seems to prevail, however, that this is the actual growth of the carcinoma in situ. The columnar epithelium is displaced, as may also be seen in the penetration into cervical glands. This property should not, however, be considered a true tendency to destroy tissue, because the same feature may be observed in normal squamous epithelium (Fig. 3).

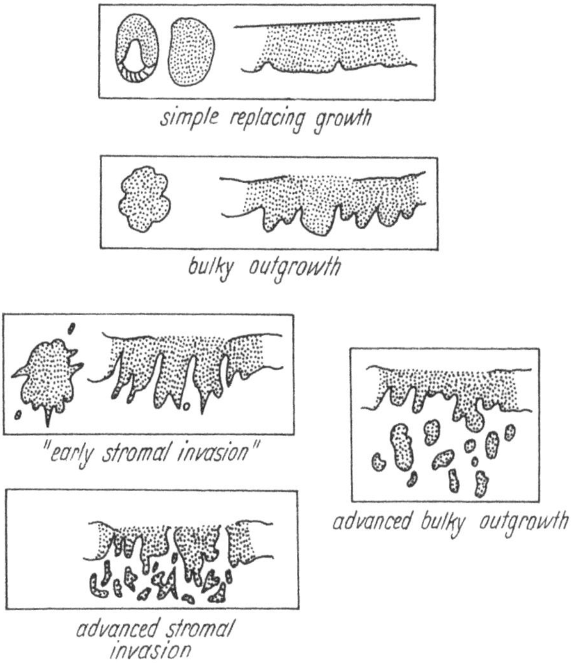

Fig. 5. Schematic classification of carcinoma in situ according to Hamperl (1959). (From: Ciba Foundation Study Group No. 3, Cancer of the Cervix. Diagnosis of early forms, pp. 2—19. London: J. & A. Churchill Ltd., 1959)

The histologic structure of a carcinoma in situ, as compared with normal squamous epithelium, is shown in Fig. 4. The change is striking and the microscopic impression is distinctly malignant; hence, the designation of "surface cancer" is understandable histologically.

Carcinoma in situ is not limited to the portio alone, but occurs as a precancerous lesion wherever there is squamous epithelium or any other kind of epithelium that can undergo squamous metaplasia (skin, larynx, pharynx, esophagus). Their appearances are practically indistinguishable.

Histological descriptions of markedly atypical epithelium may be found in papers by: Younge (1939), Wespi (1946), Novak (1947), Scapier, Day and Durfee (1952), Held (1953), Lax (1953), Büngeler and Dontenwill (1954), Hamperl, Kaufmann and Ober (1954 I, II), Büngeler (1955), Fennell jr. (1955, 1956), Feyrter (1955), Navratil (1955),

RUNGE and STOLL (1955), HAMPERL and KAUFMANN (1956), LIMBURG (1956), RANDERATH and HIERONYMI (1956), WHEELER (1956), HERTIG (1957), HILLEMANNS (1958), FRIEDELL, HERTIG and YOUNGE (1958), KOTTMEIER, KARLSTEDT, SANTESSON and MOBERGER (1959), HAMPERL (1959, 1960), BLANCHARD (1960), KAUFMANN and OBER (1960), TAYLOR (1961), FRICK, JANOVSKI, GUSBERG and TAYLOR (1963). A Symposium on the histomorphology of carcinoma in situ in Acta cytol. 1961 reveals the still present uncertainties and differences concerning the morphological diagnosis, particularly in the definition of cytomorphological intraepithelial changes (BAJARDI, DE BRUX, DUPRÉ-FROMENT, SIEGLER, SIRTORI and TAYLOR, 1961; BAJARDI, GAUDEFROY, KRIMMENAU and TAYLOR, 1961).

Whereas 30 to 40 years ago knowledge about carcinoma in situ came from incidental findings in surgical or post mortem specimens, the number of cases detected increased rapidly upon the introduction of methods of so-called early diagnosis. Attempts were made to discover in the multitude of cases a progression with transition to real cancer. At the end of 1959, we had available more than 150 cases which were serially sectioned. Using this material, HAMPERL worked out a morphological classification, which he presented at the Ciba symposium in 1959. Since that time, we have been using this classification. It is based upon the behavior of the abnormal epithelium toward the cervical stroma rather than upon nuclear anomalies, disturbances of mitosis, and so forth, in the epithelium. Fig. 5 diagrammatically illustrates the classification chosen by HAMPERL (1959, 1961).

Simple Replacing Growth

This simplest form of carcinoma in situ gives the impression that diseased epithelium replaces the normal squamous epithelium without changing the form of the latter. The possibility must be considered, however, that the cervical epithelium is undergoing metaplastic transformation into squamous epithelium. There is no unevenness at the surface. Towards the stroma, the smooth boundary of the normal squamous epithelium lies adjacent to the abnormal epithelium without any transition. The papillae of the stroma are normal. A lymphocytic subepithelial infiltration is usually noticeable, whereas it is absent in normal epithelium (Fig. 6). Carcinoma in situ during its growth behaves like normal squamous epithelium; that is, it may grow around and occlude the ducts of cervical glands. It may grow into these glands and fill them partially or totally (Fig. 3). In the latter case, isolated, smoothly outlined epithelial nests may then be seen, all of which, however, are still lying within the area of the cervical glands.

Bulky Outgrowth

In this group, there is a change at the boundary of the stroma insofar as the abnormal epithelium advances in plump projections towards the stroma, clearly visible on the surface as well as in the cervical glands. Accordingly, the papillae of the stroma become considerably deeper. The impression is gained of increased pressure within the epithelium because of the increase in nuclear density, which causes bulging as in an overfilled sack (Fig. 7). More cells appear to exfoliate on the surface, since the histologic section usually shows superficial

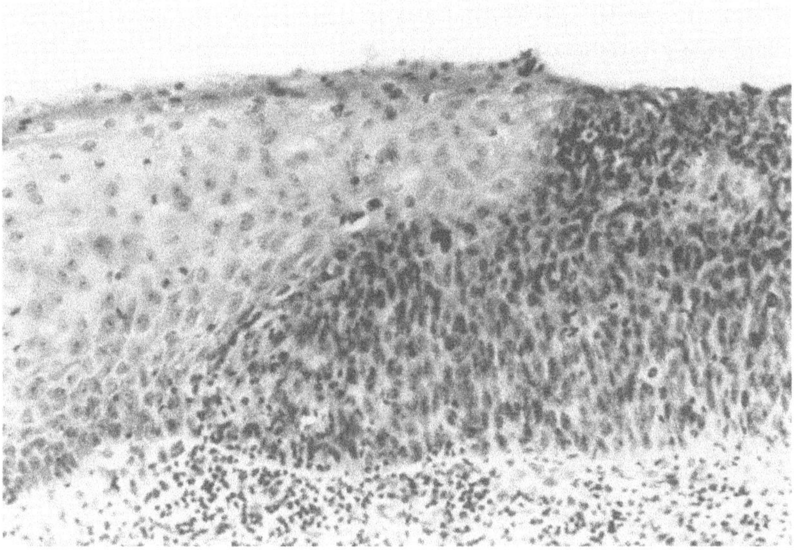

Fig. 6. Carcinoma in situ. Growth through "simple replacement", according to HAMPERL. Transition of carcinoma in situ to normal squamous epithelium. The pathologically altered epithelium is wedged beneath the normal epithelium. The subepithelial inflammatory infiltration is clearly seen in the area of the carcinoma in situ. In this case there is a sharp separation between normal epithelium and carcinoma in situ

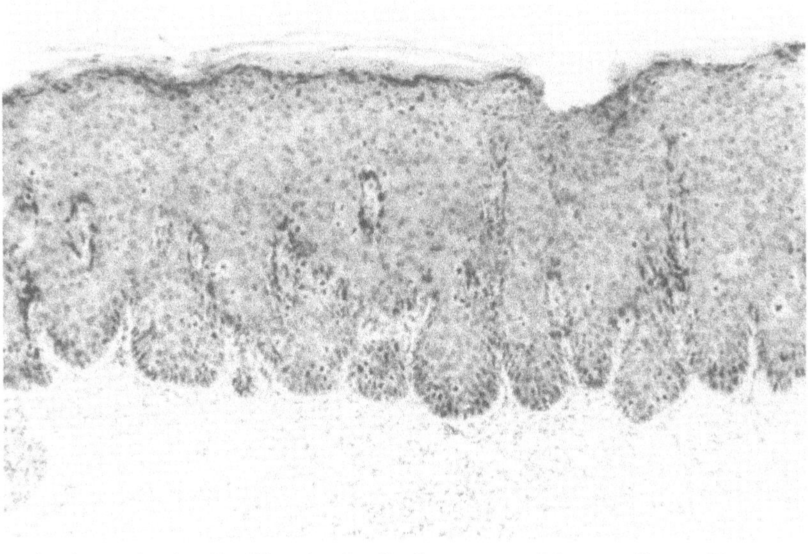

Fig. 7. Carcinoma in situ. Proliferation by "bulky outgrowth", according to HAMPERL

defects in the covering cellular layers. The epithelium growing in the cervical glands is similarly affected. It blocks its own exit and exfoliates cells in the center, leading to cystic dilatations.

Carcinoma in situ typically includes the groups "simple replacing growth" and "bulky outgrowth". It can be clearly distinguished from infiltrating carcinoma and easily recognized by its sharply defined borders.

The differentiation from the epithelial atypias known as dysplastic epithelium, basal hyperplasias, and so forth, is not uniform internationally (Fig. 8) (HERTIG

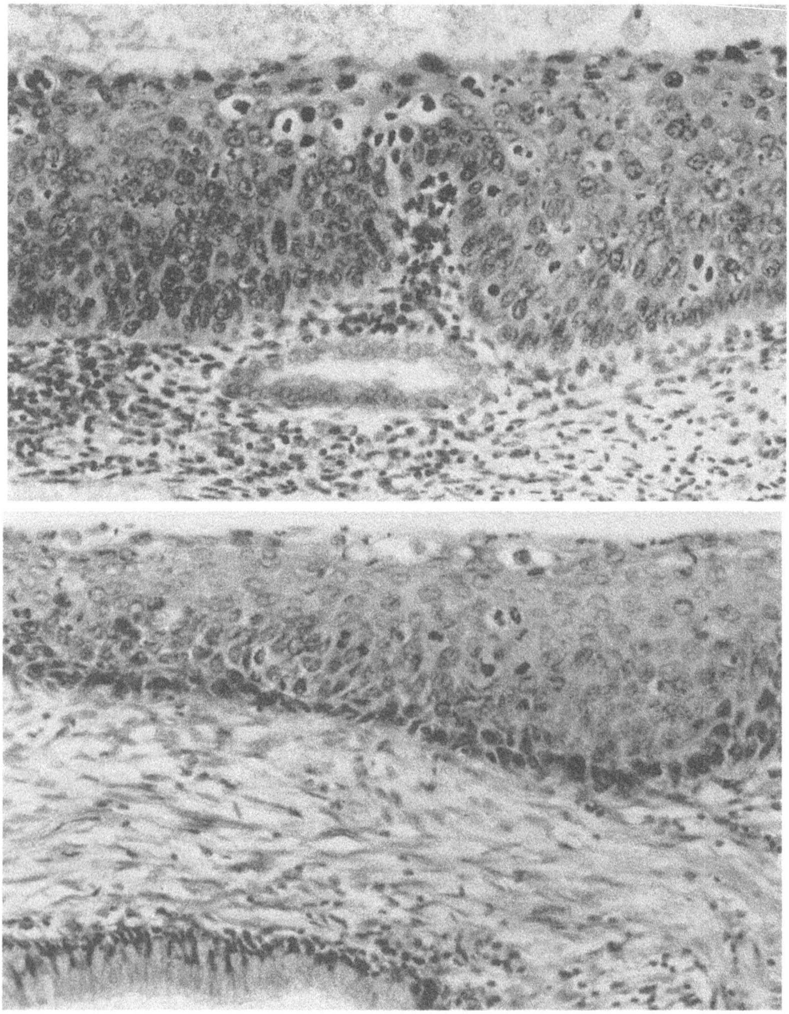

Fig. 8. Two instances of epithelial changes that are "not yet" considered carcinoma in situ. The difficulties of this distinction are obvious

and YOUNGE, 1952; MESTWERDT, 1957; ZACHERL, 1957; KRIMMENAU, 1958; BEHRENS and TIETZE, 1959; GROSS, POSPÍSIL, VIKLICKÝ and ZAVADIL, 1959; DE BRUX and DUPRÉ-FROMENT, 1960; OBER, KAUFMANN and HAMPERL, 1961; REAGAN and PATTEN Jr., 1962; LAMBERT and WOODRUFF, 1963; KOSS, STEWART et al., 1963; BANGLE, BERGER and LEVIN, 1963).

Early Stromal Invasion

In this condition, a change occurs in the behavior of the atypical epithelium towards the cervical stroma. Individual cells advance into the stroma in narrow protuberances, usually from the tightly packed cells of the epithelial nests. As soon as the cells free themselves from the narrow restriction of the abnormal epithelium, growing in slender protuberances toward the stroma, they often change

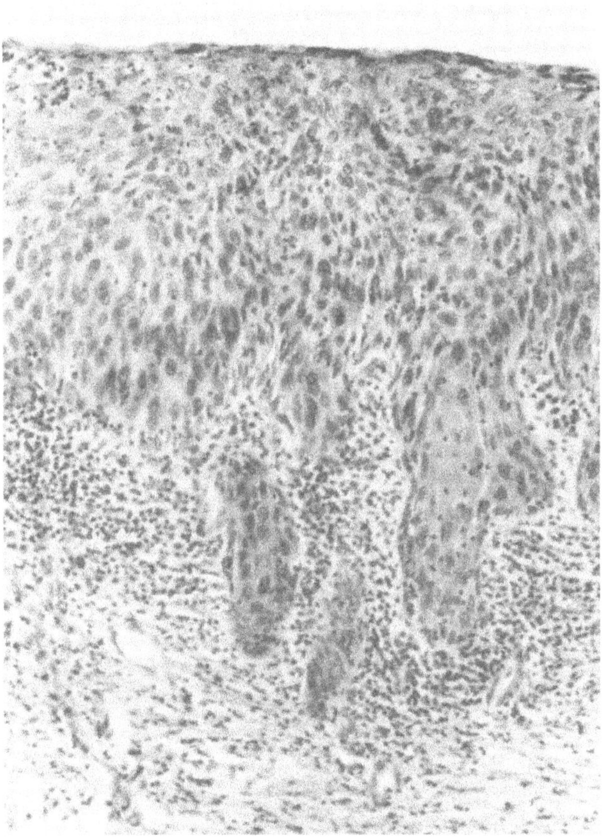

Fig. 9. "Early stromal invasion", according to HAMPERL. Beginning cellular differentiation in the outgrowing cellular projections. Inflammatory stromal reaction

their shape. They appear richer in cytoplasm and they often exhibit intracellular keratinization (Fig. 9). The accumulation of PAS-positive substances may also occur. The reaction of the cervical stroma is usually a marked leucocytic infiltration that attacks the intruding pathologic cells. If the abnormal cells have lost their connection with the epithelium, they usually succumb to the leucocytic attack. The outgrowth of cellular processes into the cervical stroma always occurs multicentrically. According to the histologic picture, the epithelial surface seems to exfoliate cells in large numbers. The histologic section shows occasionally that by loss of cells the epithelium becomes lower and stromal papillae bearing vessels reach the surface. In this case, slight bleeding from the epithelium will probably be found clinically. FENNELL (1955) described this picture as "early stromal invasion" (FIDLER and BOYES, 1959; BAJARDI, 1959). In these cases the abnormal epithelium shows its malignant property of infiltration. It is impossible to predict how long the balance between the cellular defense reaction and the invading malignant cells will continue. The group called "early stromal invasion" was named Stage Ia in the international classification in Vienna in 1961.

Advanced Stromal Invasion

In this form the malignant growth has upset the equilibrium between early stromal invasion and host reaction. The neoplastic cells invade the cervical stroma in narrow strands, forming a more or less fine network. Here, too, the

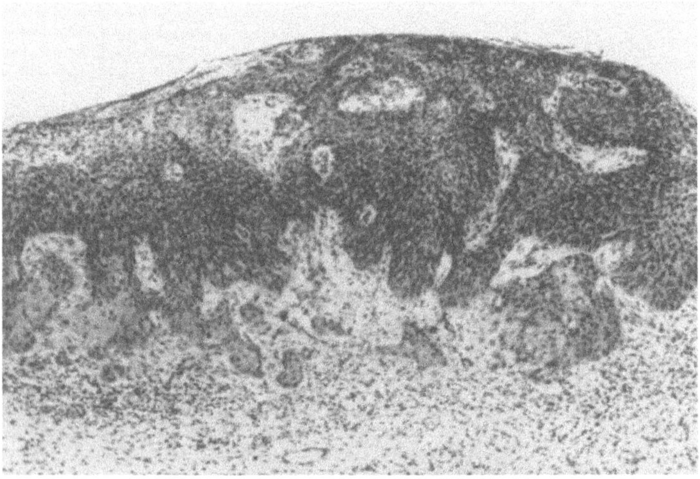

Fig. 10. "Advanced stromal invasion" (microcarcinoma), according to HAMPERL, in an ared of about 5 millimeters within a carcinoma in situ. The groups of cells that have separatea from the main epithelial mass contain more cytoplasm

development is multicentric, not originating in one neoplastic focus. The growth of a nest of neoplastic cells of this kind is, however, limited to an area of a few millimeters, whereas carcinoma in situ may occupy an area of several centimeters.

In this condition, as in early stromal invasion, the neoplastic cells liberated from the compact epithelial tissue usually develop more cytoplasm with certain signs of differentiation. The intense stromal reaction continues (Fig. 10). The surface of the altered epithelium is usually ulcerated. Several synonyms are used to describe this change: preclinical carcinoma, Stage Ib of the international classification of carcinoma of the cervix, microcarcinoma (according to MESTWERDT), or the purely descriptive term: advanced stromal invasion.

The diagnosis of advanced stromal invasion is not difficult morphologically, but it presents problems in the limitation of the term. How far can such a lesion spread and still justifiably be called microcarcinoma? In our material, we consider the upper limit of size to be that of a grain of rice or a lentil.

Advanced Bulky Outgrowth

HAMPERL delineated this special group in 1959. It is relatively small, as judged by its frequency, but it shows some peculiarities that justify this classification.

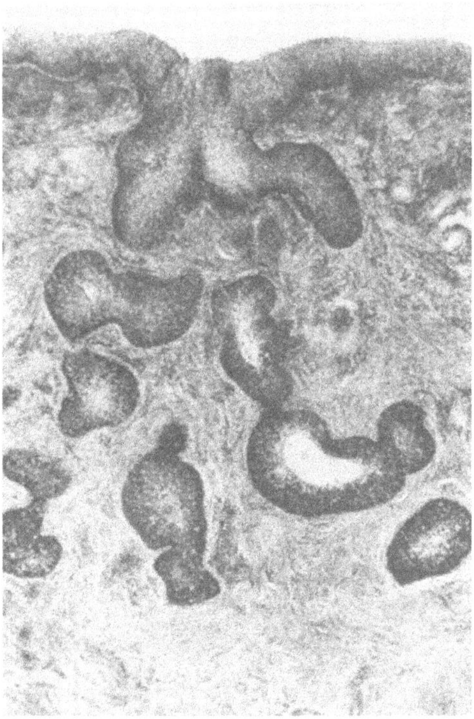

Fig. 11. "Advanced bulky outgrowth", according to HAMPERL. (From: Ciba Foundation Study Group No. 3, Cancer of the Cervix. Diagnosis of early forms, pp. 2—19. London: J. & A. Churchill Ltd. 1959)

Morphologically, the growth of the blunt projections here seems to turn into a broad infiltrating lesion (Fig. 11). This change usually involves a large area. First, the advancing blunt epithelial projections completely fill all glands; they are not limited to the existing cavities but extend beyond them. It is a peculiarity of this form of growth that there is, in general, no striking stromal reaction.

The infiltration of lymph nodes has been reported in a few cases of so-called microcarcinoma: LAX (1953), DECKER (1956), ZACHERL and SCHÜLLER (1957), SCHÜLLER (1958), FRIEDELL and GRAHAM (1959), FANGER and MURPHY (1960) and LOCK (Discussion of LATOUR, 1961).

In our clinic, the histological diagnosis in HAMPERL's classification is based on serial sections (see p. 173) according to the severest change detected.

The histologic pictures of simple replacing growth, bulky outgrowth, early stromal invasion, advanced stromal invasion with netlike infiltration and advanced bulky outgrowth are grouped together as *early stages of carcinoma of the cervix*. It is the purpose of early diagnosis to detect the disease in these stages.

Is Carcinoma in Situ the Precursor of Cervical Carcinoma?

A study of the histologic pictures within the groups described by HAMPERL gives the definite impression of a continuous process. Proof is lacking, however, since the material studied was obtained from different patients. Since it was removed *in toto*, moreover, its further development was interrupted.

The indication of continuous development may be found in the ages of the patients as well as in the morphologic picture. KAUFMANN and OBER (1960) and OBER, KAUFMANN and HAMPERL (1961) calculated the average age of the patients in HAMPERL'S classification in relation to the various stages of clinical cancer:

Table 1. (According to OBER, KAUFMANN, HAMPERL, 1961)

Type of change	Number of cases	Average age (years)	
Simple atypia, dysplasia, epithelial disturbance	32	36.1	(18—52)
Early cases:			
Simple replacing growth	182	39.5	(22—74)
Bulky outgrowth	110	42.2	(24—71)
Early stromal invasion	43	45.2	(32—64)
Advanced stromal invasion	31	45.5	(32—67)
Advanced bulky outgrowth	15	47.2	(34—62)
Clinical cancers:			
Stage I	123	46.3	(24—78)
Stage II	115	51.6	(30—81)
Stage III	68	56.5	(37—83)
Stage IV	9	60.4	(54—73)

Table 1 shows a continuous increase in the average age and could therefore perhaps be taken as an indication of a chronological sequence of the changes (HERTIG and YOUNGE, 1952; STERN, 1959; DUNN, 1960; ISBELL and GROVER, 1961).

The localization of carcinoma in situ is the same as that of clinical cancer of the cervix. Women from various social strata with early marriages, multiparas, and certain racial groups are afflicted by carcinoma in situ to the same extent as by clinical cancer. Another significant factor seems to be luetic infection (WESPI and SAUTER, 1943; LOMBARD and POTTER, 1950; WEINER, BURKE and GOLDBERGER, 1951; WYNDER *et al.*, 1954; OBER and REINER, 1955; WYNDER, 1956/57, 1957; DUNN and BUELL, 1959; HAENSZEL and HILLHOUSE, 1959; KAST, 1959; RUNGE and ZEITS, 1959; CHRISTOPHERSON and PARKER, 1960; HUBER,

1960; WYNDER and LICKLIDER, 1960; WYNDER, MANTEL and LICKLIDER, 1960; TERRIS, 1962; BOYES and FIDLER, 1963).

Another indication of the close relation of the two diseases is that carcinoma in situ often borders on areas of invasive carcinoma. OBER, KAUFMANN and HAMPERL found among 100 cases of invasive carcinoma 61 with adjacent in situ lesions (1961). BAJARDI (1962), too, believes that the in situ lesion at the margin of a clinical cancer indicates a relation between the two conditions (TREITE, 1944; HELD, 1954; GIACCAI, 1956; BURGHARDT, 1958; LANGE, 1960; BAJARDI and SIRTORI, 1961).

Finally, several authors observed the course of patients with untreated carcinoma in situ. The results, unfortunately, cannot be fully evaluated because punch biopsies were used. PAPANICOLAOU (1958) stated that this method was not ideal because each biopsy might represent total removal of the lesion, and the nature of the adjacent tissue remained unknown. AYRE and AYRE, in 1949, studied, mainly by cytology, the development of a true cancer from a preinvasive lesion (BAJARDI, 1959; BODDINGTON, COWDELL and SPRIGGS, 1960). PETERSEN (1955 and discussion at the Ciba symposium 1959) observed a group of 127 patients with carcinoma in situ for up to 8 years, either untreated or incompletely treated with radium or cautery. Of these patients, 24.6% developed clinical carcinomas up to the time that this book was written. Careful observations are available, made during the years that elapsed between the diagnosis of carcinoma in situ and of clinical cancer, by MESTWERDT and MÖNCKEBERG (1948), YOUNGE, HERTIG and ARMSTRONG (1949), RUNGE and STOLL (1955), LIMBURG (1956), MASTERSON (1956), JONES, GALVIN and TELINDE (1956/57), HÖRMANN and FREESE (1957), MORICARD and CARTIER (1957), FERGUSON and LOZMAN (1958), LANGE (1960), PETERSEN (1961), BOYES, FIDLER and LOCK (1962). FORAKER (1956, 1959) believes, on the basis of histochemical and morphological investigations, that carcinoma in situ more closely resembles cancer than normal epithelium. GLATTHAAR (1948) arrives at the same opinion on the basis of the behavior of tissue cultures of markedly atypical epithelium. The investigations by ESCHBACH and BRUCKER of DNA point in the same direction (1959, 1960).

All these observations indicate that carcinoma in situ must be considered a preliminary stage of cervical carcinoma.

Normal Epithelium of the Cervix Uteri

Two totally different kinds of epithelium meet in the cervix: the squamous epithelium of the vaginal mucosa and the columnar epithelium of the endocervix. Both epithelia not only are adjacent to each other but interdigitate within a certain area, as shown by certain colposcopic and histologic observations.

The Squamous Epithelium

The surface of the portio, or at least its periphery, is covered by nonkeratinizing squamous epithelium. Coming from the vault it stretches smoothly across the surface of the cervix. It consists of the following layers (Fig. 12):

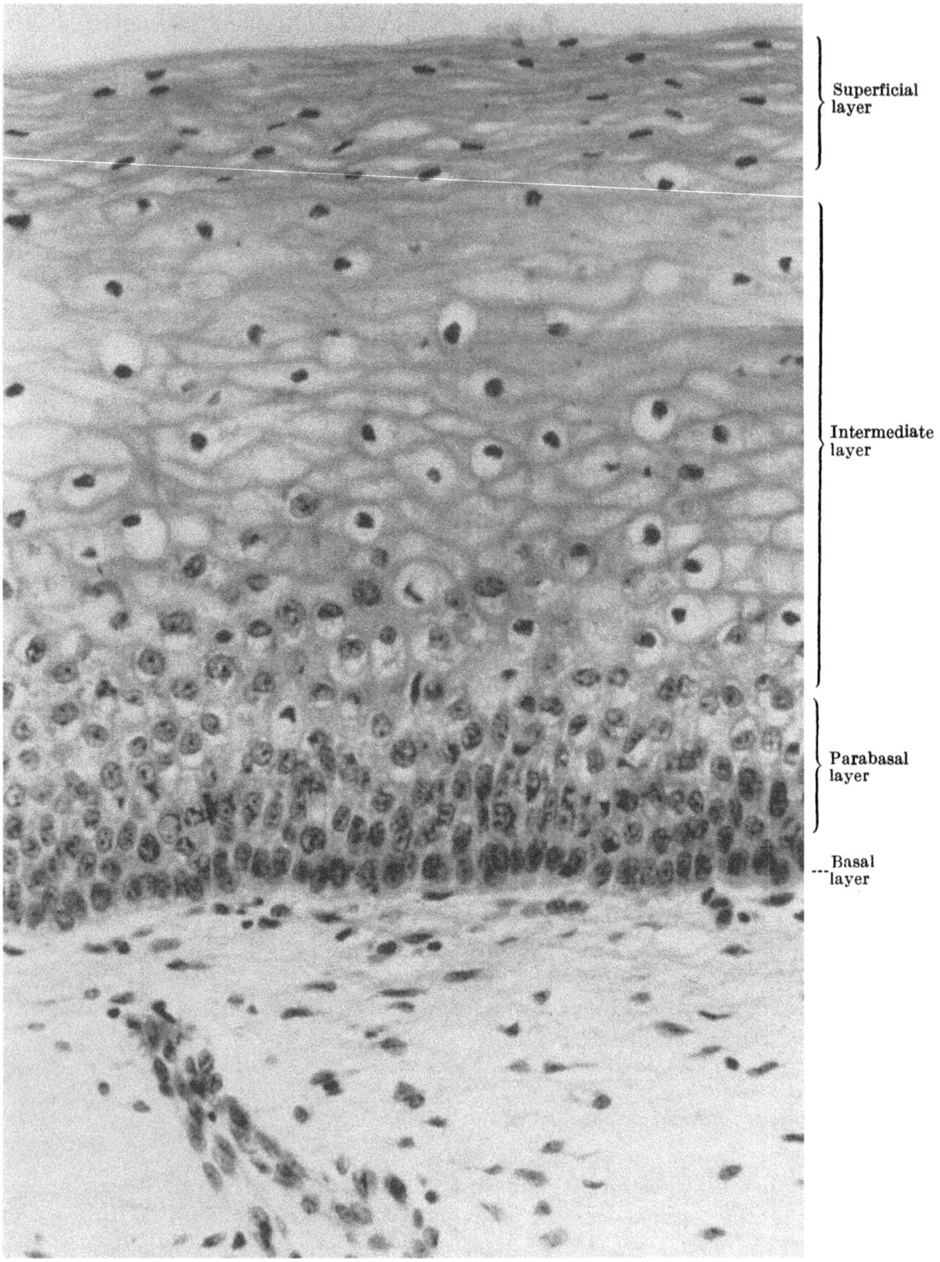

Fig. 12. Structure of normal squamous epithelium of the cervix (names of the 4 layers are along the right edge of the picture, from bottom to top)

1. The boundary with the cervical stroma is formed by a layer consisting of one row of basal cells within which mitoses can occur.

2. Above it is the so-called parabasal layer, or layer of prickle cells, which are connected with one another by intercellular bridges.

3. The intermediate layer lies above the parabasal cells, consisting of large polygonal cells with abundant cytoplasm and deposits of glycogen.

4. The most superficial layer of the squamous epithelium consists of cells that have become increasingly flattened and exhibit pyknotic nuclei. Keratinization does not occur normally.

All epithelial layers are generally well developed in sexually mature women. Stromal papillae carrying vessels reach to about half way up the squamous epithelium. Beneath the epithelium of the portio, unlike that of the vagina, there is no layer of loose connective tissue, but coarse, fibrous connective tissue

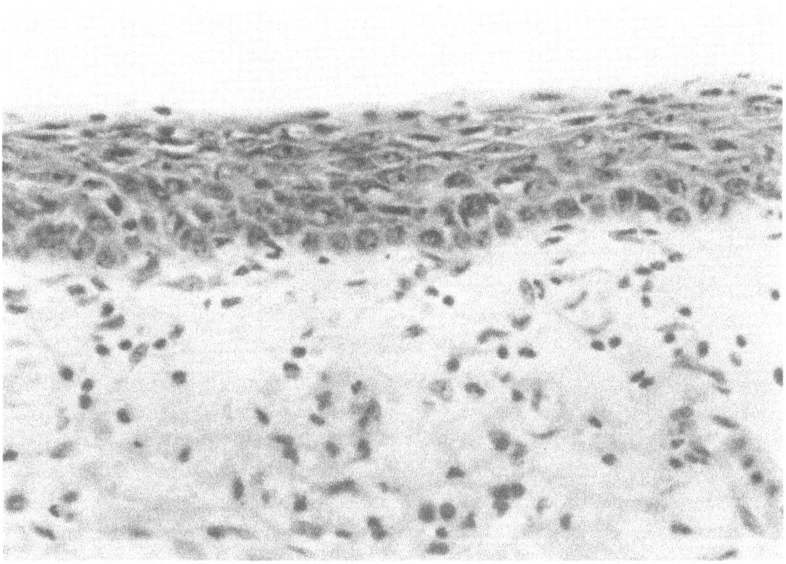

Fig. 13. Atrophic squamous epithelium of the cervix of an old woman

with relatively few vessels, allowing the squamous epithelium to attach firmly to its base. Lymph follicles may occasionally be found in the subepithelial connective tissue.

Not all layers of the squamous epithelium are always fully developed. During the cyclical changes in epithelial maturation, an epithelium consisting of only the intermediate and lower layers may be found in the presence of numerous Döderlein bacilli because of bacterial cytolysis. In senility, the epithelium becomes atrophic, consisting of only a few layers (Fig. 13).

Typical stratified squamous epithelium is very often found at a great distance from the squamous epithelial surface of the portio, amid columnar epithelium on the surface of the endocervix or even within glands. This phenomenon is known as a metaplasia in the columnar epithelium and it is called indirect squamous metaplasia in cervical glands.

The Columnar Epithelium

The endocervix is lined with columnar mucus-secreting epithelium that is present on the surface and in the cervical glands. It is a high columnar epithelium with one row of basal nuclei. The formation of mucus is marked, and dependent upon the cycle. The cervical mucus consists histochemically mainly of acid mucopolysaccharides.

All cervical glands normally open at the surface of the endocervix, discharging their secretion outwards. The glands may ramify widely, and, therefore, the area of cervical glands may have considerable depth. The extent of the area exhibits considerable individual variation. In general, hypertrophy is observed during pregnancy and atrophy in senility.

Between the cervical glands, there is loose, moderately vascular connective tissue, allowing for a certain mobility of the mucosa.

Changes in the Epithelial Boundaries during a Woman's Lifetime

Textbooks show the cervix uteri with the squamous epithelium extending over the entire surface of the portio up to the external os, where it meets the endocervical columnar epithelium. The columnar epithelium extends, accordingly, from the external os to the internal os, where it meets the low cuboidal, epithelium of the isthmic mucosa. Any other histologic arrangement, especially the presence of cervical epithelium on the surface of the portio, was formerly considered abnormal.

A portio covered by squamous epithelium appears pale red under speculum examination, and has an iridescent shimmer. It becomes obvious, merely on clinical examination of many women, that this observation cannot be made very often. Usually, a more or less distinct red spot extending around the external os is seen. This red spot may be analyzed more closely with the colposcope. It consists in many cases, of a circular area of columnar epithelium around the external os. Despite extensive colposcopic studies of the portio, however, it was still believed that the normal portio was covered by squamous epithelium.

According to systematic histological studies, undertaken by Ober, Kaufmann, Hamperl and Schneppenheim, on normal uteri from patients of all ages, certain epithelial conditions of the cervix are now known to be physiologic. This collaboration, which lasted for years, yielded the following noteworthy results:

1. The junction between squamous and columnar epithelia undergoes typical variation during a woman's lifetime (Schneppenheim, Hamperl, Kaufmann, Ober, 1958).

2. The part of the cervix that is lined with columnar epithelium always retains its length without change, despite the dislocation of its boundaries (Ober, Schneppenheim, Hamperl, Kaufmann, 1958).

3. Squamous epithelium always tries to overgrow columnar epithelium (Hamperl, Kaufmann, Ober, Schneppenheim, 1958).

4. True erosions, that is, epithelial defects, are extremely rare on the surface of the portio (Ober, 1958).

What is the Displacement of the Junction between Squamous and Columnar Epithelia?

In children, the surface of the portio is completely covered by squamous epithelium. Its boundary with the columnar epithelium is at the external os, which resembles a dimple.

At the onset of sexual maturity, the portio becomes bulkier, the vaginal fornices grow deeper, and the columnar epithelium of the endocervix enters the area of the surface of the portio, usually in a circle around the external os. This process is called formation of an ectropion, whereby the external os is transformed into an oval or even a transverse opening, as a result of the spindly flattened shape of the cervical canal (Fig. 14).

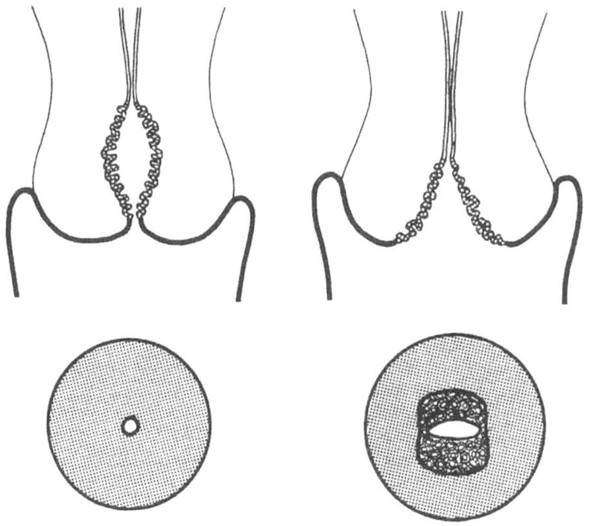

Fig. 14. Change of shape of the external cervical os resulting from formation of an ectropion of the cervical mucosa

The displacement of the epithelia is particularly marked with formation of an ectropion of the columnar epithelium during pregnancy.

After the menopause, the entire uterus undergoes involution. At the cervix, the vaginal fornices flatten out, the portio becomes narrower, and the cervical glands become some what atrophic. The columnar epithelium retracts during this involution into the cervical canal, so that the portio in old women is again covered by squamous epithelium.

Ober in 1958 reported this displacement of the boundary between squamous and columnar epithelia in relation to age. Fig. 15 demonstrates the various types of cervices observed. The epithelial displacement as described previously is shown in the left half of each diagram of the portio.

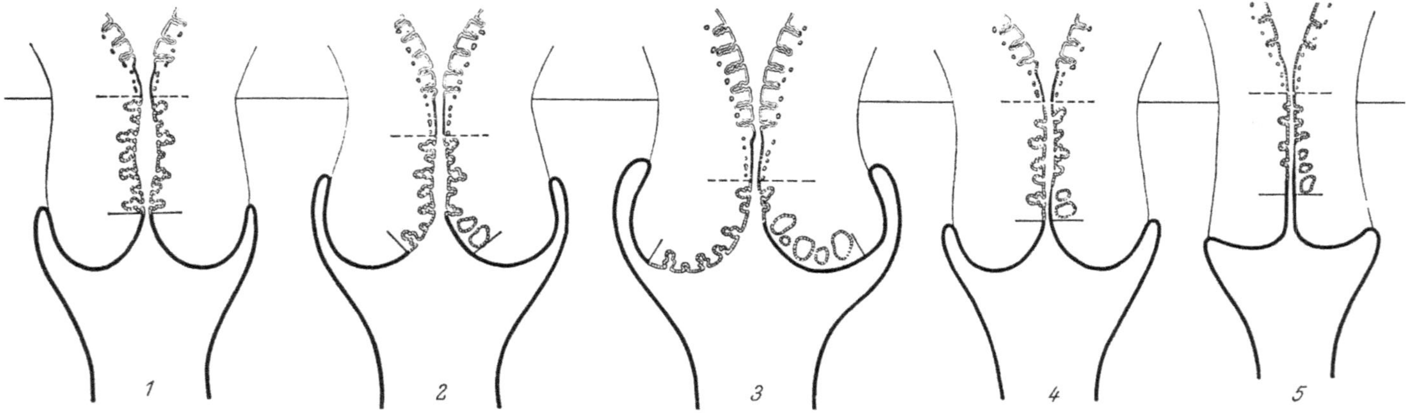

Fig. 15. Schematic representation of types of portio. Sketch 1 shows the portio of a young girl, sketches 2 and 3 the most important forms in the sexually mature woman, sketch 4 the portio in the menopause, and sketch 5 in senility. Note the change in the shape of the cervix and vaginal vault. The left half of each sketch shows the migration of the zone of cervical glandular tissue, the length of which remains constant, and the right half shows the "battle" of the glandular zone with the "ascending" squamous epithelium. The anatomic internal os is indicated by the solid line and the histologic internal os by the dotted line (OBER, 1958)

Constant Length of the Cervical Glandular Area

Ectropionized columnar epithelium does not reach the surface of the portio by active growth. It is a passive displacement of the epithelium caused by the change in cervical shape during sexual maturity, whereby the length of the tissue covered by columnar epithelium always remains constant. This length has been ascertained by OBER, SCHNEPPENHEIM, HAMPERL and KAUFMANN (1958) in serial cervical sections of normal uteri by measurement of the distance between the extreme distal and the extreme proximal cervical glands. The distance was the same in all uteri, independent of age and of the localization of the squamocolumnar junction. This finding is important since in a certain surgical procedure (conization, see p. 164) the complete removal of all the cervical glands is attempted. In view of the constant length of the cervical glandular area and its changing localization, the area to be excised varies considerably.

Squamous Epithelium Covering Columnar Epithelium

Ectropionized columnar epithelium on the portio is easily recognized macroscopically as a red spot. This phenomenon was previously regarded as an erosion. ROBERT MEYER (1923) recognized histologically that it was *not* an erosion and coined the term "pseudoerosion". Ectropionization of the columnar epithelium is a physiologic process in sexual maturity. It is largely independent of processes of gestation.

The physiologic significance of the everted columnar epithelium is not clear. Columnar epithelium opening like a funnel on the surface of the portio may perhaps provide improved conditions for migration of sperm.

Ectropionized columnar epithelium may often cause vaginal discharge. It is, therefore, not surprising that the "red spot" on the portio has been considered pathologic. The columnar epithelium on the surface of the portio actually secretes much mucus. The copious bacterial flora of the vagina finds an area of low resistance there, so that inflammation often ensues in the cervical epithelium. The epithelium in an ectropion is vulnerable, because only a single layer of cells separates the vascular stroma from the outside. Slight bleeding, therefore, is not infrequent.

The displacement of the squamocolumnar junction does not remain a mere displacement of the borderline. The squamous epithelium attempts to win back the lost territory, and from puberty through senility shows a tendency to grow over the columnar epithelium towards the external os and into the cervical canal. This phenomenon is exceptionally important, for it helps to explain practically all the benign changes and colposcopic pictures of the cervix. HAMPERL, KAUFMANN, OBER and SCHNEPPENHEIM (1958) called the spread of the squamous epithelium from the periphery over the cervical glands "aufsteigende Überhäutung" (ascending epidermidalization).

The following sequence occurs:

The squamous epithelium begins, in the presence of a circular ectropion, to overgrow the columnar epithelium in tonguelike processes. In histological section,

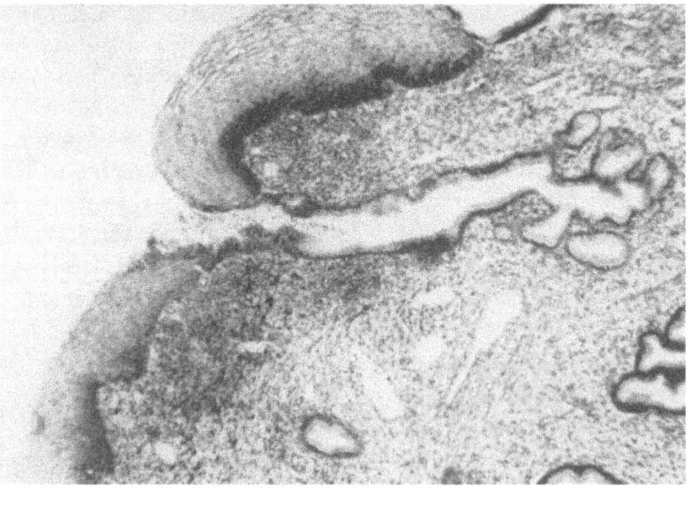

Fig. 16

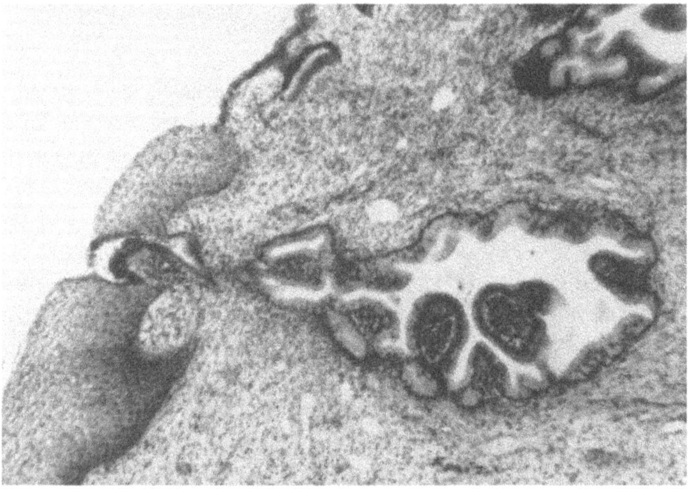

Fig. 17

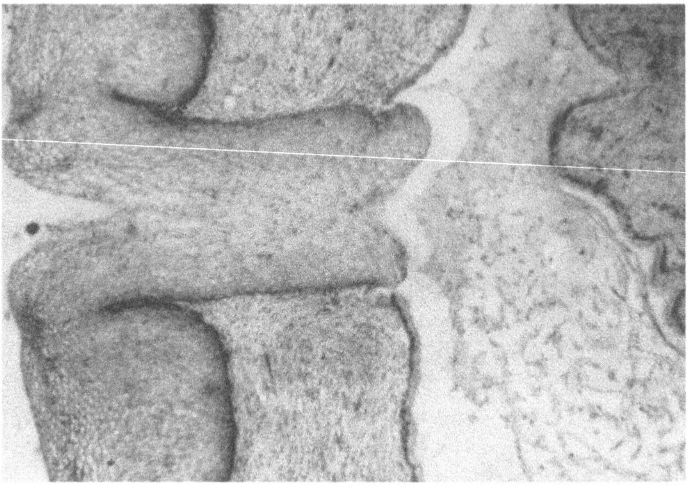

Fig. 18

Figs. 16—18. Various stages of overgrowth, up to total occlusion of the cervical glands by squamous epithelium. The occluded cervical gland in Fig. 18 lies deeply beneath the epithelial cover of the surface of the portio, and hence is not visible to the examining eye the squamous epithelium, not yet fully developed, pushes under the columnar epithelium in the manner of a plowshare. The columnar epithelium is lifted off and degenerates, but the deeper cervical glands remain viable. Squamous epithelium grows around their ducts (Fig. 16), eventually occluding them. The cervical gland thus cut off from the outside can no longer discharge its secretion (Fig. 17). The gland undergoes cystic dilatation, while its epithelium flattens out. The cystic cervical glands, long known as Nabothian follicles, may lie immediately beneath the squamous epithelium and bulge into it. Later, however, they may lie also quite deep within the cervical stroma, where they cannot be seen from the outside (Fig. 18). The process of epidermidalization in an ectropion may continue for years. The new proliferating squamous epithelium is characterized not only by its incompletely developed layers but also by its lack of glycogen (see p. 144). Knowledge of this characteristic is needed for the correct interpretation of a clinical test (iodine test) in the detection of early cases.

The contest between squamous and columnar epithelium is found in over 90% of all portios. Descending epidermidalization by endocervical squamous epithelium of metaplastic origin is undoubtedly possible also. The ascending epidermidalization is shown diagrammatically in the right halves of the pictures of the types of portios in Fig. 15.

Erosion of the Portio, a Misleading Concept

In most cases of the commonly noted red spot on the cervix uteri, there are, as apparent also in colposcopic examinations, no true epithelial defects, but rather peripheral displacements of the squamocolumnar junction. It is, therefore, incorrect to speak of an erosion of the portio. The designation of circular "erythroplakia" is more appropriate. A differentiation of the red spots with the naked eye is not possible, but the nature of the change can be observed with the colposcope.

Localization of Carcinoma in Situ

Important indications of the localization of carcinoma in situ can be gained from the knowledge of the locations of the squamocolumnar junction during a woman's lifetime.

In over 90% of cases, the carcinoma in situ is located in the vicinity of the squamocolumnar junction above cervical glands. In essence, it occupies the site that is overgrown by normal squamous epithelium in the physiologic epidermidalization, or it forms metaplastically in the endocervix. For decades (SCHRÖDER, 1959), this junctional zone has been called a "storm center". Even though the precipitating cause of carcinoma in situ is unknown, this junctional zone is exposed to unusual conditions. Young squamous epithelium receives a stimulus to grow, as shown histologically by the abundance of basal mitoses in ascending epidermidalization or metaplasia. A subepithelial inflammatory infiltration occurs frequently in this area, in turn irritating the young squamous epithelium. All transitional forms from atypical basal squamous epithelium to so called dysplastic epithelium may thus be found in the same area. Carcinoma in situ is located in the same site (Fluhmann, 1960 I, II).

From the physiologic displacement of the epithelial junctions follows the clinically important fact that carcinoma in situ during sexual maturity is located predominantly on the surface of the portio around the external os, and during the menopause and senility more proximally in the endocervix. This assumption has been confirmed in our own material. The survey specimens from 150 cases of cervical carcinoma in situ prepared by similar histologic techniques, in cooperation with Ober in 1959, were projected on a screen and sketches of the outlines were drawn. All 150 sketches were arranged according to the location of the carcinoma in situ. The most peripherally located were placed first in the row, and those lying highest within the cervical canal were placed last. The average age for the first 30 cases was 35.37 ± 1.35 years, and for the last 30 cases 47.8 ± 1.38 years. This difference is highly significant statistically (Ober and Bontke, 1959).

In this material were 20% of cases of true endocervical carcinomas in situ; 20% were located only on the surface of the portio, and 60% around the external os, that is, to some extent on the surface of the portio as well as in the cervical canal. All observations were made with uniform methods to allow comparison. Locations of carcinoma in situ as reported by others vary greatly, undoubtedly because of differing methods of diagnosis and interpretation (R. Meyer, 1941; Foote and Stewart, 1948; Pund, Nettles, Caldwell and Nieburgs, 1948; Finn, 1952; Nogales, 1953; Gusberg and Moore, 1953; Burghardt and Bajardi, 1956; Limburg, 1956; Scott and Reagan, 1956; Held, 1957, 1959; Przybora and Plutowa, 1959; Thornton jr. and Smith, 1959; Takeuchi and McKay, 1960; Cramer and Lind, 1962).

In summary:

Carcinoma in situ is an intraepithelial premalignant disease of the squamous epithelium of the cervix uteri and is to be considered a precursor of cervical carcinoma. The location of this change involves the squamocolumnar junction. Knowledge of the physiologic epithelial displacements on the cervix during a woman's lifetime permits conclusions regarding the possible location of carcinoma in situ in individual cases.

Symptomatology and Clinical Findings

To understand the symptoms of the early stages it is best to consider them in comparison with those of the clinical carcinomas.

Pathologic discharges develop in clinical cancer of the cervix from exophytic rather than endophytic growths. A brownish, hemorrhagic secretion, a watery pink discharge, postcoital bleeding, metrorrhagia or, in older patients, postmenopausal bleeding, are the signs noticed by the patient and the cause of her consulting a physician. Detailed information has been repeatedly given in order to direct the woman's attention to the danger indicated by these signs (WINTER, 1942). In practice, however, one is frequently horrified to note extensive clinical findings with a very short history. For this reason, LÖNNE suggested, as far back as 1938 and 1942, that the signs just described be called not "early signs" but "first signs", because the concept of an early sign may frequently carry the wrong prognostic implication, namely that the lesion has been discovered in good time. It has been known for a long time, furthermore, that clinical carcinomas may produce only very few symptoms and signs at first.

Table 2

Author	Symptoms in early cases			
	No symptoms	Nonspecific	Blood-stained discharge (diagnostic symptoms)	Number of cases
ACHENBACH, JOHNSTONE and HERTIG (1951)	20 (33.3%)	20 (33.3%)	20 (33.3%)	60 (100%)
LIMBURG (1956)	99 (36.9%)	91 (34.0%)	78 (29.1%)	268 (100%)
KOFLER and KREMER (1960)	22 (19.1%)	64 (55.7%)	29 (25.2%)	115 (100%)
FRIEDELL, HERTIG and YOUNGE (1960)	89 (37.9%)	64 (27.2%)	82 (34.9%)	235 (100%)
RIVA, HEFNER and KAWASAKI (1961)	45 (30.2%)	48 (32.2%)	56 (37.6%)	149 (100%)
MEYBERG (1962)	37 (57.8%)	—	27 (42.2%)	64 (100%)
THEISS (1963)	100 (25.6%)	144 (36.8%)	147 (37.6%)	391 (100%)
Total	412 (32.1%)	431 (33.6%)	439 (34.3%)	1282 (100%)

For early cases even fewer indications may, therefore, be expected. The morphology of carcinoma in situ makes it clear that there is a greater tendency toward degeneration on the surface than in normal squamous epithelium. Vascular anomalies are usually not demonstrable histologically, whereas they can often be discerned with direct light through the colposcope.

Many authors have stressed the lack of symptoms of carcinoma in situ. Some observations published in recent years have been assembled in Table 2. The selection of authors was made on the basis of the relative comparability of their numerical data. With a few exceptions, in approximately one third of patients there are no symptoms whatsoever. In other words, these women feel entirely well. Another third of the patients may complain of nonspecific symptoms that occur in many other gynecologic disorders as well. Only the last third may develop certain diagnostic symptoms.

We shall now describe the variety of symptoms encountered in our own material.

As part of a dissertation by THEISS (1963), the symptomatology of the early stages of carcinoma of the cervix in the Women's Clinic at the University of Cologne and in the Evangelical Hospital, Weyerthal (Cologne), was surveyed and compared with the symptomatology of clinical cervical carcinomas (Table 3).

Table 3

Dysplastic epithelium	Carcinoma in situ	Microcarcinoma	Carcinoma of the cervix I	Carcinoma of the cervix II—IV
36[a]	293[b]	62[c]	213	348
	391		561	

[a] 25, [b] 136, [c] 43 } From the Evangelical Hospital Cologne-Weyerthal

Tables 4 and 5 reflect the symptomatology individually and in summary. It is at once apparent that the early cases differ from the invasive cancers because of their fewer and less specific symptoms.

The histories of 391 early cases and 561 carcinomas were examined to study the symptoms of the disease. The women who felt perfectly well were considered "symptom-free". Whitish-yellow discharge, abdominal pains, menorrhagia, and incontinence or prolapse were classified as "nonspecific symptoms". Brownish, blood-stained discharge, contact bleeding, metrorrhagia, postmenopausal bleeding, and loss of weight were considered "diagnostic symptoms". Whenever a woman mentioned more than one sign, the gravest was used.

The patients *without symptoms* were examined gynecologically during prophylactic check-ups in sterility and antenatal clinics, and 100 early changes were detected with the methods for early diagnosis. There were, however, eight clinical cancers also, which had produced no symptoms.

Patients with *nonspecific symptoms* usually consulted a physician because of these complaints. Malignant disease could be demonstrated in 46 of these patients clinically on speculum examination. An epithelial atypia was recognized in 144 cases through the routine application of methods for early diagnosis. The symptoms in these cases were so unremarkable and so common in gynecologic practice that the examining physician had no suspicion of a malignant growth. In retrospect also, the combination of early epithelial change with these nonspecific symptoms appears to be accidental.

Table 4

	Dysplastic epithelium	Carcinoma in situ	Microcarcinoma	Carcinoma I	Carcinoma II—IV
Without symptoms	8 (22.2%)	75 (25.6%)	17 (27.4%)	8 (3.8%)	— (0%)
Nonspecific Symptoms	18 (50.0%)	115 (39.25%)	11 (17.8%)	18 (8.4%)	28 (8.0%)
Whitish-yellow discharge	9	50	7	6	7
Abdominal pains	8	46	3	10	15
Incontinence/Prolapse	—	10	1	—	3
Menorrhagia	1	9	—	2	3
Diagnostic symptoms	10 (27.8%)	103 (35.15%)	34 (54.8%)	187 (87.8%)	320 (92.0%)
Brownishblood-stained discharge	3	27	12	21	22
Contact bleeding or spotting	2	25	7	40	25
Metrorrhagia	4	38	11	58	69
Postmenopausal bleeding	1	13	4	66	199
Weight loss	—	—	—	2	5
Total	36 (100%)	293 (100%)	62 (100%)	213 (100%)	348 (100%)

One third of all early cases had so-called *diagnostic symptoms*, such as were present in about 90% of all clinical cancers. The specific signs of the clinical cancers are explained by the presence of a tumor. Upon attaining a certain size, malignant tissue on the portio causes, through necrosis and friability, a brownish blood-stained discharge, contact and intermenstrual bleeding, and postmenopausal bleeding. Loss of weight may also be interpreted as incipient cachexia.

The question arises, however, whether the diagnostic signs in the early cases actually were caused by the epithelial disease, or whether they should be regarded as "lucky" accidents, inducing the examining physician to make a careful search for malignant disease. The answer is difficult, especially in retrospect. The early cases at the Women's Clinic of the University were examined once more with the special purpose of ascertaining whether the diagnostic signs were causally related to the epithelial atypia. In three quarters of the material, the leading symptom could be explained by another lesion in the genital tract. In addition to the epithelial atypia, the patients had uterine myomas, endometriosis or endometrial or cervical polyps, or had been receiving inadequate endocrine treatment or had decubital ulcers from pessaries. Without the use of methods of cancer detection the presenting signs could have been explained satisfactorily by some other genital disease. These cases have not been summarized numerically since individual cases are controversial.

Table 5

Symptoms	Early cases	Invasive cancers (clinical and only histologically detected)[a]
Without symptoms	100 (25.6%)	8 (1.4%)
Nonspecific symptoms	144 (36.8%)	46 (8.2%)
Diagnostic symptoms	147 (37.6%)	507 (90.4%)
	391 (100%)	561 (100%)

[a] Definition according to Ober, Kaufmann and Hamperl (1961).

No lesion other than epithelial atypia was present in one quarter of the cases with diagnostic signs. It may, therefore, be assumed that the blood-stained discharge was caused by the disease. It is noteworthy that the proportion of such cases is substantially higher in microcarcinomas than in carcinomas in situ.

In summary, it can therefore be stated that out of 391 early cases, 37.6% exhibited suspicious signs in the form of bloody discharge, whereas in only about 11% could the epithelial atypia be considered the cause for the abnormal bleeding. On the other hand, 90% of 561 clinical cancers had suspicious clinical symptoms.

The clinical findings of carcinoma in situ may be discussed briefly because they are practically nonexistent. The macroscopic examination of the portio without the use of aids (colposcopy or iodine test) provides no indications of an epithelial atypia. If the carcinoma in situ is situated on the surface of the portio, it is not elevated above the level of the normal epithelium and it does not stand out because of differences in color. It cannot, therefore, be seen with the naked eye. Intraepithelial carcinoma does not usually exhibit a particular tendency to bleed on contact nor can it be depressed with a probe, because the cervical stroma remains intact. If the lesion is situated within the cervical canal, moreover, it is outside the range of inspection. Only large areas with leukoplakic surfaces or prominent mosaic areas can be seen with the naked eye. (More about these lesions and the frequency of carcinoma in situ on p. 133.)

Table 6

Gross findings on portio	Dysplastic epithelium	Carcinoma in situ	Micro-carcinoma	Total
Not suspicious	33	246	50	329 (84.4%)
Equivocal	3	25	2	30 (7.7%)
Suspicious	—	22	10	32 (7.9%)
Total	36	293	62	391 (100%)

Table 7

ACHENBACH, JOHNSTONE, HERTIG (1951)	91%	Early cases of cervix uteri were not suspicious macroscopically
PETERSEN (1955)	69.8%	
CARTER, CUYLER *et al.* (1956)	88.5%	
ERICKSON, EVERETT, GRAWES et al. (1956)	90%	
PARKER, CUYLER et al. (1960)	85.7%	
KOFLER and KREMER (1960)	45.3%	
RIVA, HEFNER and KAWASAKI (1961)	97.4%	

Table 8

Macroscopic findings on the portio	Early cases	Invasive carcinoma (clinical and only histologically detected)[a]
Not suspicious	329 (84.4%)	24 (4.3%)
Equivocal	30 (7.7%)	19 (3.4%)
Suspicious	32 (7.9%)	46 (8.2%)
Cancer	—	472 (84.1%)
Total	391 (100%)	561 (100%)

[a] Definition according to OBER, KAUFMANN, HAMPERL (1961).

THEISS surveyed the gross findings concerning the portio, on the same material, using this terminology:

Surface of the portio not suspicious macroscopically.

Surface of the portio equivocal.

Surface of the portio suspicious macroscopically.

These observations were collated (Table 6).

In only 7.9% of all early cases was clinical suspicion aroused, with all the subjectivity inherent in such examinations. OBER and BÖTZELEN (1959) found 18 out of 56 early cases macroscopically suspicious, indicating a higher percentage. The difference can probably be explained by the fact that THEISS used the first findings shown in the case history, whereas OBER and BÖTZELEN used only the findings of experienced colleagues.

Similar observations were reported by other authors (Table 7).

The direct comparison of early cases with invasive carcinoma is of interest, for it forcefully demonstrates that the diagnosis of invasive cancer can be reached largely on the basis of examination by speculum and the naked eye (Table 8).

It is, however, noteworthy that among the invasive cancers, too, a diagnosis on first examination was not possible in 15.9%.

In summary, it should be stated that, with regard to clinical findings, the early cases of cervical carcinoma cannot be detected by the usual speculum examination because of lack of macroscopic evidence. Special methods of early diagnosis therefore had to be developed for detection of this lesion.

Cytology

Historical Introduction

The history of early detection of cancer by diagnostic cytology is inseparably linked with the name of Papanicolaou.

Papanicolaou was born in 1883 in Coumi, Greece, studied in Athens and Munich, and worked in New York from 1913. There is nobody more qualified than he to describe the development of the cytodiagnosis of cancer. The following paragraphs therefore represent most of the text of a lecture on the history of cytodiagnosis that he delivered at the International Congress for Cytology in Brussels in 1957[1]:

"The earliest report on the microscopic examination of a body fluid is, presumably, that of Donne in 1838, on fresh smears prepared from human colostrum. This was the year Schleiden published his classical paper on 'Phytogenesis', which laid the foundation of the 'cell theory' as applied to plants. The term 'cell theory', however, was introduced one year later by Theodore Schwann in his epoch-making work, 'Microscopic investigations on the accordance in the structure and growth of plants and animals'. The names of these two great men stand out in the history of the science of Cytology, yet, according to several historians, the principles of the cell theory, as applied to plant and animal tissues, had been defined by some of their predecessors.

Microscopic examinations of fresh sputum specimens were reported in 1843, by Walsche, who was presumably the first to observe tissue fragments expectorated from malignant growths of the respiratory tract and then Lancereaux in 1856, in a case of a primary carcinoma of the lung: Beale in 1860, who demonstrated cancer cells in the sputum of a case of cancer of the pharynx; and Hampeln in 1876 and 1887, in the cases of a sarcoma and an alveolar carcinoma of the lung. Similar observations were made by several other investigators during the late 19th and early 20th Centuries.

The earliest observations on record in the exfoliative cytology of the female genital tract are those of Pouchet in 1847. In contrast to previous investigators, who turned their attention chiefly to the detection of cancer cells or fragments of malignant tissue, Pouchet confined his studies to normal cytology. Being an advocate of a spontaneous ovulatory process, he sought evidence in favor of it in a study of the modifications of the vaginal secretion during the different stages of the human menstrual cycle. The only early reference I was able to find on the examination of uterine discharge for evidence of cancer is a rather negative report given in a paper by Dickinson in 1869, in which he states that (quote): 'In cases of cancer of the uterus I have often examined the discharge but never succeeded in finding anything diagnostic of the disease' (unquote).

In urine, the oldest reference of a microscopic examination is that of Sanders in 1864, who found small fragments originating from a cancer of the bladder in the urine of a 43 year old man. A similar observation was made in 1869 by Dickinson.

In pleural or peritoneal exudates, exfoliated tumor cells were observed in fresh unstained smears first by Luecke and Krebs in 1867, and later by Quincke in 1875, and Boegelick in 1878. It may appear strange that although the cytologic study of exudates and transudates was the last in chronological order, it soon became the most favored application in the diagnosis of cancer and other pathologic conditions. Toward the end of the 19th Century the cytologic

[1] Published in: Acta Un. int. Cancr. (Brux.) **14**, 249—254 (1958).

method of diagnosis gained many new friends and ardent supporters, particularly among pathologists, as a result of advancements not only in the field of optics but also in the development of special techniques for processing, fixing, and staining the specimens and the smears. EHRLICH in 1880 and 1882, introduced the use of dry smears fixed by heat and stained like blood smears, a method which found wide application. WIDAL, like EHRLICH, also worked with dry smears, but fixed them in alcohol-ether and stained them with thionin-eosin-hematein, Zinna's blue and Ehrlich's triacid. He and his co-workers gained wide recognition toward the end of the century for their pioneer studies on exudates. Vital staining was used by JOSEFSON in 1901. QUENSEL in 1919, introduced a supravital staining procedure, which he had used previously in the examination of urinary sediments. In a subsequent paper in 1928, he described his Methylene-Cadmium-Sudan staining technique, with which he could make an excellent differentiation of the various cellular types.

BAHRENBERG in 1895, was presumably the first to introduce a technique for embedding sediments and sectioning them for examination. A method consisting of fixation in formalin and embedding in celloidin or paraffin, which has been extensively used by later investigators, was decribed by MANDLEBAUM first in 1900 and then in 1917. SEECOF and BOETHS (1924), BOCK (1925), and ZEMANSKY (1928), employed the paraffin block method. FOORD, YOUNG and WETMORE (1929), used both smears and sections of the sediment, but expressed their preference for the latter. On the other hand, 'Cytodiagnosis' found an enthusiastic advocate in KOENIGER (1908). An enlightening discussion on the cytologic method of diagnosis, as applied to exudates and transudates, may be found in the publications of ZADEK (1933), MCDONALD and BRODERS (1939), and WIHNAM (1948).

Next to the microscopic study of effusions, the one which received greatest attention for its potentialities in cancer diagnosis was that of sputum. To cover the large number of papers pertaining to this application and to review the findings and the many staining and other technical procedures used by the various investigators during this most fertile period covering the later part of the 19th and the early years of the 20th Centuries would be far beyond the scope of this presentation and the time allotted for it. BEJANCON and DE JONG in 1913, were perhaps the first to use fixation in sputum smears. However, the development of a 'wet film method' comparable to the one used today was the achievement of DUDGEON and PATRICK in 1927. DUDGEON and WRIGLEY in 1935, reported that, in a series of 58 cases of suspected malignant growth, sputum examination by the wet film method established the diagnosis in 68% of proved cases of carcinoma of the lung or larynx. In his outstanding monograph published in 1944, WANDALL states that by using the wet film method of DUDGEON and PATRICK, with a minor modification introduced by GLOYNE in 1936, he was able to demonstrate neoplastic cells in the sputum of 84 out of 100 patients with primary lung cancer.

Looking into these remarkable accomplishments, one wonders why the cytodiagnosis of cancer did not receive greater attention on the part of the clinicians as well as the pathologists. What were the factors which held back for such a long time its rightful recognition and with it the full unfoldment of exfoliative cytology?

One of these factors was perhaps the introduction of the cell block technique by BAHRENBERG in 1895, and the wider utilization of the improved technical procedure described by MANDLEBAUM in 1900 and 1917. Many pathologists began to use cell block sections in preference to smears since the evaluation of the latter was based on criteria which were less familiar to them and required special training and long experience.

The lack of a simple, adequate, and well standardized technique for the preparation, preservation, and staining of cytologic smears might have been another contributory factor. Such a technique has been developed in the course of investigations initiated some 40 years ago on the basic morphology of the cyclic changes in the reproductive organs of the guinea pig. It was then that the vaginal smear was introduced as a means of identifying the various stages of the oestrous cycle in this animal. Its use was soon extended to women, first, in the study of the menstrual cycle and of problems related to the morphology and physiology of the female organs of reproduction, and then, in the diagnosis of cancer of the uterus, especially of the cervix. Two significant steps in the development of the smear have been: 1. its protection from the damaging effects of drying through its immediate fixation and subsequent preservation in a solution of 95% alcohol and ether and 2. the introduction of alcoholic cytoplasmic staining solutions which provide the smear with greater transparency.

It was in 1940 that I first realized the urgent need for a method of staining that would be more sensitive than the aqueous solution of eosin and waterblue which was used until that time in our laboratory. In reviewing smears from cases of carcinoma of the cervix and adenocarcinomas of the endometrium, which were interpreted and reported as negative, I noticed that in many instances malignant cells, though present in some of the smears, were missed during the first examination because of the lack of translucence which was due to the deep staining of the cellular and other components of the smear. An intensive search was thus set in motion, which lasted for approximately two years. During this time a new stain or staining procedure was tested practically every day in our laboratory to the despair of my faithful assistants who finally lost their patience and threatened a sit-down strike unless this nonsense stopped. The end result of this search was the development of the two alcoholic stains OG6 and EA36, the formulae of which were published in 1942. It surprises me that these stains are still in use because my work was entirely empirical and I thought that by this time new revolutionary methods would have been devised by cytochemists and other investigators better qualified for such work than myself. I was very glad to see Dr. EBNER'S paper on this program and I expect to learn a great deal from his analysis of the cytochemical background of my staining procedure.

The publication of this staining method was soon followed by a monograph on the, 'Diagnosis of Uterine Cancer by the Vaginal Smear', published in 1943, by HERBERT F. TRAUT and me. It immediately aroused the interest of gynecologists and other medical men in the great potentialities of this diagnostic procedure. A previous paper presented by me at the 1928 Conference on Race Betterment, in which the usefulness of the smear method in the detection of cancer of the uterus was described under the title, 'New Cancer Diagnosis', was almost totally ignored chiefly because of its brevity and its insufficient documentation but also because of the fact that the gynecologists of that time were largely preoccupied with problems related to the cyclic manifestation of morphologic changes in the vaginal and cervical epithelium, and their correlation with the ovarian and uterine cycles. My monograph, in 1933 on 'The Sexual Cycle in the Human Female as Revealed by Vaginal Smears', contained only a brief reference to malignant cytology. However, the many investigations conducted during those most productive years on the normal exfoliative cytology of the female sex organs have been of immense value in that they provided us with a yardstick for measuring and evaluating more intelligently the morphologic changes brought about by the onset of malignant or other pathologic processes. They also contributed to the advancement of gynecological endocrinology and to the study of problems related to amenorrhea, sterility and menopause by throwing new light on the correlation of the ovarian and uterine changes during the various phases of the normal menstrual cycle and their dependence upon the hypophyseal and other hormonal secretions.

These basic contributions coupled with the specific technical procedures introduced in the course of these studies formed a vigorous root which brought fresh sap and new strength to the tree of exfoliative cytology. Its growth in the past fifteen years has indeed been phenomenal. Its unique value in clinical diagnosis and in medical and biological research is now fully appreciated. Its use is no longer limited to the female genital system but extends to practically all organs of the body. At present, the cytologic method of cancer diagnosis finds its most successful application in the following organs: uterus, particularly the cervix, lung, esophagus, stomach and rectum, bladder and the pleura and peritoneum. In these organs the diagnostic accuracy of the method proved to be very high. In other organs, like the kidney, the prostate and the breast, the difficulty in obtaining adequate material for examination has been a limiting factor in the wider use of the method. However, even in these organs the presence of cancer has, in many instances, been revealed primarily by the cytologic examination.

The swift expansion of the cytologic method in its use in the diagnosis of cancer was due in large measure to the endorsement and support given to it by the American Cancer Society and the United States Public Health Service. The first Cytologic Conference, which was held in Boston in 1948, was organized under the sponsorship of the American Cancer Society. It was then that Cytologists and Pathologists had their first encounter around a conference table. The ensuing enlightening discussion paved the way for a better understanding which has since developed into close cooperation and friendship between these two groups. Exfoliative Cytology, in its use in cancer diagnosis, is now accepted as a requirement in the Board examination for specialty certification in Pathology in the United States and is recognized as an integral part of a large and steadily increasing number of pathology laboratories. The enthusiastic endorsement of Exfoliative Cytology by clinical men, not only those belonging to specialized fields of medicine but also by family physicians and general practitioners, has been another potent stimulus to its wider utilization. The role of the gynecologists has been particularly important in this respect since the cytologic method of diagnosis has always been and still is most extensively used in the female genital system. The bond uniting cytologists, pathologists, gynecologists, and other clinicians and surgeons is actually embodied in the Constitution of the Inter-Society Cytology Council, which was founded in 1952. It is felt that the coordination of the cytologic activities of representatives of these various groups will greatly help toward the solution of the many problems with which Exfoliative Cytology is still confronted.

By far the most important feature of Exfoliative Cytology is that it has furnished us with the means of detecting cancer in its incipiency. This has been its greatest contribution to Science and Humanity. Much of our knowledge of the cytology and histopathology of early cancer has been derived primarily from investigative work done on the cervix, an organ which readily lends itself to both cytologic and pathologic exploration. The many intra-epithelial carcinomas or carcinomas-in-situ thus far uncovered through the use of cytology have provided the pathologist with excellent material for the study of the histogenesis of cervical carcinoma, and the clinician with the opportunity to attack cancer more effectively at an early, curable stage.

A very advantageous feature of the cytologic method is that it makes possible a day-by-day follow-up, without surgical intervention, of the progressive as well as the regressive morphologic changes occurring in spontaneous or experimentally induced malignant tumors. Furthermore, it permits an evaluation of the results of operative procedures and of the action and effects of various modes of treatment, including radiation, in experimental and clinical studies.

By virtue of its particular usefulness in the early diagnosis of malignant disease, the cytologic method has become an important investigative tool in preventive medicine. Its dependability and value have already been convincingly demonstrated by several mass-screening projects sponsored by the United States Public Health Service and the American Cancer Society involving large sections of the population for the purpose of detecting unsuspected carcinomas of the uterine cervix.

The study of the exfoliative cytology of early malignant lesions of the cervix has revealed the existence of several distinct patterns which add greatly to the diagnostic as well as the prognostic value of the method. Variations in the cytologic pattern of smears have also been described in cases diagnosed pathologically as borderline or potentially malignant. The final evaluation of the significance of these changes can be best achieved through the correlation of cytologic and pathologic findings by the combined efforts of pathologists and cytologists, each group following its own path of investigation, yet both working in close cooperation toward the attainment of the same goal.

The most serious handicap in the wider utilization of Exfoliative Cytology in the diagnosis of cancer is perhaps the lack of an adequate number of well trained cyto-pathologists and cyto-technologists. Such training requires proper instruction and study in a qualified cytology laboratory for a period of at least one year. Owing to the existing shortage of adequately trained personnel the practice of cytology in many laboratories is at present greatly hampered. To correct this situation the American Cancer Society and the United States Public Health Service have recently launched an intensive campaign in a coordinated effort to expedite education and training in this special field.

In evaluating cytologic smears the use of strict criteria of malignancy is strongly recommended in order to prevent false positive interpretations, which may harm not only the patient, but also the reputation of the clinician, the laboratory and the method itself. Reports positive for cancer must be confirmed, whenever possible, by biopsy or curettage. There are, of course, instances in which a confirmation is not feasible. In such cases the surgeon finds himself in a dilemma as to whether he should decide for or against an exploratory operation. His confusion is apt to be even greater when the correctness of a cytologic report positive for cancer is refuted by negative histopathologic findings. What should he do then? To ignore the cytologic report, particularly when it comes from a reputable laboratory, may deprive him of the only opportunity to save the life of the patient. On the other hand, to proceed with major surgery or other radical treatment in the face of negative histopathologic findings implies a grave responsibility. One should, however, take into consideration that the histopathologic examination of a surgical specimen is usually based on a relatively limited number of sections, in which an existing malignant lesion, particularly if early and small, may not be shown at all. There are indeed several cases on record in which a subsequent examination of further histologic sections has proven the presence of an early cancerous lesion, which could not be seen in the originally examined slides. With this in mind, one may be justified in stating that the issue is not one of cytology versus histopathology but rather of positive versus negative findings. A positive report rendered by a well qualified cytology laboratory might not be fully honored, but should under no circumstances be entirely ignored.

The intense interest in Exfoliative Cytology now exidenced in all parts of the world is most gratifying and is a most auspicious omen for its future. I am particularly happy to witness here at this meeting the enthusiastic participation of so many oustanding men of Science, representative of long-established and time-honored European and other world-famed institutions. Exfoliative Cytology is thus becoming a symbol and a bond uniting all of us under the banner of the far-embracing ideal of better understanding and closer cooperation. With such an inspiring incentive, we may look forward to greater conquests in the days to come."

Papanicolaou dedicated a large part of his life to the early detection of cancer. The last weeks of his life were occupied with the preparations for taking over an institute for cytodiagnosis in Miami, Florida. During these activities, he died in 1961 at the age of 78. As indicated in Papanicolaou's statements, cytodiagnosis was first recognized and accepted in America at the beginning of the nineteen forties. Because of the war, Germany was isolated from any international exchange of ideas, and the development of cytodiagnosis was therefore delayed. Colposcopy, successfully used for decades, seemed to produce equally good results. Igel in Berlin was the first, in 1947, to report on his experiences with cytodiagnosis, but he did not receive much attention. The method nevertheless gained wider use and recognition. In Germany the success of cytology is linked with the names of Boschann, Limburg, Navratil, Smolka, Soost, Stoll, Wied, Zinser and others. Cytodiagnosis today is considered a routine investigation in all gynecologic examinations. In some parts of the Federal Republic, support by the state guarantees the establishment of cytodiagnostic laboratories to make possible the handling of the influx of submitted material. Despite undeniable progress we are still far from capable of screening the entire female population, because of organizational and financial problems and especially because of shortages in staff.

Who should be Screened?

Discussion of the localization of the carcinoma in situ showed that it changes, during the life of a woman, according to the physiologic displacements of the cervical epithelium. The pathologic transformation of the epithelium may occur at any age in sexually mature and menopausal women. The results of numerous investigations in various parts of the world indicate that the average age of patients with carcinoma in situ is about 5—10 years lower than that of patients with clinical cancer (Cuyler, Kaufmann *et al.*, 1951; Wespi, 1952; Gorga *et al.*,

1953; SCHUBERT, 1954; PETERSEN, 1955; WHEELER, 1956; NIEBURGS and PUND, 1957; ANDERSON, 1959; v. MIKULICZ-RADECKI, 1960; OBER, KAUFMANN and HAMPERL, 1961; KAUFMANN, 1963).

OBER and BONTKE in 1959 calculated an average age of 41.44 years in 150 early cases, with a scatter from 19 to 64 years. The material, supplemented by THEISS, including the cases of the Evangelical Hospital of Cologne-Weyerthal, indicated an average age of 42.4 years in 391 early cases, with 2 patients younger than 20 and one older than 70 years. A graph of the age distribution in the same series showed a percentage rise after the 30th year of life, as compared with the age distribution of the cervical carcinomas (Fig. 19).

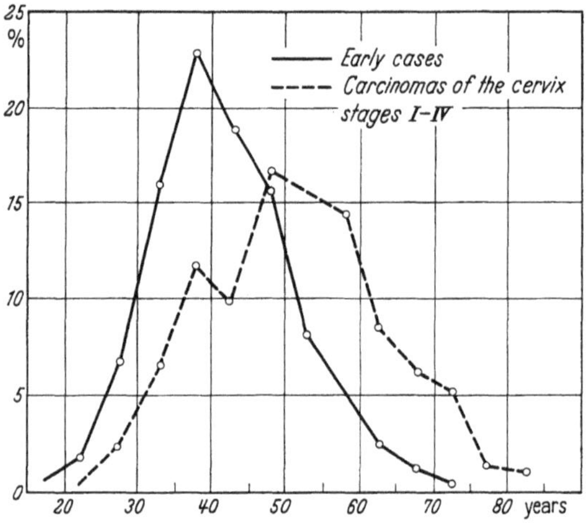

Fig. 19. Age distribution of early cases and clinical carcinomas. The graph is based on 391 early cases and 561 clinical carcinomas (THEISS, 1963)

The appearance of an early change may therefore be expected in women of any age. The number of women visiting cancer prevention clinics is infinitesimal in comparison with the total female population. Progress would be achieved if at least in every gynecologic examination methods of early diagnosis were applied routinely. About 300,000 women live in Cologne. Each year about 6% of them visit a gynecologist or a gynecological clinic for various reasons. If a speculum is inserted, as should be mandatory in examination by a specialist, methods of early diagnosis may easily be included. Patients generally find it difficult to have a gynecologic examination. They should in every case be given the chance of early cancer detection regardless of the symptoms that prompted the visit to the doctor. We advise, every patient above 30, moreover, to request a regular check-up. Only a very small fraction follows that advice.

Obstetric patients who have not been examined vaginally after a normal delivery and puerperium present a problem. Examination of these patients for early detection should become part of antenatal or, at least, postnatal care, since most of them may not see a gynecologist again for years, and an appointment 2—3 months postpartum might cause administrative difficulties (OSBOND and NICHOLSON-JONES, 1962; JANISCH and ULM, 1963). More will be said later about possible erroneous diagnoses regarding the cervix in pregnancy and the puerperium. In view of our knowledge about the age distribution of early stages of malignant disease of the cervix, every woman over 30 should be advised to have regular gynecological examinations and every gynecologist is expected to examine his patients with methods for early diagnosis. It is difficult to decide to what extent this requirement should apply also to general practitioners. One can scarcely expect a general practitioner to perform a pelvic examination on a woman who consults him because of heart trouble, first, because he does not have enough time, and, second, is not, under present conditions, paid for this special service. Clear instruction of the patient by her family physician to undergo examinations by a specialist may perhaps help.

Documentation from Data on Early Diagnosis

Today new concepts in medicine are only rarely gained from individual observations and intuitive speculation. Information is obtained by biologic methods or statistical analysis of large numbers. Individual observation has been increasingly replaced by the study of groups.

Following science and industry, medicine adopted the methods of modern documentation and statistics. Statements based on extensive material could thus be tested for accuracy and corroborated with the help of applied statistics.

We, too, were confronted with the problem whether we should limit ourselves to the daily diagnosis of the incoming material or whether we should collect the material for subsequent systematic evaluation. After pilot studies we decided on documentation by manual punch cards. The following considerations led to this decision.

At the time there was no documentation by mechanical punch cards in the area of the University of Cologne. An annual yield of 3,000—4,000 cards was expected. Individual inquiries should be answered as quickly as possible in our own laboratory. The installation of the Hollerith system in our own laboratory appeared too costly.

Further problems arose in conjunction with material that should be included and how completely it should be recorded. It was necessary to restrict the material included to that which within medical limitations conformed to strict standards of statistics and documentation.

The material had to be collected in accordance with the requirements of the documentation. All questions were phrased to allow answers as unequivocal as possible. Only the most essential numerical data were requested. Subjective information given by patients, for instance the date of the last menstrual period, was not included. With regard to cytology and colposcopy, the findings of only those colleagues were included who had, after a sufficiently long period of training, gained enough experience to ensure the uniformity of the material. No findings of colleagues in training were included.

All concepts of cytology, colposcopy, and histology were standardized as far as the material permitted. A uniform evaluation of findings was obtained by frequent comparison of findings and discussions among the individual doctors.

The inclusion for documentation of many medical data, findings, and diagnoses, is very difficult or entirely impossible, because statements may be too subjective and not directly comparable with other similar statements. In contrast to this subjective information is the objective information essential to adequate documentation. Concepts like "hard", "relatively hard" and "soft" data have come into use (PIPBERGER and FREIS, 1960).

The patient's age, number of deliveries, and age at menarche and menopause are examples of, "hard data". Laboratory and clinical findings, cytology, colposcopy, iodine test, and histology provide "relatively hard data", since errors inherent in the method or interpretation may occur. A large part of medical information includes "soft data", for example information about abortions, regularity or irregularity of the cycle, clinical evaluation of the cervical surface or the zone of atypical transformation of the portio, and so forth.

It was the aim of the preparatory documentation to collect mainly "hard data" and to omit all questionable data.

For more than 7 years all the data of early detection have been evaluated according to the same system, which we shall describe below:

A report on the method of documentation was made in 1959 in collaboration with BÖTZELEN. Only minor modifications have been introduced since then. The 3,000—4,000 cards entered annually can be easily evaluated, but analysis of the total of 15,000 cards becomes cumbersome. With this order of magnitude, the mechanically punched cards are undoubtedly superior to the system of manual punches.

We need three forms for documentation:

1. Clinical form (Fig. 20);
2. Status card (Fig. 21);
3. Punch card (Fig. 22).

1. Clinical Form (Fig. 20)

These forms are kept in the gynecological wards in pads with sheets of carbon paper between them, and are thus always completed in duplicate. The examining doctor who performs an examination for early diagnosis also fills in the clinical questions on the accompanying form. The questions concern personal data, menstrual cycle, pregnancies, data on surgical operations and irradiation, the clinical findings on the portio, and the clinical diagnosis. To minimize the number of erroneous entries, the questions were constructed so that entries could be made by placing crosses in the appropriate sections. Inclusion of time references (for example, date of the last menses) was omitted, since no hormonal diagnosis was included in this project.

Either the completed form accompanies the cytologic specimens or the findings of colposcopic examination are inserted in the appropriate space. In the laboratory, the forms are given the same number as the slides and transferred to status cards (Fig. 21). The cytologic report is inserted after microscopic examination of the specimens. One copy remains in the laboratory and the other is returned to the patient's file.

This clinical form contains data about the patient that are important for the early diagnosis of cancer. The report is intended only as an answer to the clinician. The details that are important for the documentary evaluation of the findings of early diagnosis, however, appear only on the status and punch cards that remain in the card index in the documentation room.

Women's Clinic
Cologne University

Date 2/4/63   432/63   **Cytology** **Colposcopy**

Name	Given name	Ward	Patient's file No.
Berger	Hilde	III	

Age	Date of birth	Has patient attended before?	Year	Patient's old file No.
40	8/15/22	yes	1957	1217/57

Present menstrual status:		Previous treatments:	
before menarche		Operation:	
primary amenorrhea		removal of cervix	/
regular cycle	X	removal of uterus	/
irregular cycle		supravaginal hysterectomy	/
secondary amenorrhea		removal of one ovary	/
menopause		removal of both ovaries	

Number of deliveries	2	Pregnant at present?	~~yes~~ no	Ra/X-radiation:	
				carcinoma dose	/
Number of abortions	0		month	Ra-menopause	/
				X-castration	/

Clinical diagnosis:	Macroscopic finding on the portio:	
Discharge	not suspicious	X
	inflammation	
	suspicious area	
	polyp	
	bleeding on contact	
	hemorrhage from endocervix	

Cytologic finding:	Remark:
degree: 3	
class: IV	
Colposcopic finding:	

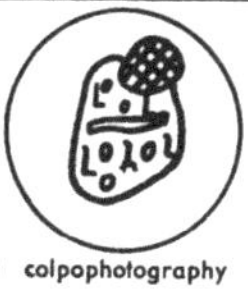

Vascular, closed transformation zone.
At 12 o'clock, mosaic area

Iodine test: iodine-negative
sharp edges

(X) colpophotography

Fig. 20. Clinical form. The personal data in this figure and also in Figs. 20 and 21 are fictitious

2. Status Card (Fig. 21)

The status card reproduces all clinical data and provides space for five cytologic, three colposcopic, and two histologic reports. Colposcopic and histologic reports are put into in words. Histologic findings are entered only if they are significant for early diagnosis. The characteristic cytologic findings, however, are indicated by crosses during the examination of the slide, with space reserved for certain, mainly pathologic, cellular patterns and admixtures of bacteria and cells. The diagnosis is based on the characteristics indicated by crosses and is classified by degree and group (for details see normal and abnormal cellular

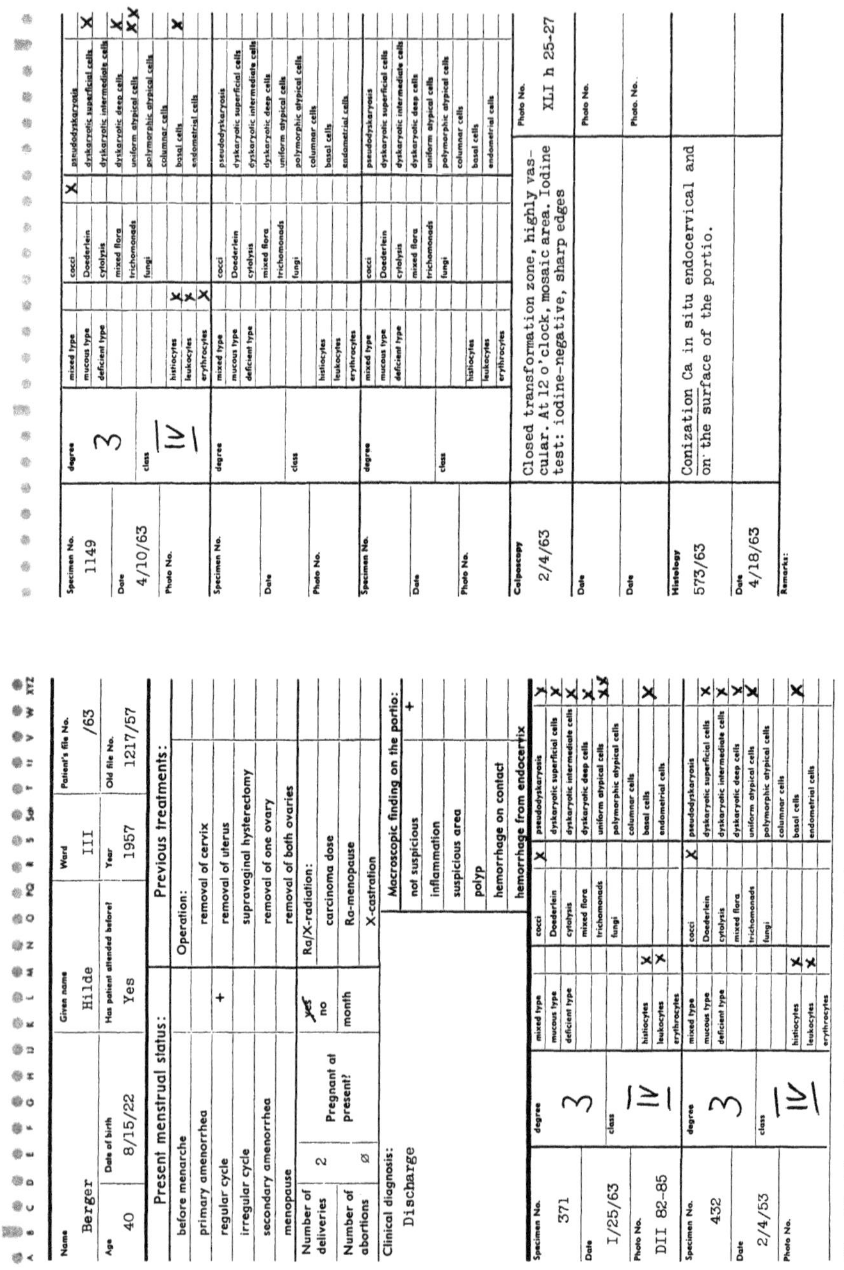
A B C D E F G H IJ K L M N O PQ R S Sch T U V W XYZ

Name	Given name	Ward	Patient's file No.
Berger	Hilde	III	/63

Age	Date of birth	Has patient attended before?	Year	Old file No.
40	8/15/22	Yes	1957	1217/57

Present menstrual status:		Previous treatments:	
before menarche		Operation:	
primary amenorrhea		removal of cervix	
regular cycle	+	removal of uterus	
irregular cycle		supravaginal hysterectomy	
secondary amenorrhea		removal of one ovary	
menopause		removal of both ovaries	
Number of deliveries 2	Pregnant at present? ~~yes~~ no	Ra/X-radiation:	
Number of abortions ø	month	carcinoma dose	
		Ra-menopause	
		X-castration	

Clinical diagnosis: Discharge

Macroscopic finding on the portio:	
not suspicious	+
inflammation	
suspicious area	
polyp	
hemorrhage on contact	
hemorrhage from endocervix	

Specimen No. 371; Date I/25/63; Photo No. DII 82-85; degree 3; class IV
histiocytes X; leukocytes X; cocci X; pseudodyskaryosis X; dyskaryotic superficial cells X; dyskaryotic intermediate cells X; dyskaryotic deep cells X; uniform atypical cells XX; basal cells X
(also: mixed type, mucous type, deficient type, erythrocytes, Doederlein, cytolysis, mixed flora, trichomonads, fungi, polymorphic atypical cells, columnar cells, endometrial cells)

Specimen No. 432; Date 2/4/53; Photo No.; degree 3; class IV
histiocytes X; leukocytes X; cocci X; dyskaryotic superficial cells X; dyskaryotic intermediate cells X; dyskaryotic deep cells X; uniform atypical cells X; basal cells X

Specimen No. 1149; Date 4/10/63; Photo No.; degree 3; class IV
histiocytes X; leukocytes X; erythrocytes X; cocci X; dyskaryotic superficial cells X; dyskaryotic deep cells X; uniform atypical cells XX; basal cells X

Specimen No.; Date; Photo No.; degree; class

Specimen No.; Date; Photo No.; degree; class

Colposcopy		Photo No.
2/4/63	Closed transformation zone, highly vascular. At 12 o'clock, mosaic area. Iodine test: iodine-negative, sharp edges	XLI h 25-27
Date		Photo No.
Date		Photo. No.

Histology	
573/63	Conization Ca in situ endocervical and on the surface of the portio.
Date 4/18/63	

Remarks:

Fig. 21. Front and rear view of the status card

patterns on p. 57, 68). For purposes of comparability and reproducibility of reports the indication of certain characteristics by crosses appears to be essential. The current number of the specimen, the date when taken, and the number of the photograph in cases in which photomicrographs were made, also are entered on the status cards.

At the upper edge of the card, the first three letters of the patient's name are impressed, allowing for alphabetical order within the general card index.

3. *Punch Card (Fig. 22)*

The card in use has a combination of punches along the edge and over the surface. In the areas of perforation along the edges are 20 symbols for general categories, and in the large punched area are 105 individual symbols. The reports

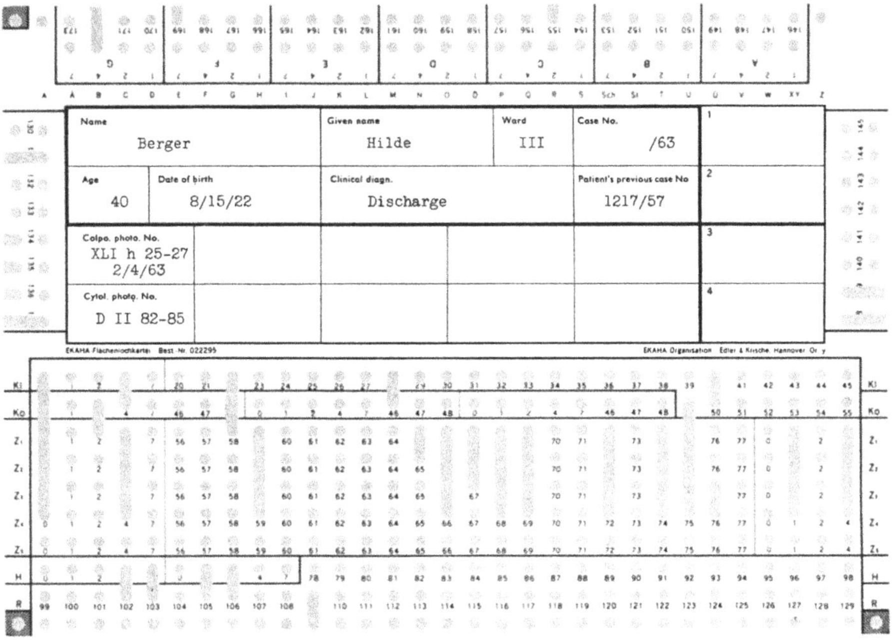

Fig. 22. Punch card

on the status card are transferred by means of a code (see code list) to the punch card. Space is left in the center for uncoded data (name, age, clinical diagnosis, etc.). The patient's name is impressed at the upper edge of the card (first letter deep, the next two letters shallow) for the alphabetical arrangement of the cards. The lower part of the card is occupied by the punch holes, where all findings entered on the status card may be recorded (five cytologic, three colposcopic, and one histologic report, etc.). The data that appear only once (e.g. age) are punched into the additive system; all other data, which may include several characteristics of one group, are punched in direct coordination. These two coding systems have been chosen to save space. About 1/6 of the possible punch holes may be left free. On the sides next to the uncoded text, are two double rows of punch holes for symbols of more general categories to facilitate the preliminary sorting of the cards.

Code[1]

Upper Edge: First 3 letters of name. First letter deeply impressed, next two shallow.

Slit-punch area: Row Kl, Ko, Z1—Z5 and H

I. Clinical Findings Row Kl

Age 0—19	1
20—24	2
25—29	3
30—34	4
35—39	5
40—44	6
45—49	7
50—54	8
55—59	9
60—64	10
65—69	11
70—74	12
75 and older	13
Menstrual status	
before menarche	20
primary amenorrhea	21
regular cycle	22
irregular cycle	23
secondary amenorrhea	24
menopause	25
Parity 0	26
1	27
2	28
3	29
4	30
5 and more	31
Abortions 0	49
1	50
2	51
3 and more	52

Operations	
Removal of the cervix	32
Removal of the uterus	33
Supravaginal hysterectomy	34
Removal of one ovary	35
Removal of both ovaries	36
Ra/X radiation	
Carcinoma dose	37
Ra menopause	38
X castration	39
Clinical finding on the portio	
not suspicious	40
inflammation	41
suspicious area	42
polyp	43
bleeding on contact	44
bleeding from endocervix	45
Iodine test	
iodine-positive	46
iodine-light	47
iodine-negative	48

II. Cytology Row Z1—Z5

Grade 4	1
4—3	2
3—4	3
3	4
3—2	5
2—3	6
2	7
2—1	8
1—2	9
1	11
Class I	1
II	2
II w	3
III	4
IV	5
V	6

Types	
mixed type	56
mucous type	57
deficient type	58

Microbiology	
cocci	59
Doederlein	60
cytolysis	61
mixed flora	62
trichomonads	63
fungi	64

Pathologic cells	
pseudodyskaryosis	65
dyskaryotic superficial cells	66
dyskaryotic intermediate cells	67
dyskaryotic deep cells	68
uniform atypical cells	69
polymorphic atypical cells	70

[1] Simplified reproduction without technical details of the punching.

Others	histiocytes	74	columnar cells	71
	leukocytes	75	basal cells	72
	erythrocytes	76	endometrial cells	73

III. Colposcopy Row Ko

Positive findings

exophytic, endophytic, IV a-area, adaptive vascular hypertrophy 1

Suspicious areas

matrix areas: leukoplakia, punctation, mosaic 2
matrix-like areas = resembling matrix areas 3
atypical transformation zone 4
other colposcopically suspicious findings 5

Benign findings

ectopy 6
ectopy with transformation zone 7
open transformation zone 8
closed transformation zone 9
vascular transformation zone 10
portio covered with normal squamous epithelium 11
cervical polyp 12
other colposcopically benign findings on the portio 13
colposcopic findings of different localization 14

IV. Histology Row H

Findings on the portio

squamous carcinoma 01
microcarcinoma 02
carcinoma in situ 03
borderline case of carcinoma in situ 04
dysplastic epithelium 05
metaplasia, ascending epidermidalization, cervicitis 06
cervical polyp 07
papilloma 08
adenocarcinoma of the portio 09
other forms of carcinoma of the portio 10
other histologic findings on the portio 11
insufficient findings because of artifacts 12

Corpus and appendages

adenocarcinoma 13
adenoacanthoma 14
carcinoma of the tubes 15
ovarian carcinoma 16

Other sites

carcinoma of the vagina 17
carcinoma of the vulva including Paget's disease 18
carcinoma of the urethra 19
urethral polyp 20
sarcoma at any location 21
other histologic findings 22

V. More general categories

Left side, numbers 130—137	shallow impressed	deep impressed	
clinical diagnosis	suspicious	positive	130
cytology	suspicious	positive	131
vault smear in cases where portio is absent	yes		132
smear from other sites	yes		133
cytologic photograph	yes	good	134
colposcopy	suspicious	positive	135
colposcopic findings available	1	2 and more	136
colposcopic photograph	yes	good	137
Right side, numbers 138—144			
histology	suspicious	positive	138
histologically evaluated	insufficiently	completely	139
phase-contrast photograph	yes	good	140
pregnancy	suspected	confirmed	141
mammary secretion	negative	positive	142
endometrial secretion	negative	positive	143
hormone assay	yes		144

VI. Row R

card completely filled 99
second card started the same year 100
years 1957—1962 . . . . 103—108

Reserve 77, 78—98, 101, 102, 109—129 and 145

In general, one card is enough for one patient per year; It is rarely necessary to start a second card for the same patient within the same year.

The evaluation of the punch cards is made with the mechanical sorting equipment of the Edler & Krische Company. The cards for a particular year are not arranged within the annual grouping.

A report on the experience with the card files of material from almost 15,000 cases follows (Rissmann, Kern and Zu Eulenburg, 1964).

The information pertaining to a symbol of the more general category of the marginal punch area (e.g., how many patients within the total material were subjected to colposcopy) is obtained through manual use of a pin. If about 150 cards are pierced at a time through the marginal hole with the symbol for "colposcopy", all cases examined with the colposcope drop out. About 4,000 cards can thus be analyzed in $1^1/_2$ hours. It therefore takes about 5 hours to learn how many of the 14,100 patients were examined by colposcopy. After this preselection, only the pile of the 4,787 cases thus selected rather than the total number of 14,100 is sorted for further detailed information in the field of "colposcopy".

Details, for example the nature of the colposcopic findings, must be ascertained with the help of the equipment by placing the pin in the appropriate symbols. Here too, however, an economical procedure is possible. By pinning first those symbols that are expected to appear frequently, the cardpiles to be sorted are gradually decreased. By selecting first, for example, the colposcopic finding "Closed transformation zone" and secondly "Portio covered with normal squamous epithelium" about 50% of all cards are dropped out. It would be wrong first to pin "Matrix areas" and to place 4,787 cards into the sorting equipment for this purpose. Much time is saved in the sorting procedure by appropriate choice of the sequence of frequency to be expected.

Not more than 300 to 350 cards should be worked on at one time in the selection equipment. If the cards are too tightly packed, the selector does not reach every single card and some may stick together. If this difficulty is kept in mind, even inexactly punched holes or attached so-called "card savers" will not upset the selection. Errors caused by incorrectly punched cards practically never occur, since there is a double check in comparing the findings of the status card with those of the punch card. A faulty ejection of cards is mechanically impossible with the selection equipment.

The number within the individual card packs has to be counted by hand, for the selection equipment, unlike the mechanical method, does not count the ejected cards. This procedure is undoubtedly time-consuming and tiring. By adding up all card packs, the accuracy of the counting may be checked, for it must add up to the known sum.

Further additional information, for example, "Which cytologic reports (Papanicolaou class II, IIw, III, IV/V) are associated with the available colposcopic findings?" is obtained in the most time-saving way by analyzing the card packs according to colposcopic data. According to the cytologic findings, one obtains, for example, four card packs from 1,346 cards (colposcopic finding: closed transformation zone). After counting by hand, 1062 cards correspond with class II, 193 cards to class II with repetition, 20 cards to class III, and 61 cards to class IV-V. Ten cards remain, showing that in ten cases the cytologic findings are inconclusive (incorrect smear technique, inadequate staining, and so forth). The numbers add up to 1,346, proving the count correct. Repetition of the selection can be omitted upon such verification.

In our experience, the source of error lies less often within the status and punch card index than in the uncoded entries of the clinical forms. The uncoded text is, therefore, critically examined in the laboratory, and, if necessary, corrected after further inquiry. In this connection the simplest possible arrangement of the clinical form has proved most useful, that is, entirely unequivocal questions to be answered merely with a cross. The least exact part of this form is the heading "Clinical Diagnosis" in the uncoded text. We have refrained from coding this category because on reexamination of the same patient by different gynecologists variable entries may be made.

The introduction of a punch card index in the study of early diagnosis of cancer has proved valuable in the analysis of an annual load of 3,000—4,000 cases. Complex questions can be answered by the card index at any time, for instance the age distribution of early cases, the frequency of early cases in the clinical material, the comparative accuracy of various methods after histologic diagnosis, the number of false negative and false positive reports, and many more.

Despite these favorable experiences, the future of modern documentation lies in the mechanical treatment of data because within a few years the capacity of a manual system will be exceeded by the rapidly increasing material.

With mechanical treatment of the data the entire material may evaluated directly by the mathematician, facilitating especially the resolution of problems of correlation.

Cost and Maintenance of Early Diagnosis

There is considerable lack of information about the costs of material and personnel for the installation and maintenance of a cytological laboratory. The bottleneck is exclusively in the field of diagnosis. A person experienced in cytodiagnosis is able to screen smears from about 40—60 patients (80—120 slides) per day. Examination of the slides is tiring, and attention flags after 1—2 hours at the microscope. On an average, 4—6 minutes are needed for one smear (two slides). Three to four hours are required, therefore, to examine 40 smears. Medical technicians after appropriate training can be used for screening (Clauss, 1958).

Half a year of daily practice in diagnosis under experienced guidance is the minimal period of training in cytologic diagnosis required of someone without histological experience. Papanicolaou suggested one year (see also Philipp, 1957; Antoine, 1959; Navratil, 1959 and Zinser, 1959).

A competent medical technician can handle many more slides per day. Planning her work systematically, she can stain, cover, and label about 100 smears (200 slides) per day. This number each day means 25,000 smears a year.

A number of that magnitude is scarcely needed for the institution itself. Boschann (1958) has given a clear report on the organization of a cytological laboratory, including material sent in; see also Ulm (1959), Weber (1961) and Zinser (1959 I, II, 1961, 1962). With about 5,000 patients examined cytologically in a large gynecologic clinic, there will be about 6,000 smears a year including repeated smears. With roughly 250 work days a year, there will be 24 smears a day, and, hence, the need for about $2^1/_2$ hours of microscopic work per day. The technician can use the remaining time to record the findings and prepare the smears.

This aspect has been mentioned in order to demonstrate that cytodiagnosis within a gynecological department is, at least with regard to staffing, entirely possible.

Costs of Installation and Maintenance of a Cytological Laboratory

The following figures illustrate the costs of a cytological laboratory with the simplest equipment.

Original Installation (prices 1962) (4.0 [approx.] DM = $ 1.00; 1967)

1. Laboratory furniture		6000.— DM
2. 1 Standard microscope		2330.— DM
3. Glass and other equipment:		
35 specimen glasses, 15 cm high, ∅ 10 cm round	288.75 DM	
2 funnels 10 cm ∅	3.60 DM	
2 funnels 5 cm ∅	2.— DM	
12 Hellendahl cuvettes	37.20 DM	
1 measuring cylinder 1000 ml	6.50 DM	
1 measuring cylinder 500 ml	4.50 DM	
2 measuring cylinders 100 ml	4.00 DM	
1 measuring cylinder 50 ml	1.65 DM	
3 pipettes 10 ml	4.95 DM	
5 pipettes 1 ml	6.75 DM	
10 glass bottles 2000 ml	27.50 DM	
4 glass bottles 1000 ml	17.50 DM	
2 small dishes for cover slips 20 ml	10.— DM	
1 Petri dish	1.75 DM	
1 glass rod	1.25 DM	
1 bottle for distilled water 10 liters (plastic)	26.— DM	

5 staining stands	120.— DM	
2 laboratory alarm clocks	37.50 DM	
2 forceps, various	11.50 DM	
1 pair of scissors	9.70 DM	
		622.60 DM
4. 1 typewriter		556.— DM
5. 20 folders for slides at 2.85 DM each		57.— DM
6. 50 cabinets for slides at 5.80 DM each		290.— DM
7. 2 table lamps		84.— DM
		9939.60 DM

Current Expenses for Personnel Per Year:

1 female medical technical assistant full-time (21 years old, BAT VII)	6362.40 DM
1 cleaning woman 2 hours per day (2.01 DM per hour gross, 50 weeks × 5 days = 250 days)	1005.— DM
	7367.40 DM

Current Expenses for Material per Year:

1. Glassware (slides and cover slips)		1210.— DM
2. chemicals		
isopropyl alcohol	780.— DM	
petrol-benzene denatured alcohol	858.— DM	
xylene	156.— DM	
ether	327.60 DM	
acetone	8.— DM	
mounting medium	61.60 DM	
Harris hematoxylin	153.— DM	
Eosin EA 31 Papanicolaou Polychrome Merck	276.— DM	
Orange G, OG 6 Merck	156.— DM	
hydrochloric acid normal	33.80 DM	
		2810.— DM
3. filter paper, fluted filters		143.15 DM
4. stationery (note pads, schedules, pencils, letter paper, envelopes, and carbon paper)		760.— DM
5. repairs, spare parts, electric bulbs		200.— DM
		5123.15 DM

The equipment of the laboratory costs roughly 10000.— DM. The recurrent annual expenses are 7367.40 DM for personnel and 5123.— DM for materials. Current annual costs for the running of the laboratory are therefore 12000 to 13000 DM, if no payment is made for the diagnostic service.

If the annual costs are calculated on the basis of 5,000 patients a year, the cytological examination of an individual patient costs, on the average, 2.50 DM. At a rate of detection of about 1.7% of early cases and small cancers, the cost for each detected case is about 150.— DM.

The cost of the installation and maintenance of a modern filing system for early diagnosis varies (Stoll and Riehm, 1954; Halfpap and Hosemann, 1959;

Wagner and Stegmann, 1959; Waschke, 1959; Wildner, 1959; Stoll, 1960, and Zechner, 1960). We mention, for example, the special punch card system introduced by us, with its status cards and clinical forms.

10,000 clinical forms in duplicate with carbon paper	700.— DM
5,000 status cards	475.— DM
5,000 punch cards	375.— DM

About 0.31 DM must therefore be taken into account per patient for this additional registration. There are, furthermore, the initial costs of the notching pincers, the slit puncher for the perforation of the corresponding areas, and the equipment for sorting.

The colposcopic examination of a patient is considerably cheaper. There are no current annual expenses after the purchase of one or two colposcopes. The need for repair of the colposcopes is extremely small. The reagents, acetic acid and iodine solution, can certainly be charged to the clinical department.

The Methods of Cytology

The value of cytodiagnosis, its accuracy, and the number of mistakes made with it depend to a very significant extent on the correct technique of obtaining the specimen. Cytodiagnosis is unjustly discredited through careless or incorrect technique. The cytodiagnosis of cervical carcinoma has attained its level of success because the location of the developing cancer is easily accessible to the naked eye and to instruments. Certain basic technical details must, nevertheless, be given careful attention. The following requirements must be met for the cellular material sampled:

1. Viable cells should be obtained carefully from the epithelium.
2. Smears must comprise cells from all epithelial surfaces of the cervix in which a pathologic transformation of the epithelium is possible.

The method for satisfying these requirements is as follows (Kern, 1960):

Instruments. To prepare a cytologic smear one needs:

1. A pair of gynecological specula to separate the vaginal walls.
2. Two applicators, 20 cm long, 3—4 mm thick, tightly but thinly wrapped with cotton at one end to a length of 2—3 cm. These applicators are prepared by the assisting personnel.
3. Two grease-free slides marked by a diamond pencil with the patient's name before the cellular material is taken. We use plain slides. Slides frosted at one end on which the name may be written with a pencil are available, but they are expensive, and blurring or fading of the writing in the staining jars may occur. A name that has been etched with a diamond pencil cannot be removed from the glass.
4. A Hellendahl cuvette with liquid fixative.
5. Accompanying form (see above).

Other authors recommend the wooden spatula of Ayre (1944), or the glass pipette of Papanicolaou (1949), or a lavage instead of the applicators. Since the wooden spatula of Ayre adapts well to the external os, it removes cellular material from an important region. It has two drawbacks, however. It does not penetrate far enough into the cervical canal, and rather large strips of epithelium are often mechanically torn off. Ayre (1947, 1949) himself called this method of removal a "surface biopsy" (Schüller, 1955; Bajardi, 1960). It invites bleeding, on the one hand, thus interfering with the subsequent colposcopic examination, and on the other hand, bulky cellular aggregates result, rendering the microscopic evaluation more difficult. A combination of Ayre's spatula (for the surface of the portio) with the cotton-tipped applicator (for the cervical canal) eliminates the first disadvantage. Horn and Ashworth in 1957 designed a wooden spatula with differently shaped ends. One end scrapes the surface of the portio; the other allows deep penetration into the cervical canal.

Removal of cellular material with a glass pipette from the posterior fornix must be considered inadequate, because it furnishes only secretion with cells already shed that do not, therefore, satisfy the requirement for fresh material. Miller and v. Haam in 1961 were able to demonstrate the superiority of the abrasive technique, as compared with that of aspiration. McLaren and Attwood arrived at the same conclusion in 1961. Similar statements can be made concerning various lavage procedure that have been described. The Cytophor of Langreder (1958, 1959) may be mentioned here as one example: the isotonic solution used to rinse out the vagina is collected in Cytophor and the cells obtained are allowed to settle to the bottom and are then examined in a smear. We have had no experience with this method but we do not believe that its reliability approaches that of the direct smear. It appears, furthermore, to be much more time-consuming.

Platinum loops for the removal of cells are out of the question, because they remove far too little material and may injure the epithelium (Langreder, 1954; Majewski, 1956).

Other procedures definitely to be rejected are those in which the patient herself or a assistant removes secretion from the vagina without exposure of the portio; a smear obtained from inserted tampons appears to be equally inadequate (Brunschwig, 1954; Papanicolaou, 1954; Jaeger, 1957; Tietze, 1958; Pomerance *et al.*, 1959; Soost and Nevin, 1959).

The Patient. Certain precautions are recommended before taking a cytologic smear:

The patient should abstain from vaginal douches for several days (Petracca, 1962). No medications (particularly contraceptives) should be inserted vaginally. The patient should not have had intercourse, and she should not be bleeding at the time the smear is taken.

These requirements are justified, but cannot always be fulfilled in practice. It would be necessary to refrain from taking the smear during this first gynecologic examination and many patients would have to be given reappointments. A considerable number of the patients would probably not come again. Therapeutic vaginal douches as a treatment for discharge, or procedures on the portio such as electrocoagulation, punch biopsy, and curettage should not be performed for several weeks before the smear, because the pattern of the smear would thereby be altered. Return to normal of the epithelium cannot be expected before 4 to 6 weeks, especially after electrocoagulation.

Vaginal douches are rarely taken by our patients. It may be difficult to collect sufficient material if all the secretion has been washed out of the vagina shortly before the gynecologic examination, usually with astringent solutions. Collection of sufficient cellular material by direct smear should, nevertheless, be attempted. If remnants of vaginal tablets or suppositories remain in the vagina, they must be carefully removed before collecting the cells.

Bleeding patients present a more difficult problem. No smear can, of course, be made during massive hemorrhages (for example abortion). If the bleeding is light, however, the blood can be carefully removed with a gauze tampon and a direct smear then be made from the surface of the portio. In that case, the smear from the cervical canal is usually more extensively contaminated with blood. In women with a heavy mucous discharge, which is often found not only in the posterior vaginal fornix but also over the entire surface of the portio, the secretion must be removed by careful swabbing before the direct smear is made. The same precautions apply to the lochia of women in the puerperium.

At the time of ovulation, the cervical canal is filled with the typical gelatinous secretion that reduces the yield of cells. An attempt may be made, in that case, to remove the secretion first, but is often not possible because of the viscosity of the mucus. In such a situation, the smear may have to be repeated at another phase of the cycle. Another possibility is an attempt to precipitate the mucus with acetic acid and to remove it, and then to make a rather vigorous direct smear a few minutes later. The acetic acid does not affect the evaluation of the subsequent smear. In old women the cellular yield is frequently very small. In such cases, the Ayre spatula often yields more material than the cotton-tipped applicator.

Hemorrhages, heavy discharge, or lochia create possibilities for erroneous cytodiagnosis, but if one heeds the principle of removing disturbing secretions carefully and then collects cells from the epithelium, it is undoubtedly better to perform the smear than to dismiss the patient without cytologic examination.

Technique of Removal. The cytological smear should be made at the start of every gynecologic examination before the bimanual palpation. The vagina is held apart with specula that are dry or only slightly moistened with water. The portio and vaginal walls are carefully inspected; disturbing secretions or bloody contaminants may then be gently removed (see preceding paragraph); and the entire surface of the portio is wiped with a cotton-tipped applicator (Fig. 23). Some pressure may be applied, for injuries can scarcely be caused by the cotton-tipped applicator. A light smear produces too few cells. By moving the blades of the specula the portio can be slightly tilted or moved laterally to produce good contact between the applicator and the epithelial surface. The cotton-tipped applicator is removed without touching the vaginal walls and stroked uniformly over three-fourths of the surface of the prelabeled slide, which is then put into the fixative (ether-alcohol) while the smear is still moist. Desiccation of the secretions before fixation must be avoided or the cells cannot be evaluated microscopically. The applicator is discarded. Another is then inserted as deeply as possible into the cervical canal, often with the cotton tip almost disappearing (Fig. 23). While the applicator is rotated several times, it is drawn along the entire lining of the cervical canal with light pressure; the canal can be dilated considerably, especially in multiparas. A second smear is prepared in like manner and also fixed immediately. The endocervical smear is sometimes followed by scant bleeding. Spreading of the cellular material in a uniformly thin layer is successfully accomplished with the cotton-tipped applicator. Distortion of cells through spreading rarely occurs as described by authors who use wooden spatulas.

The whole procedure takes scarcely 2 minutes and therefore is not much of a burden to the physician. The accompanying form is filled out after completion of a thorough gynecologic examination.

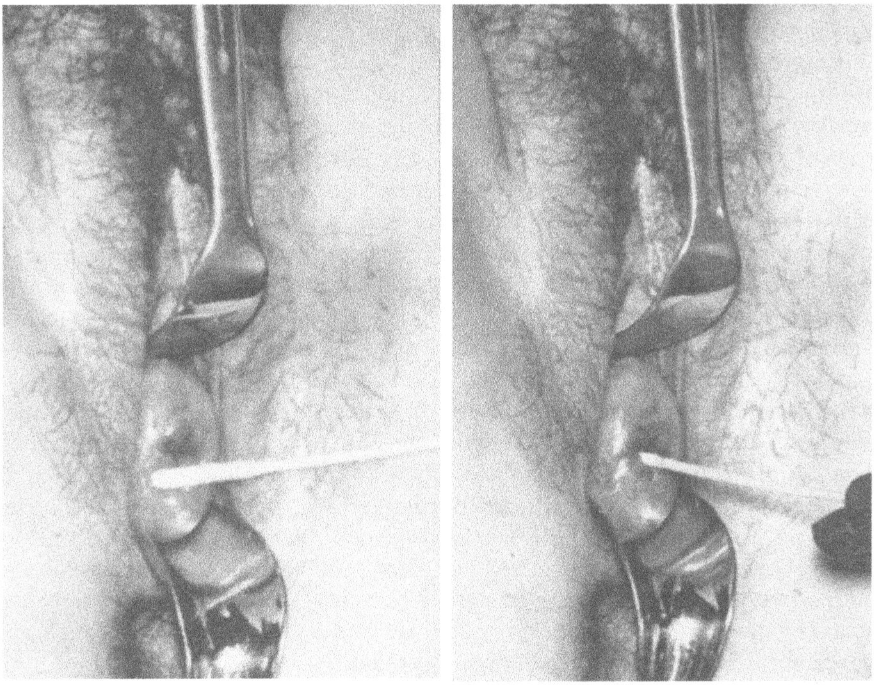

Fig. 23. Technique of collecting cells. The left half of the picture shows the preparation of the smear from the surface of the portio, and the right half from the cervical canal. (For technical photographic reasons, a prolapsed portio was chosen) (KERN, 1960)

If, despite the technique of removal described above, the diagnosis meets with difficulties, making a repeat study advisable, evaluation of the bacterial flora and the hormonal status may provide suggestions for treatment that are recommended to the clinician before the smear is repeated (see p. 55, 56).

We remove, as shown, the cellular material in contact with the surface of the portio and the cervical canal. Originally exfoliative cytology was concerned with the examination of cells already shed into the vaginal pool of the posterior fornix. AYRE (1946 I, II), ISAAC and WURCH (1952 I, II), WIED (1956), NIEBURGS (1956), SOOST (1958), TRIFON (1958), WIED and BAHR (1959), SONG, FANGER and MURPHY (1959), BICKENBACH and SOOST (1960), FERGUSON and MATZ (1960), Symposium Acta cytologica (1960 I—IV) and KOSS (1961) called attention to the fact that the yield of pathologic cells from the posterior vaginal fornix is not optimal. We searched for the most favorable region for obtaining the cells in 50 cytologically positive patients (KERN, 1961 I, II). Three smears from each patient were prepared: from the posterior vaginal fornix, from the surface of the portio, and from the cervical canal. When the histologic material was available in the form of survey slides of the cervix, the cellular yield from each of the three regions was again checked and related to the localization of epithelial changes. The result was unequivocal. About half of the malignant growths would have been overlooked after isolated removal of cellular material from the posterior vaginal fornix. This failure to find cells must be attributed to the fast autolysis that the cells undergo at body temperature in the presence of bacteria. In contrast, failures were minimal at the other two regions of sampling. The smears from the surface of the portio and the cervical canal complemented each other, thus preventing any oversight in this material, provided the smears were carefully prepared from the surface of the portio as well as from the cervical canal. The intracervical smear should be considered especially valuable, because it affords the only possible way of recognizing changes that occur high within the cervix, generally in older women (about 20% of the early changes). If malignant cells are found only in the cervical smear, a lesion in the cervical canal is suspected. Cytologic smears otherwise do not provide any indications of localization.

Fixation. Fixation of the slides takes place, as mentioned previously, in a 1:1 mixture of ethyl ether and 96% ethyl alcohol. This fixation has been successful with PAPANICOLAOU'S stain, as described below. None of the other common fixatives used for tissues (formaldehyde, etc.) are suitable for cytodiagnosis. The shortest time of fixation is 20 minutes. There is no upper limit (SOOST, 1958).

The customary glass cuvettes are not covered hermetically, and the mixture therefore evaporates slowly. Since ether is more volatile than alcohol, the proportion of the mixture changes in favor of the alcohol, and the fixation deteriorates. The fixative solution, therefore, has to be completely changed. The correct proportion of the mixture cannot be restored by refilling. This fact must be pointed out repeatedly, especially to the nursing personnel.

Transportation. If the cytodiagnosis is performed in a laboratory in the same building, the slides are delivered in their fixative. For the practicing physician, however, the problem of sending the slides to the laboratory must be considered. Because the fixative solutions are highly inflammable, they cannot be mailed. It is generally recommended that the slides be removed from the ether-alcohol mixture after at least 20 minutes, mounted with glycerol, and then protected with a cover slip before sending them on (AYRE and DAKIN, 1946; PAPANICOLAOU, 1956/57; SOOST and PICHLMAYR, 1959). We do not, for several reasons, consider this procedure advantageous and we suggest the following method:

The slides are taken from the fixative after at least 20 minutes; the remaining liquid is allowed to drip off, and the uncovered slides are placed in slide folders or boxes, with care that they do not touch one another. The slides dry in a few seconds and may then be sent out. Upon arrival at the laboratory, they are again put into ether-alcohol and passed through the staining sequence as usual. The results are not different from those with slides that have not been dried. Similar satisfactory experience has been reported by BUCHHOLZ (1959) and BOSCHANN (1960).

The procedure of mounting the slides with glycerol causes the physician who sends them out much more trouble. The slides often are stuck together on arrival in the laboratory. With attempts to separate them some of the cellular material is often detached. The glycerol must be removed from the slides by leaving them for hours in 70% alcohol. Residues of glycerol subsequently disturb the staining. Dry transportation avoids all these troubles. A minimal fixation time of 20 minutes is required for a perfect stain, but it is best to prolong this period. PAPANICOLAOU and BRIDGES recommended in 1957 that the moist unfixed smear be covered with a drop of Diaphan before sending it off. We have no experience with this method.

Staining. The method recommended by PAPANICOLAOU seems to be rather cumbersome, but no other stain has proved superior, although many authors have made numerous attempts to improve it.

Acridine orange fluorescent staining has been used on a wider scale during the last several years. (For our experience with this stain see p. 76.) All other methods are essentially modifications of the PAPANICOLAOU stain, none of which we have tested (SHORR, 1940, 1941; ZINSER, 1950, 1954; CRAMER and STAMM, 1950; WIED, 1951; WURCH and ISAAK, 1951; STEMMER, 1953; GABOR and SZEGVÁRI, 1958; GRÜNBERGER and KREMER, 1960; MASIN and MASIN, 1960; WAGNER, 1960; WAGNER, KALMUS and STEGMANN, 1961).

Basically, the PAPANICOLAOU stain (1942) consists of a nuclear stain, hematoxylin, which has to be well differentiated and blued, and a polychrome cytoplasmic counterstain. The latter begins with Orange G (OG 6), with which especially epithelia that tend to keratinize are stained orange, and ends with staining in Polychrome EA 36 or EA 31. These designations vary with the manufacturer. This polychrome counterstain consists of a mixture of eosin, light-green, and Bismarck brown. Although the chemistry of the cytoplasmic stain is not entirely clear, it can be stated that mature superficial cells stain "acidophilic" with eosin, whereas less mature epithelial cells take a "basophilic" blue to blue-green stain. The nuclear and cytoplasmic stains are performed in sequence, through descending and ascending series of alcohols, to allow for the aqueous and the alcoholic media of the stains. We use the following staining technique with consistent results:

1. After fixation (20 minutes minimum, no upper limit) another rinse with ether-alcohol (1:1).
2. Descending alcohol series, 1 minute each (90%, 80% and 70%).
3. Rinse in distilled water. All slides must be made uniformly wet (with water) to achieve a uniform nuclear stain in the next phase of the procedure.
4. Nuclear stain in Harris' hematoxylin, 15—20 minutes. The stain must be filtered once a day. No overstaining is permissible with the nuclear stain, because hyperchromasia may thus be simulated. Nuclear hyperchromasia is of importance in the diagnosis of pathologic nuclei.
5. Rinsing off the excess stain in distilled water.
6. Brief differentiation in 3% HCl-alcohol.
7. Blueing of the nuclear stain in tap water. Again, the slides are to be made wet quickly and uniformly by the blueing tap water, or else the HCl-alcohol causes patchy, continued differentiation, resulting in uneven nuclear stain.

8. Short rinse in distilled water.

9. Ascending alcohol series (50%, 70%, 80%, 95%) 1 minute each.

10. First cytoplasmic stain in Orange G, 6—10 minutes. Since this cytoplasmic stain can easily be rinsed off again,

11. Dip briefly in 95% alcohol and

12. Transfer into Polychrome cytoplasmic dye EA 31 (mixture of eosin, light-green, and Bismarck brown). Stain 3—5 minutes (always half the time of step 10).

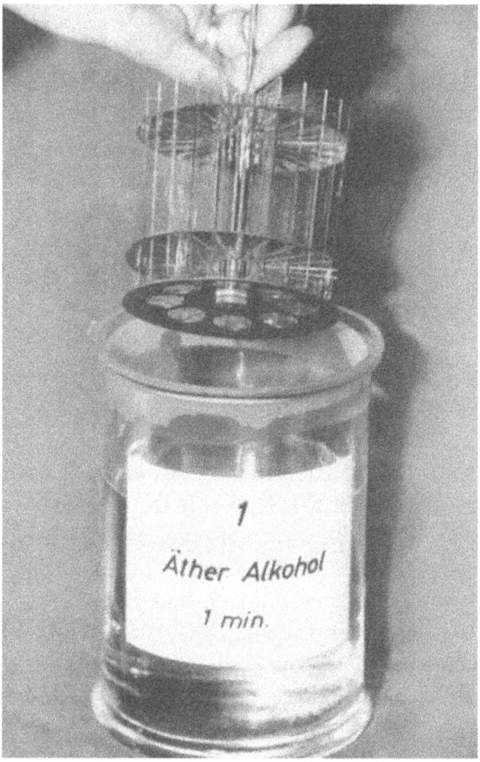

Fig. 24. The staining stand we use is made of metal and holds 24 slides for one entire staining sequence. All round staining jars are closed with fitted covers to prevent evaporation of the solutions

Allow the slide holder to drip off thoroughly upon removal from the dye solution. While dripping, the slides become more intensely red, apparently under the influence of the oxygen in the air. This phenomenon must be allowed to proceed to completion, for in this manner an excellent shade of stain of the cytoplasm is achieved.

13. Very brief rinse in 95% alcohol; allow to drip off again thoroughly, and allow slides to "redden" again in the air.

14. Another thorough rinse in 95% alcohol, then transfer to absolute alcohol (twice), then to alcohol-xylene (1:1), and into xylene.

15. Cover with Caedax or Eukitt.

About 1 hour is needed for this stain. We use round staining vessels with fitted covers to prevent excessive evaporation of the solutions. The round metal stand shown in Fig. 24 has been used successfully for transportation of the slides.

The alcohols of the staining sequence in steps 1, 2, 9, 11 and 13 are prepared with denatured ethyl alcohol. For step 14, however, isopropyl alcohol is recommended; otherwise, the slides become quite green.

One difficulty arises during the use of the dyes. The Harris hematoxylin nuclear stain can be used for months without changing the staining time. The cytoplasmic stains, on the other hand, are used up relatively quickly and must be renewed every 4 to 6 weeks. During that time, the staining periods must be continuously prolonged and at the same rate. The alcohols have to be renewed every 6 to 8 days.

Another problem is the variability of the dye solutions as manufactured by the producers. The staining produced by a new batch from the same firm can be different. Dye solutions with the same name produced by different firms often create quite variable staining effects. We use the dye solutions of Gurr (England) and Merck (Darmstadt) with relatively consistent results.

The Papanicolaou stain, unfortunately, does not last through the years. The slides fade after a few weeks if left exposed to light. The stain fades after 6—8 months in slide boxes. If old slides are to be reexamined, the cover glasses can be removed with xylene and the slides restained satisfactorily, after having been taken through the descending alcohol series and decolorized for several hours in HCl-alcohol.

What May Render Cytodiagnosis Difficult Despite Proper Preparation of the Specimen and What can be Done About it?

If the previously described instructions are heeded, the slide will permit successful diagnosis in the great majority of cases. There are cases, however, in which the diagnosis is difficult and in which the conditions should be improved, before a smear is repeated.

Cytodiagnosis may become complicated in serious inflammations, generally with a marked disturbance of the vaginal flora, and in smears of epithelium atrophic because of age.

Inflammations. In cervicitis and vaginitis the material obtained often consists mostly of leukocytes, even though the discharge has been removed before the smear is taken. The squamous epithelial cells that are of interest in early diagnosis are few and show signs of the inflammation (see p. 65). The patients appear in the office usually because of the discharge and are, therefore, easily persuaded to undergo treatment. If the smear is not contaminated by specific microorganisms (see p. 63), and cocci prevail, we initiate a so-called cleansing treatment, involving the insertion of tampons, e.g. with an estrogenic ointment for 3 days. The treatment temporarily effects a substantial decrease of bacteria and leukocytes; contact smears can then be taken under improved conditions. Systemic antibiotic treatment should be avoided because of the danger of producing resistant strains. Similar success is achieved with an estrogenic creme in senile vaginitis, which is usually nonbacterial.

Trichomonads and threads of *Leptothrix* may be easily recognized in the cytologic smear. Both are often accompanied by inflammatory signs. We apprise the clinician of these findings and he initiates specific treatment. In trichomoniasis the patient's partner should be treated simultaneously to prevent reinfection. Since the man can be treated per os, no difficulties will be encountered. If treatment for vaginal discharge is planned anyway, the smear can be repeated upon termination of treatment.

Smears from Atrophic Epithelium. The beginner in cytodiagnosis finds it especially difficult to distinguish with sufficient precision the atrophic epithelia

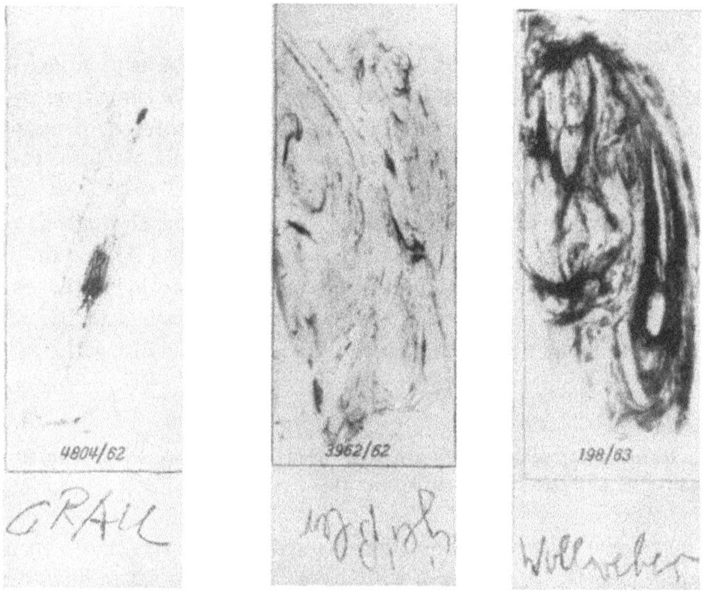

Fig. 25. Macroscopic picture of smears. At right, too much material has been put on the slide, and on the left, too little. The smear in the center was prepared correctly

from the pathologic cells in menopausal women. The ratio of nucleus to cytoplasm often appears to be increased. In this instance, short-term hormonal treatment of the vaginal epithelium will suffice to make the distinction. In old women, who are often very reluctant to permit gynecological treatment over a period of several days, an injection of estrogen (e.g. 1×5 mg estradiol benzoate = Progynon B oleosum) and repetition of the smear after 3 days are recommended. The dose must not be sufficiently great to stimulate the endometrium to bleed.

The following mistakes are generally made when cytologic smears are prepared:

Careless removal from the pool of secretions in the posterior vaginal fornix.

Secretion, unevenly, usually too thickly, applied to the slide.

Too little material.

Material allowed to dry.

These difficulties render the results of cytodiagnosis very questionable. Observation of the following rules produces good results:

Careful removal directly from the epithelia of the cervix at the start of a gynecologic examination.

Elimination of contaminants (blood, discharge, mucus) before making the smear.

Immediate fixation of the smear while it is still moist.

Fig. 25 shows the macroscopic appearance of smears in which mistakes in the technique are clearly evident.

The Appearance of the Normal Cell

The cytological smears for early cancer detection are taken from the surface of the portio and from the cervical canal. Contact is made with squamous and columnar epithelia. Exact knowledge of the picture of a smear taken under normal conditions is prerequisite to the clear differentiation of pathologic cells from normal cells. The correct interpretation of numerous nonmalignant conditions is particularly important; for example, epidermidalization or inflammatory phenomena with all their cellular and bacterial contaminants. Excellent discussions of normal cytodiagnosis of the vaginal smear can be found in Ayre; Boschann; Koss and Durfee; Papanicolaou; Papanicolaou, Traut and Marchetti; Pundel; Schmitt; Smolka and Soost, and Zinser.

Cells Shed by the Squamous Epithelium

The vagina and most of the surface of the portio are covered with nonkeratinizing squamous epithelium.

The epithelium is clearly stratified in the sexually mature woman (Fig. 12). Above the basalis is the so-called layer of spiny cells, or the parabasal layer, which is characterized by intercellular bridges. It is followed by the intermediate layer containing glycogen, and finally, by the superficial cells, which are grouped into discernible outer and inner layers. With the squamous epithelium thus composed, detachment of cells with the cotton-tipped applicator, mainly from the outer and inner superficial layers of the epithelium, is feasible.

The estrogen-sensitive vaginal epithelium in a normally menstruating woman is subject to various growth stimuli during a cycle. Generally higher levels of estrogen are associated with more nearly complete maturation of the epithelium. Physiologically, such conditions obtain at the time of ovulation. The percentage of superficial cells in the smear reaches its maximum at that time. Hormonal cytodiagnosis, to be discussed here only as far as required for understanding the appearance of the normal cell, has developed because of the hormonal sensitivity of the vaginal epithelium, which far surpasses that of the endometrium (Murray, 1938; Stoll, 1961).

Epithelial Cells of the Outer and Inner Superficial Layers. These cells appear in the cytologic smear as large, polygonal, usually flattened cells about 50 μ in diameter. The cytoplasm of the *outer superficial cells* is eosinophilic and sharply delimited at the periphery. Strongly blue to brown perinuclear granules are present at times. With higher levels of estrogen, the eosinophilic cells lie isolated, without folds, on the slide. At other phases of the cycle they usually diminish in number in favor of the inner superficial cells. The nuclei of these cells are round to oval and small, about 5 μ in diameter. Complete pyknosis of the nucleus, which exhibits no structure at all, is typical (Figs. 27, 35, 39).

The maturation of the squamous epithelium proceeds normally only up to the outer superficial cell, but occasionally true keratinization occurs with loss of the nucleus. In that case, yellowish or orange-colored flakes without nuclei are found in the smear, in which an unstained "shadow" is discernible in the place of the nucleus (Fig. 28). These structures, which frequently appear with a prolapse of the uterus, have no significance. In the absence of a prolapse, a particularly thorough scrutiny of the slide is indicated, because the flakes may originate from a leukoplakia, which must always be given special attention.

The cytoplasm of the *inner superficial cells* is basophilic, and the contour is sharp. Granulations do not usually occur in the cytoplasm. These cells, according to the time of the cycle, are spread flat and isolated, or lie wrinkled in groups (Fig. 39). The volume of the cytoplasm is usually somewhat smaller than that of the eosinophilic superficial cells. The nucleus is larger (ca. 9 μ) and round to oval, and it exhibits no pyknosis. The chromatin is relatively dense. The proportion of these two cellular types varies in typical manner during a cycle. These changes can be seen most clearly in smears from the posterior third of the lateral vaginal wall, the location of the smear preferred for hormonal cytodiagnosis. Smears from the surface of the portio exhibit the cyclical variations somewhat less distinctly, but one must become familiar with them too.

In addition to the cellular types just described, cells from deeper strata of the squamous epithelium, down to the basal layer, are found in the sexually mature woman. These cells do not originate from normal squamous epithelium, which could never be destroyed by the cotton-tipped applicator down to the basal layer. The cells from deeper strata in the sexually mature woman originate from incomplete epidermidalization or metaplastic squamous epithelium of the cervix uteri.

If the everted columnar epithelium (see p. 21) is overgrown by squamous epithelium, the latter does not advance in a completely differentiated front, but pushes ahead first in a single layer and later in several or many layers over the columnar epithelium. The development of metaplastic squamous epithelium is similar. The lower the epithelium, the less completely is it differentiated.

The epidermidalization of the portio is most frequent in sexual maturity. It plays no role in the short cyclic processes. Accordingly, deep cells are very often found in smears from the surface of the portio. These smears are, therefore, not used for accurate hormonal analyses of the vaginal epithelium.

Only when ovarian function decreases or completely subsides, that is, in the climacteric, after the menopause, and in senility, is the structure of the squamous epithelium of the whole vagina and the surface of the portio changed to the extent that complete differentiation no longer occurs. In the first few years after the menopause, the so-called mixed type is often found, namely a cellular smear in which cells of all strata are present in about equal numbers.

As a woman ages, cells of the intermediate, parabasal, and basal layers come to dominate the picture. Finally, in old women, only cells of the basal type are found; they may, furthermore, exhibit a certain atrophy (Fig. 13, 26).

In the study of the deeper cells of the squamous epithelium in the smear it is important to imagine the changes in the cell after it has been separated from the epithelial tissue. The epithelial cells are polygonally interdigitated, or, in the parabasal layer, are connected by intercellular bridges. If they are separated from the epithelial tissue, all protoplasmic processes retract and the cells become round. Only exceptionally are cells fixed in a condition in which minute protoplasmic processes, the former intercellular bridges for example, may be discerned.

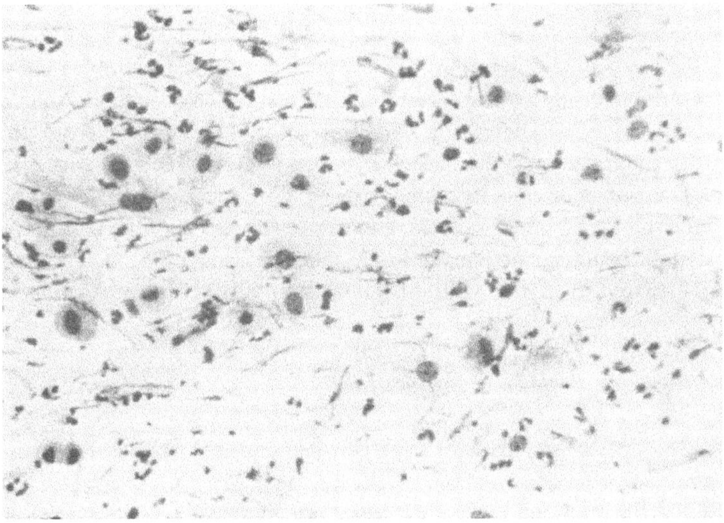

Fig. 26. Atrophic cells from an old woman with typical artifacts of the smear

Epithelial Cells of the Intermediate Layer. The cells are usually oval to round and of medium size, about 40 μ in diameter. The cytoplasm is always basophilic. With proper cytoplasmic differentiation using the Papanicolaou method, the intermediate cells stain a slightly deeper blue than the inner superficial cells. The cell boundaries are sharply outlined. The cytoplasm appears homogenous. The nucleus is round and of medium size, about 9 μ in diameter, with a fine but clear chromatin structure. Nucleoli can often be discerned as well as the Barr body at the nuclear membrane. The cells of the intermediate layer usually lie together, spread flat, in irregular groups (Fig. 40).

Epithelial Cells of the Deep (Parabasal and Basal) Layers. The cells from the deep layers of the squamous epithelium usually appear completely round in the smear. Remnants of intercellular bridges in the form of delicate protoplasmic projections are occasionally found among the parabasal cells. The diameter of the parabasal cells is about 30 μ and that of the basal cells about 20 μ. The cytoplasm of both cellular types is always basophilic and with good staining more intensely blue than that of the intermediate cells and that of the inner superficial layer. The cell boundaries are sharply outlined. The cytoplasm is never folded or rolled up but always spread flat. If fresh batches of dye are used, the cytoplasm of the deep epithelial cells stains blue-green. Apparently, the light-green in the polychrome dye is very quickly used up, because this effect disappears after the batch has been in use for a few days. The nuclei of the epithelial cells from the deep layers are round and relatively large (10 μ in diameter). The chromatin is sharply outlined, and the nucleoli and Barr body are usually visible. Parabasal and basal cells often lie together in groups or in rows like strings of pearls (Fig. 41).

There is a certain difference between the deep cells from epidermidalized mucosa of the sexually mature woman and the basal cells of the old woman. In young women, strongly basophilic, swollen cells are found. In old women, on the other hand, only weakly basophilic cells appear, with a narrow rim of cytoplasm and a relatively dark nucleus. The cytoplasm may, under certain conditions, be entirely absent. Smears of atrophic, senile epithelium, furthermore, tend to contain artifacts, as nucleus and cytoplasm lend themselves to considerable stretching and distortion. In addition, the nuclei exhibit slight deviations from their round shape. Faulty diagnoses may be caused by overstaining with hematoxylin (Fig. 26).

The total number of cells in a smear from old women is considerably reduced. These cellular pictures cause trouble, especially for the beginner, and are at times difficult to tell from certain pathologic cellular types. A temporary hormonal restoration (see p. 56) of the vaginal epithelium solves the problem.

Cells Shed from the Columnar Epithelium

The normal epithelial surface of the cervical canal is the columnar epithelium, which can spread over the surface of the portio more or less extensively. It is a columnar epithelium of one layer with basal nuclei and marked secretion of mucus. The luminal epithelial surface has cilia (Schüller, 1960). The surface of the endocervix is very extensive because of the many glands formed there. The quantity, composition, and consistency of the mucus produced undergo typical cyclic changes. Leukocytes and histiocytes migrate easily through the epithelium. Consisting of a single layer, and therefore very thin, it is quite vulnerable to contact. Bleeding ectopies are known, especially during pregnancy, as well as slight bleeding when the endocervical smear is taken.

Rather few columnar epithelial cells are found in the smear from the surface of the portio and the endocervical canal, despite the macroscopically great vulnerability of its columnar epithelium. The epithelial cells apparently are able to cling to the cervical tissue because of the stickiness of the mucus. Their form may vary considerably if they have been separated from the epithelium. Rarely do they keep their original shape. They usually lie in groups of three to four cells. The cytoplasm usually flows around the nucleus after the cell has been isolated, causing the outline of the cell to look oval or round (Fig. 27). The cytoplasm may occasionally be absent or it may be drawn out into a long tail. The cytoplasm is stained blue with the Papanicolaou method. The nucleus of the columnar epithelial cell is large and vesicular with a delicate chromatin structure. Nucleoli can often be discerned.

Especially if their original shape has been lost and the nuclear stain has been too intense, columnar epithelial cells may sometimes be mistaken for certain pathologic cellular forms (SMOLKA, 1961) (see p. 73) (Fig. 27).

Other Cells of the Vaginal Smear

There are, in addition to the epithelial cells just described, mainly cellular elements of the blood in the smear. The mixture of the epithelial cells with these cells may be, to a varying extent, dependent on the phase of the cycle, but may

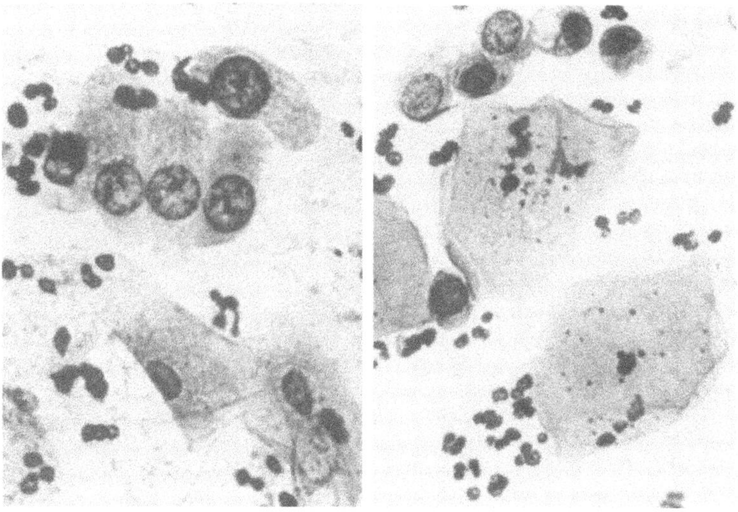

Fig. 27. Columnar epithelial cells in the cytologic smear. In the left half of the picture are morphologically well-preserved cells; at the right are rounded cells that could, under certain conditions, be mistaken for uniform atypical cells

also be the expression of an inflammation in the vagina and cervix (STOLL and MUTH, 1952).

Leukocytes. Leukocytes with segmented nuclei are found in almost all smears; during the menses they are more numerous in the cervical smear than in that from the surface of the portio. This distribution is, of course, not maintained in inflammation. The leukocytes are present in various states of preservation. Some are found quite intact, with a distinct cellular outline and a segmented nucleus, but usually only the nuclei are found, whereas the cytoplasm is missing. The nuclei, however, may have been elongated and distorted during spreading of the smear. In most severe bacterial infections only shadows of nuclei are found, that is, blurred forms that barely take the blue stain (Fig. 28). This alteration of neutrophils is seen quite often in smears from the posterior vaginal pool (WIED, 1957). The leukocytes are well preserved if the smear has been taken directly from the epithelium; their state of preservation, therefore, permits conclusions regarding the care that was taken in preparing the smear.

Leukocytes overshadow the picture of the smear in severe inflammation. Lymphocytes appear there as well. They are clearly discernible, but of minor quantitative importance compared with the polymorphonuclear leukocytes.

Erythrocytes. Red blood corpuscles are normally found in the premenstrual and postmenstrual smear, but frequently are also well preserved in cervical smears because of the vulnerability of the epithelium. Microscopic bleeding can also appear in inflammation through diapedesis. The rather marked presence of blood in smears from clinical carcinomas is typical (Fig. 44).

Well-preserved erythrocytes with the typical shape of small, biconcave disks appear red with the Papanicolaou stain. If the hemoglobin has been leached out,

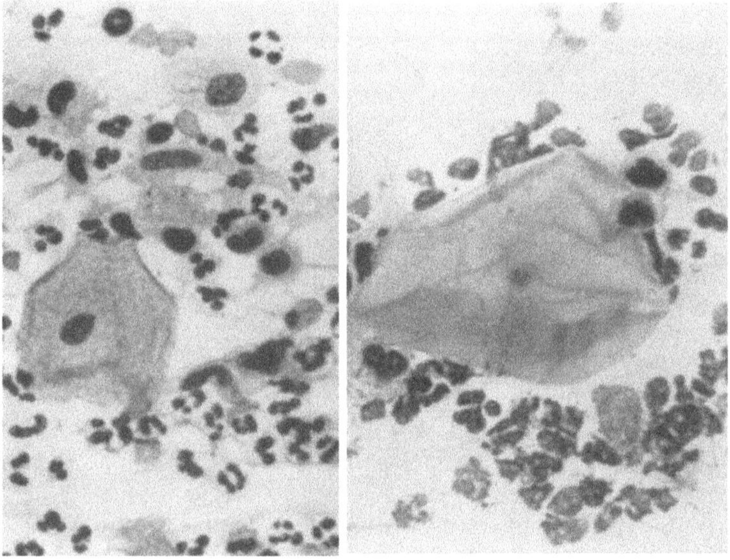

Fig. 28. On the left, well-preserved polymorphonuclear leukocytes among numerous histiocytes, conspicuous because of their kidney-shaped nucleus. On the right, an anuclear flake amid ghosts of leukocytes, which are produced by autolysis

red rings or completely colorless round shadows remain. They may then, occasionally, take on a delicate greenish-blue tinge.

Unless the admixture of blood causes a definite dilution of the material to be examined, making the detection of epithelial cells difficult, the evaluation of a smear is generally not disturbed by erythrocytes.

Histiocytes. An additional and rather variable cellular type, the histiocyte, remains to be mentioned. This type includes cells of the blood stream and connective tissue that, because of their ameboid motility, penetrate epithelia and often appear in large numbers, especially in the cervical smear (Fig. 28) (Papanicolaou, 1952, 1953; Graham, 1961). Some are round with a kidney-shaped nucleus, resembling monocytes. Others are spindly, with an elongated nucleus, and are arranged in rows. There are many intermediate forms. Cells with two or more nuclei frequently occur. All of them are somewhat larger than a normal neutrophilic leukocyte, and always smaller than basal cells, a feature enabling them to be distinguished from these other cells. Their cytoplasm sometimes stains basophilic, but more often it does not stain at all. It is frequently vacuolated or granular. These cells are not significant in cancer detection, except that under certain conditions it is difficult to tell them from pathologic cells arising from carcinoma of the corpus.

If, for any of several possible reasons (after curettage, electrocoagulation, treatment with radium, punch biopsy, and so forth), granulation tissue develops on the portio and in the cervical canal, *giant cells* may appear in the smear. The shape of these cells varies greatly and their cytoplasm is pale and basophilic. The number of their nuclei varies.

It is often difficult in a smear to differentiate endometrial cells from histiocytes. The former are found mainly around the time of menstruation. They are small cells with a round nucleus and basophilic cytoplasm; they are usually arranged in clusters.

Microorganisms

Microorganisms appear in the vagina physiologically as partners in symbiosis. In addition, microorganisms inhabit the vagina as nonpathogenic saprophytes, and as pathogens that can cause a severe inflammation.

The microorganisms mentioned below are usually stained only a pale blue by the Papanicolaou method, but they are clearly recognizable. Acridine orange fluorochroming provides an excellent method for demonstrating them (see p. 78).

In bacteriological examinations of the posterior third of the vagina, numerous saprophytic microorganisms are found. The conditions under which they become pathogenic and cause severe inflammations have not yet been fully ascertained. The antibacterial defense is always weakened during menstruation and all gestational processes (WIED and CHRISTIANSEN, 1953).

Döderlein's Bacilli. These bacteria are small rodlike forms of varying length, staining light blue by the Papanicolaou method. Döderlein's bacilli dominate the normal vaginal flora. By forming lactic acid, they create an environment with a pH of 4.0. Needing glycogen for their subsistence, they cause lysis of the intermediate cells, which contain glycogen. If the Döderlein flora is copious, the phenomenon of bacterial cytolysis can be observed, that is, the cytoplasm of the epithelial cells is dissolved bacterially and the bare nuclei remain (WIED and CHRISTIANSEN, 1953, 1953/54). If the bacilli of Döderlein are present in the vagina, the growth of other bacteria is suppressed by the acidic environment. A normal flora of Döderlein's bacilli is never found in clinical carcinomas, but it may occur in early cases (Fig. 30).

Other Bacteria. Other bacteria (short, plump, or comma-shaped rods) are rarely found with the small bacilli of Döderlein. Spherical cocci appear most frequently and may completely crowd out the normal vaginal flora. Of increasing significance as a cause of discharge is *Haemophilus vaginalis*. Morphologically, it is a short, plump little rod. No diagnosis can be reached from the Papanicolaou smear. The organism seems to react in various ways to the bacterial contaminants.

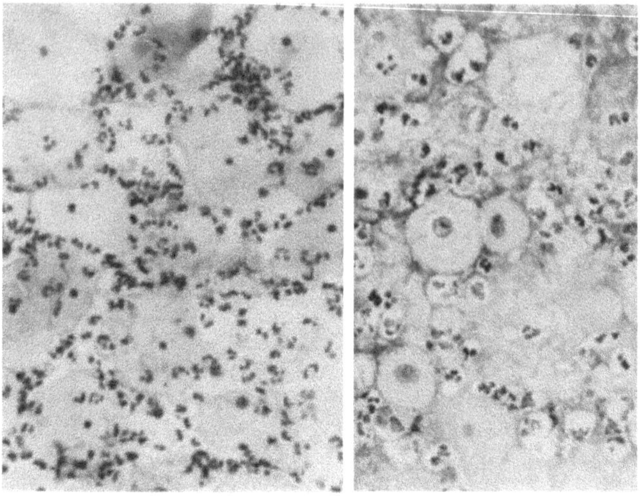

Fig. 29. Changes in smears caused by severe infection with cocci. On the left, pronounced eosinophilia of all epithelial cells. On the right, intensely washed-out appearance of the cells. The evaluation of the smear is made difficult, *in both cases*, by the coccal infection

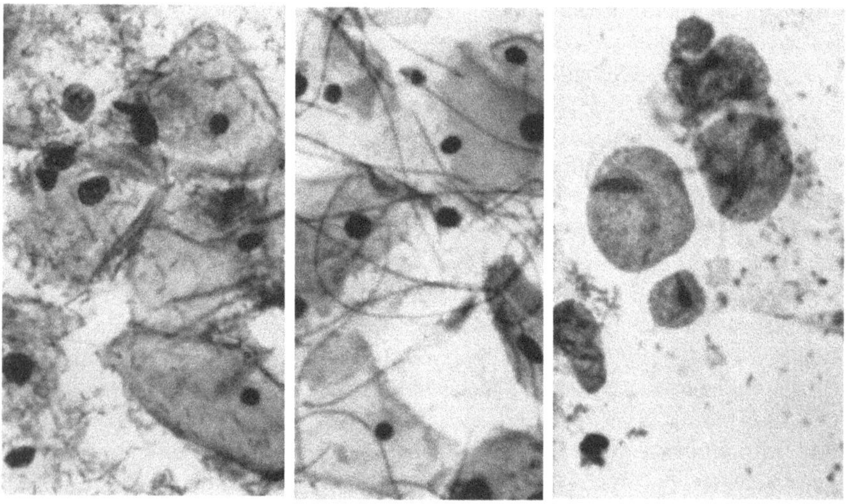

Fig. 30. Examples of microorganisms in the cytologic smear. On the left, DÖDERLEIN's flora. Bare nuclei can be recognized, brought about by lysis of the cytoplasm. In the center, threads of *Leptothrix*. On the right, well-preserved trichomonads

At times a massive leukocytic exudate is found with the bacteria. In other smears, however, the slide is covered with cocci; all epithelial cells on the slide are covered with them and their outlines are blurred because of them, but almost no leukocytes can be detected in the slide. A pseudoeosinophilia of all epithelial cells is usually found then, in which the cells of the outer as well as the inner superficial layers and of the intermediate layer are stained red (Fig. 29).

Bacterial contamination of the vagina occurs quite frequently. The patients usually complain of a yellowish, watery and acrid discharge.

Leptothrix. Invasion of the vagina by threads of *Leptothrix* can vary greatly in extent. Single threads are occasionally found in the whole smear. They appear pale blue with the Papanicolaou stain (Fig. 30). Single threads in the cytologic smear do not seem to be significant clinically, as they are in general incidental findings. These microorganisms do not cause difficulties in diagnosis.

Trichomonads. Invasion by trichomonads seems to be increasing recently. As BEDOYA, RICO, and RIOS (1956) have been able to demonstrate, these unicellular organisms establish themselves in the vagina of the woman and the urethra of the man, whence they are quickly disseminated. They are oval to round unicellular organisms, equipped with one to three flagella. Organelles are clearly visible within their cytoplasm (Fig. 30). They appear in varying numbers in the vagina, with or without bacterial infection. With the Papanicolaou stain they are usually recognized as roundish or oval gray-blue shadows. In the presence of considerable numbers of cocci, they are often difficult to find, because the cocci are then superimposed on them. If they appear in increased numbers, the foamy, yellowish discharge develops clinically. More information about the invasion of trichomonads is available from LISTON and LISTON (1939), MASCALL (1954), CHAPPAZ and co-workers (1955), PUNDEL and SCHWACHTGEN (1956, 1957), KORTE (1957), RIBA (1957), ZINSER (1957) and MICHALZIK (1959). Whether trichomonads are responsible for nuclear and cellular changes will be discussed below.

Nuclear and Cellular Changes Induced by Inflammation

The appearance of neutrophilic leukocytes and microorganisms in the cytologic smear is not necessarily always connected with a clinically demonstrable inflammation of the vagina and cervix (MEYBERG, 1960). The same fact applies also to the relation of the normal squamous epithelia to leukocytes and microorganisms in the cytologic smear. At times the structure of the squamous epithelial cells and their affinity for stain are not affected, but at other times the changes in them may be so great that the beginner may find it difficult to differentiate them from malignant cells. We believe, however, that a clear differentiation of cellular and nuclear changes from true epithelial diseases is feasible. The more intensely and persistently the noxious inflammatory stimuli affect the squamous epithelium, the more frequently will the changes appear in the epithelial cells. What kinds of changes are these and which microorganisms produce them?

The cell membrane becomes blurred and washed out in superficial cells of the inner and outer layers and in the intermediate cells, particularly in the presence of severe infection with cocci. A so-called pseudoeosinophilia develops (see Fig. 29). That is, cells that are normally stained basophilic by the Papanicolaou method become eosinophilic. A perinuclear halo can be discerned in superficial cells in the presence of a marked leukocytic contamination; that is, a cytoplasmic zone around the nucleus does not stain with eosin. AYRE calls this cellular form a "halo cell" and believes it represents a "precancerous tendency" (1960). KEAN and DAY (1954) describe these cells mainly in infections with trichomonads. The nucleus of superficial epithelial cells may exhibit a slight distortion of its roundness in the presence of severe inflammation (Fig. 31).

In the cellular nuclei of the intermediate layer too, inflammation may be recognized by a minor loss of roundness, by a beaded nuclear membrane, and by a coarsening of the chromatin. A polychromasia of the cytoplasm is typical of these cells as well as of those from the deep layers of the squamous epithelium. The border of the cell is basophilic, and the perinuclear zone acidophilic (Fig. 31).

Nuclear changes are most pronounced in basal and parabasal cells. Their number is usually increased in severe inflammations, since the superficial epithelial layers may be partially destroyed. The nuclear chromatin, which has become

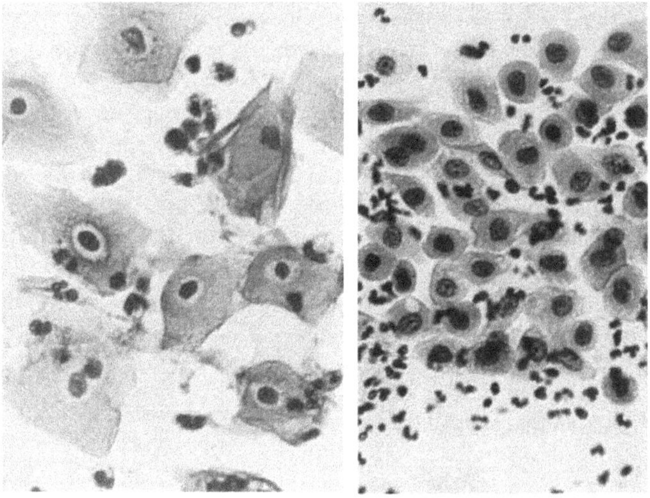

Fig. 31. Inflammatory changes in the cells of the cervical smear. On the left, well-developed perinuclear halos with slight loss of roundness of the nucleus of superficial cells. On the right, polychromasia of the cytoplasm and slight loss of roundness of the nucleus, resulting from inflammation of the parabasal and basal cells

denser, may become more so, producing the effect of hyperchromasia. The nuclei may exhibit loss of roundness, but they are never substantially enlarged (Fig. 31). The normal relation of nucleus to cytoplasm is important in all nuclear changes in inflammation, since it makes possible the differentiation from malignant cells (Blumenthal and Hecht, 1956). The polychromasia of the cytoplasm is typical. Often all degrees of nuclear disintegration may be recognized (Fig. 32), which one rarely sees in the nuclei of malignant cells.

Finally, in inflammation vacuoles form in the cytoplasm mainly of the intermediate and deep cells (Fig. 32).

Other authors (Bechtold and Reicher, 1952; Lindenschmidt and Stoll, 1958; Koss and Wolinska, 1959; Michalzik, 1959; Ferreira do Amaral, Menezes and Schneider, 1960), consider trichomonads to be particularly responsible for the nuclear changes. Even though trichomoniasis is becoming more widespread, it does not seem to have attained the extent described in the Spanish literature. We have to date, in infections with trichomonads, never observed a nuclear change sufficiently marked to lead to false diagnosis of carcinoma in situ or invasive carcinoma (see p. 83). Neither Slate, Merritt and Kennedy (1960) nor Frost (1962) could find cellular and nuclear changes typical of infection by trichomonads. If doubts actually arise, a clarification of the true character of the cells must be attempted by appropriate cleansing treatments.

A distinction between acute and chronic inflammation, as is feasible histologically, is not clearly made in the cytological smear. Polymorphonuclear leukocytes are always the predominant expression of the inflammation. We have never seen a predominantly lymphocytic exudate that would have justified the diagnosis of chronic inflammation, nor has the increase of eosinophilic leukocytes in the

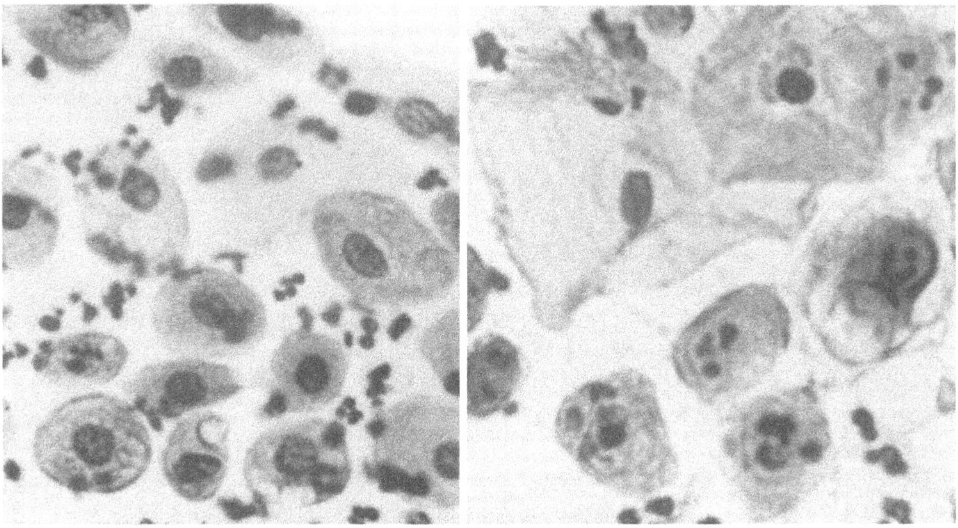

Fig. 32. On the left, cytoplasmic vacuoles in parabasal and intermediate cells. On the right, nuclear disintegration in cells of the parabasal layer

smear ever been conspicuous. The suggestion of chronic inflammation is best given by the increased shedding of deep cells with appropriate nuclear changes, and by the unphysiologic maturation of the squamous epithelium. The latter is indicated by small, markedly eosinophilic cells with pyknotic nuclei, a miniature variety of mature superficial cells. These cells are found also among mixed types of menopausal smears.

In summing up, we can make the following statements about the influence of inflammation as seen in the cytologic smear: inflammatory changes in the cytologic smear are manifested by contamination with leukocytes and microorganisms. The cells of the squamous epithelium sometimes have blurred cytoplasmic outlines, and exhibit pseudoeosinophilia and polychromasia. The effects of inflammation on the nuclei are revealed by slight enlargements, loss of roundness, and coarsening of the chromatin network (Figs. 39—41). All of these phenomena should disappear with appropriate anti-inflammatory treatment; if they do not, they must be investigated until their true significance has been ascertained.

The Appearance of the Pathologic Cell

In this chapter the types of cells shed in epithelial atypias and carcinomas of the cervix will be discussed.

This will not be an exhaustive presentation of the cytology of carcinomas of the corpus, or of tubal and ovarian carcinomas, for these carcinomas can be diagnosed better and more surely by means other than cytology.

In contrast, for carcinoma in situ and preclinical cancer of the cervix, cytology is the method of choice.

We distinguish two basic kinds of pathologic cells:

1. Dyskaryotic cells.
2. Atypical cells.

The dyskaryotic cells have a pathologic nucleus, but their shape still permits comparison with normal epithelial cells. The atypical cells have such abnormal nuclei and cytoplasm that they do not resemble any normal cell of the squamous epithelium.

Dyskaryotic Cells (Dyskaryoses)

Papanicolaou coined the term dyskaryosis in 1949, and fortunately chose a very appropriate designation (karyon = nucleus). It is, indeed, mainly the nucleus that is altered in the dyskaryoses. We distinguish dyskaryoses in superficial, intermediate, and deep cells, that are analogous to those in normal squamous epithelium. The most important features of a dyskaryotic nucleus are *enlargement, loss of roundness*, and *hyperchromasia*.

Dyskaryoses in Superficial Cells. The nucleus of these cells is substantially enlarged, usually to several times the normal size. The enlargement exceeds by far that described in inflammatory changes. The nuclear shape has lost its roundness and frequently exhibits bizarre corners and edges. The nucleus is distinctly hyperchromatic, but need not become pyknotic as do mature normal cells. The nucleus, is, however, always substantially more hyperchromatic than the nuclei of normal inner superficial cells.

The form of the cytoplasm of these cells markedly resembles that of a normal superficial cell, despite the deviations. The cell is polygonal and usually flattened; the cellular boundaries are occasionally blurred and may be drawn out into long processes. The cell is generally smaller than normal. The differentiation of the cytoplasmic stain between the inner and outer superficial cells is not pronounced.

Fig. 33. Dyskaryosis in superficial cells. In the specimen in the right half of the picture, perinuclear halos have formed

Fig. 34. Dyskaryosis in intermediate cells. The nuclear change and the deformation of the cytoplasm are clearly visible. The normally basophilic intermediate cells often stain eosinophilic after undergoing dyskaryosis

Fig. 35. Dyskaryosis in parabasal and basal cells, respectively. In both pictures, the pathologic cells lie next to normal superficial cells

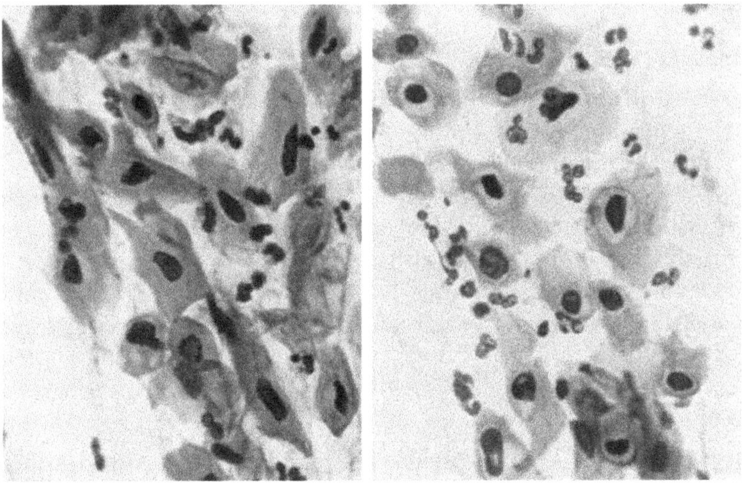

Fig. 33

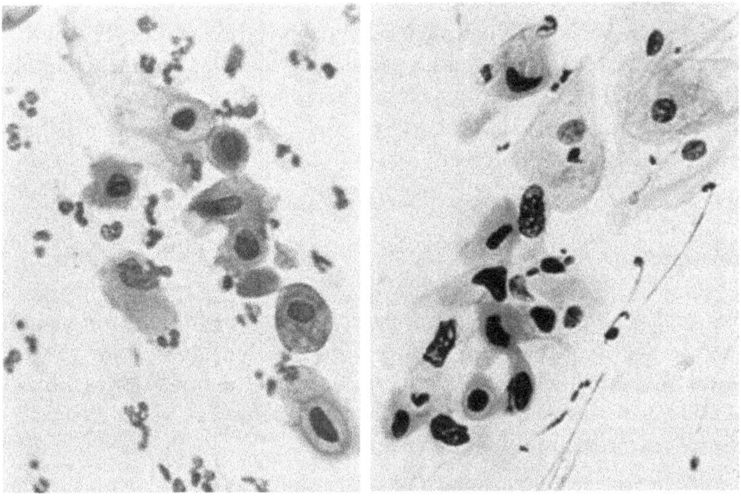

Fig. 34

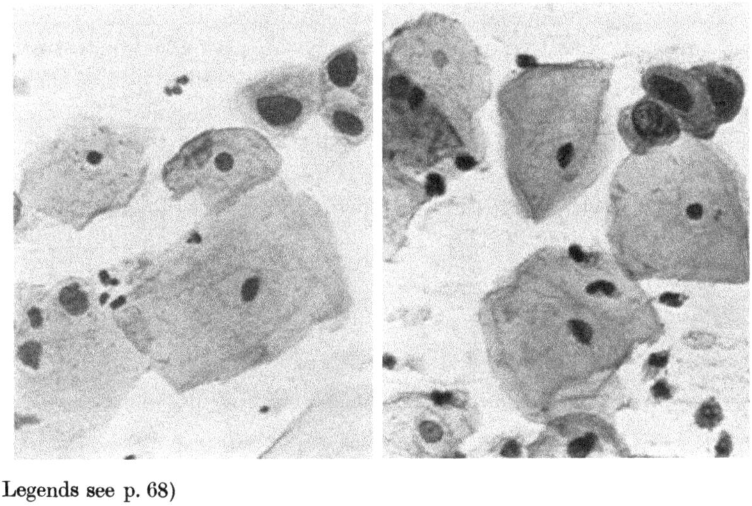

Fig. 35

(For Legends see p. 68)

The dyskaryotic superficial cell is strongly eosinophilic and often assumes an intense orange color. Perinuclear halos may occur around the enlarged nucleus, as in inflammation (Figs. 33, 39).

Dyskaryoses in Intermediate Cells. The nuclei of cells from the intermediate layers of the squamous epithelium are enlarged to about double their size; the loss of roundness is pronounced. There too the hyperchromasia important for the diagnosis of "dyskaryosis" is striking; all transitions may occur, from a dense chromatin pattern to the formation of clumps to complete pyknosis. The cytoplasm is relatively well-preserved, with regard to its extent and shape, but its response to cytoplasmic stains varies between basophilic and eosinophilic. The eosinophilia of the cytoplasm is pathologic in this cellular layer, and its frequency is increased in dyskaryoses. The cytoplasm stains uniformly within an individual cell, however. Polychromasia of the cytoplasm occurs only in cells altered by inflammation (Figs. 34, 40).

Dyskaryoses in Deep Cells. The nucleus is only slightly enlarged in deep cells but has clearly lost its roundness, and it is markedly hyperchromatic with a clumped chromatin pattern. Nuclear details are not discernible. The cytoplasm is well preserved. It is always basophilic, often very blue, and usually homogeneous, but sometimes granular. Polychromasia or vacuoles rarely occur in the cytoplasm. In the smear, the dyskaryotic parabasal and basal cells, like normal cells, are arranged in groups or rows (Figs. 35, 41).

Pseudodyskaryotic Cells

Without first going into an interpretation of the cellular types, a pathologic cellular change will be described that can be differentiated from the true dyskaryoses, and that also occurs in all layers of the squamous epithelium. Typical of the pseudodyskaryoses is the marked swollen nucleus with a certain loss of roundness *without* pronounced hyperchromasia.

Pseudodyskaryoses in Superficial Cells. The nucleus in inner and outer superficial cells is enlarged to several times its normal size, appearing inflated. The enlargement often exceeds by far that of true dyskaryosis. The nucleus often has an indented kidney shape and shows numerous infoldings of its membrane. Suggested or completed formations of double nuclei are frequent. The chromatin is coarsely reticulated and granular. The nuclear membrane is prominent. The shape and tinctorial characteristics of the cytoplasm are well preserved, as is its differentiation. The cytoplasmic mass, however, may be substantially larger, resulting in giant cells (Figs. 36, 39).

Fig. 36. Pseudodyskaryoses in superficial cells. The nucleus is substantially enlarged, is not hyperchromatic, and shows a slight loss of roundness

Fig. 37. Pseudodyskaryoses in intermediate cells at two different magnifications

Fig. 38. Various forms of pseudodyskaryoses in basal and parabasal cells, next to normal superficial cells

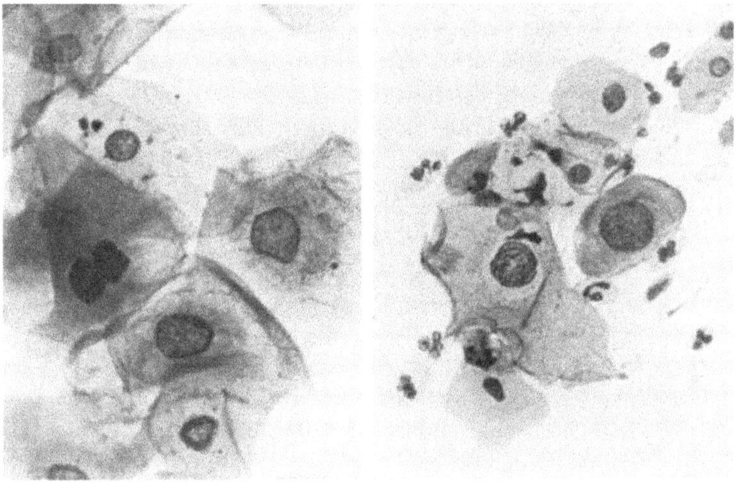

Fig. 36

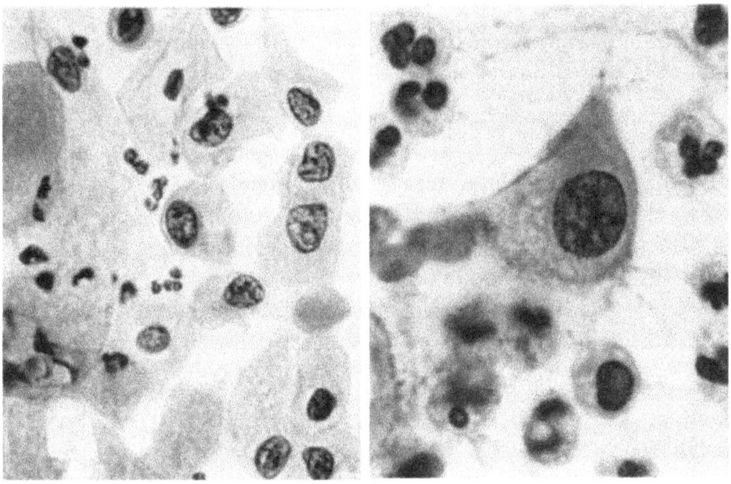

Fig. 37

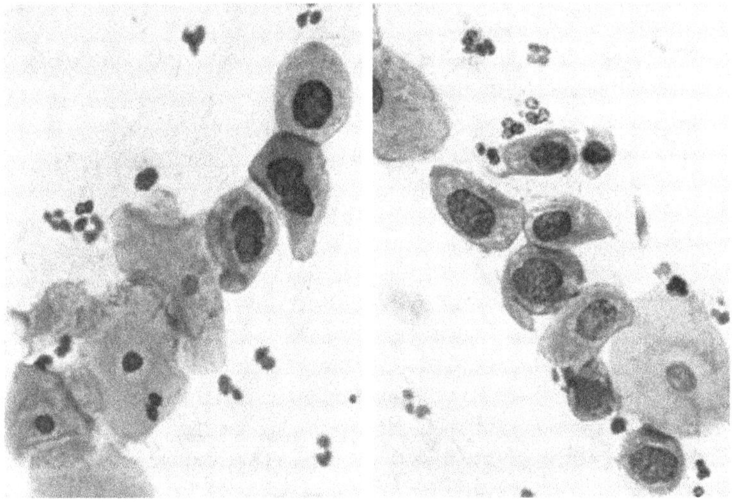

Fig. 38

(For Legends see p. 70)

Pseudodyskaryoses in Intermediate and Deep Cells. In the cells of the intermediate and deep layers of the squamous epithelium, a pseudodyskaryotic nucleus is conspicuous, mainly because of its marked enlargement, which exceeds that in true dyskaryosis. There is no hyperchromasia. The loss of roundness of the nucleus is slight and the nuclear membrane is prominent. The nuclear interior appears inflated. The cytoplasm of these cells is not changed (Figs. 37, 38, 40, 41).

Up to this point cellular changes have been described in cells of the squamous epithelium. In view of the importance of their correct diagnosis and differentiation from inflammatory changes, the principal characteristics will be briefly summarized and described schematically.

Superficial Cells (Fig. 39)

Inflammation. Pseudoeosinophilia, perinuclear halo, blurred cellular boundaries, slightly enlarged nuclei with some loss of roundness.

Pseudodyskaryosis. Occasional giant cells. Inflated nuclei with coarse chromatin pattern. Prominent nuclear membrane.

Dyskaryosis. Cells often smaller than normal. Deformed cytoplasm. Marked eosinophilia or orangeophilia. Staining of cytoplasm of outer and inner superficial cells not differentiated. Enlarged, hyperchromatic nuclei with loss of roundness.

Intermediate Cells (Fig. 40)

Inflammation. Blurred cellular boundaries, polychromasia of the cytoplasm, slightly enlarged nuclei with a little loss of roundness.

Pseudodyskaryosis. Mainly normal cytoplasm. Inflated, considerably enlarged nuclei with slight loss of roundness.

Dyskaryosis. Cytoplasm may stain basophilic or eosinophilic. Nuclei are enlarged and markedly hyperchromatic, and show loss of roundness.

Deep (Basal and Parabasal) Cells (Fig. 41)

Inflammation. Polychromasia of the cytoplasm. Slightly enlarged, mildly hyperchromatic nuclei with a little loss of roundness.

Pseudodyskaryosis. Normal, basophilic cytoplasm. Inflated nuclei with slight loss of roundness.

Dyskaryosis. Normal, basophilic cytoplasm. Enlarged, markedly hyperchromatic nuclei with loss of roundness.

Atypical Cells

The designation "atypical" is not entirely appropriate, because it reflects too vague a judgment. The designation "malignant" would be more to the point. Since cytologic nomenclature was introduced about two decades ago, a change now does not seem practical. "Atypical" cells are those that have no analogy with normal cells in the smear; generally, they can be easily recognized as pathologic. Two categories of pathologic cells belong among the atypical cells. One is conspicuous because of its uniform appearance; the other comprises a wide variety of cells with marked pathologic changes.

The nomenclature of these cells varies. The first, or uniform group of cells is called embryonic atypical, basal atypical, differentiated atypical, or undifferentiated atypical; the second group of cells is called undifferentiated atypical, atypical with loss of differentiation, or differentiated atypical. We have avoided this confusion in nomenclature by using the purely descriptive designations "uniform atypical" and "polymorphic atypical".

Uniform Atypical Cells. This type of cell is about as large as a basal cell. The nucleocytoplasmic ratio is markedly increased. The nucleus is large and round to oval. The dense nuclear membrane causes the nucleus to appear prominent. The

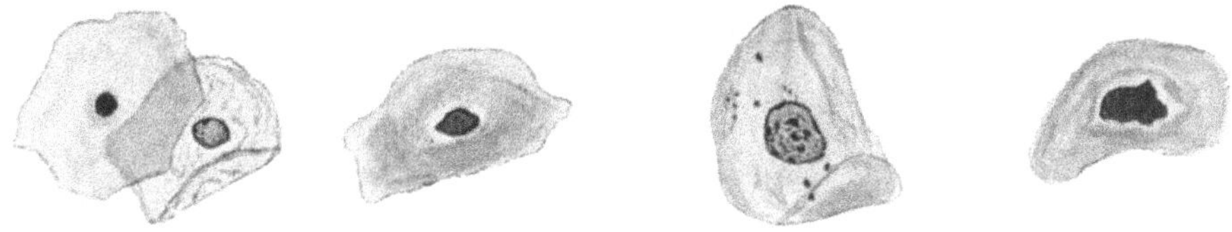

Fig. 39

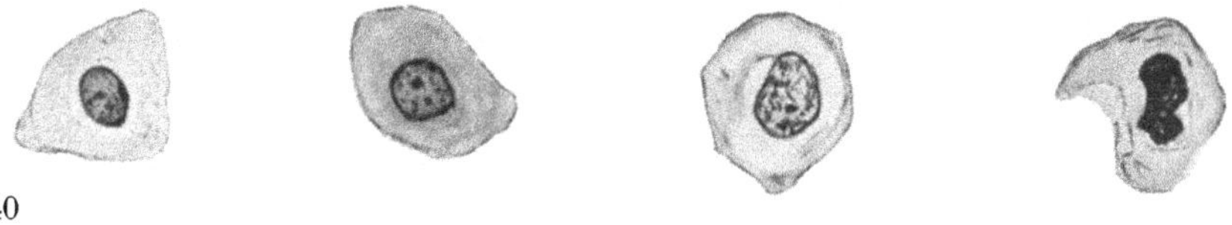

Fig. 40

Fig. 41

Fig. 39. Outer and inner superficial cells

Fig. 40. Intermediate cells

Fig. 41. Parabasal and basal cells

Figs. 39, 40 and 41 from left to right: Nuclei and cytoplasm of normal compared with inflammatory, pseudodyskaryotic, and truly dyskaryotic cells. (Aquarelle. The cells were drawn from color photomicrographs)

chromatin pattern has wide meshes but somewhat coarse threads. A few nucleoli may usually be discerned. The cytoplasmic border is narrow and its relation to the nucleus is comparable to that in a lymphocyte. The contour of the cytoplasm is mainly sharp, but in some places it is drawn out into projections. Occasionally the cytoplasm is absent entirely or only in part. It is palely basophilic, partly granular, and partly vacuolar. The cells may appear in the smear singly or in groups (Fig. 42).

Overstained columnar epithelial cells with rounded cytoplasmic borders may sometimes be mistaken for uniform atypical cells.

Polymorphic Atypical Cells. This cellular group presents a polymorphic picture that one immediately recognizes in the smear as atypical. Shape and size of the cytoplasmic mass and of the nuclei vary greatly (Fig. 43).

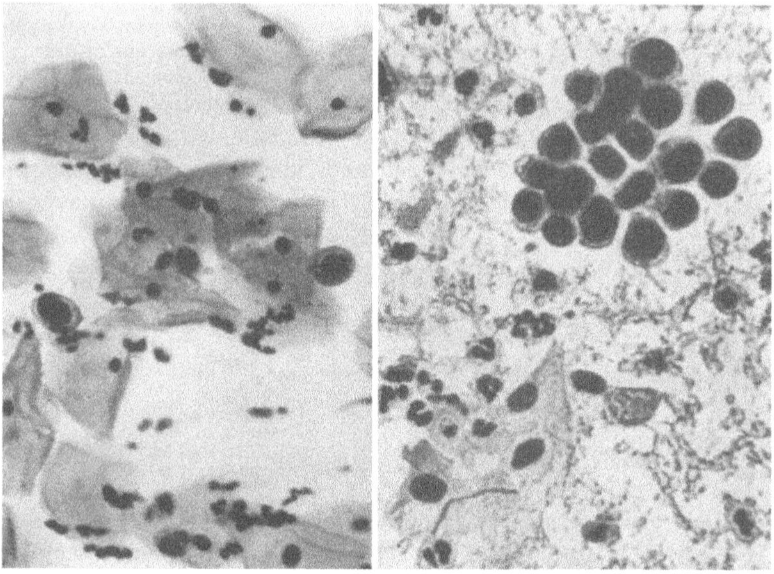

Fig. 42. Uniform atypical cells. In the left half of the picture a few of these cells are scattered among normal superficial cells. On the right, an agglomeration of uniform atypical cells more highly magnified. The chromatin pattern is actually not so dense as it appears in the black and white print

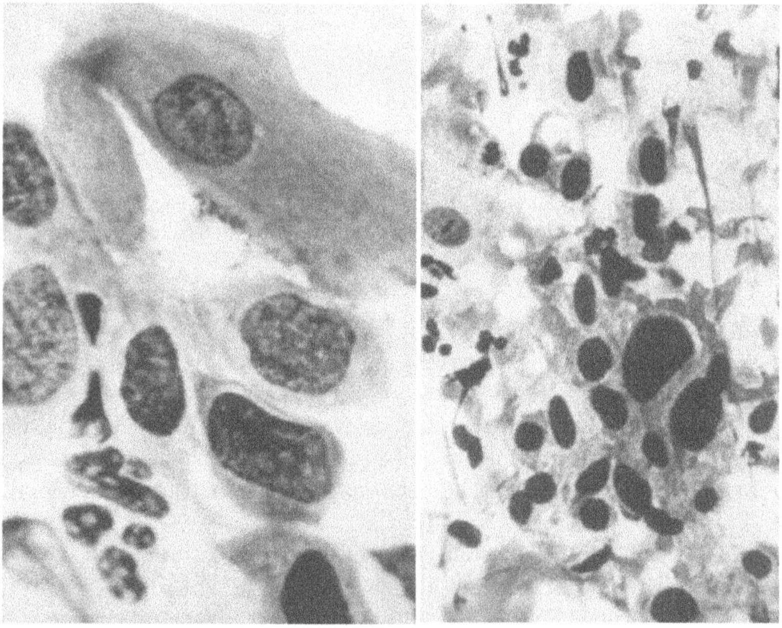

Fig. 43. Polymorphic atypical cells. The polymorphism of nuclei and cytoplasm is clearly shown in both examples

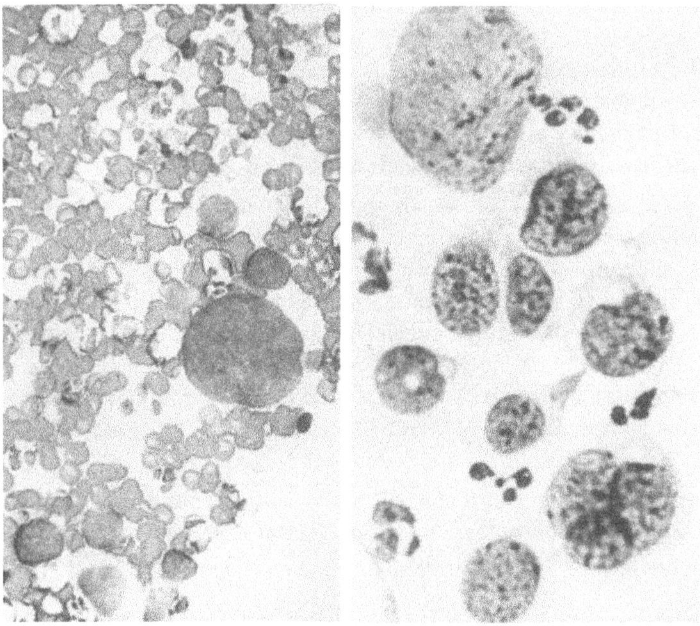

Fig. 44. Predominantly "naked nuclei" of polymorphic atypical cells. On the left, only palely stained neoplastic nuclei of various sizes among erythrocytes. On the right, the affinity for stain of the neoplastic nuclei, which readily undergo autolysis and heterolysis, is disturbed

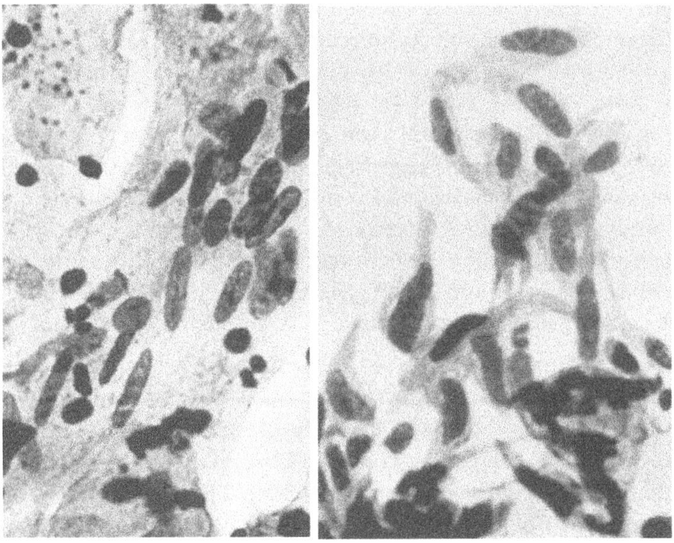

Fig. 45. So-called spindle cells in a positive smear. They are considered polymorphic atypical cells

The cytoplasm may be similar to that of an epithelial cell. It may be drawn out into grotesque shapes, or it may be absent entirely or only in part. If there is no cytoplasm at all, only bare nuclei remain, appearing quite different from the bare nuclei resulting from cytolysis by Döderlein bacilli (Fig. 44). If nuclei of columnar epithelial cells are denuded of cytoplasm, they may be distinguished from the bare nuclei of neoplastic cells because of their inconspicuous chromatin pattern. Often their nuclei have a honeycomb structure. The cytoplasm is usually basophilic, but it may also be smudgy and eosinophilic. The nuclei always have a clumped chromatin-pattern, and their shape and size vary.

Inadequate affinity of the entire cells for stain is often typical. The lack of staining makes them appear as mere shadows. In these cases, the nuclei stain a pale violet and appear clearly pathologic because of their polymorphism. These cells are subjected to rapid autolysis, which is the cause of poor affinity for stain. We consider all the pathologic special types described by Papanicolaou to be forms of polymorphic atypical cells. The so-called spindle cell is one of them. It has a nucleus that is drawn out like a spindle, and cytoplasm of similar shape (Fig. 45) (de Brux, Rauzy, Dupré-Froment, 1958; Fidler, 1958; Graham, 1958; Siegler, 1958).

Another type in this group is a cell with a small, round, pyknotic nucleus and an extremely narrow cytoplasmic border. These cells suggest adenocarcinoma if they appear singly in larger numbers.

Acridine Orange Fluorochrome Staining in Gynecological Cytodiagnosis

The preceding description of the cellular picture has been presented on the basis of the Papanicolaou stain. Acridine orange fluorochrome staining has found its place in recent years as a competitive method with broader application, mainly through the work of F. D. and L. v. Bertalanffy (Bertalanffy and Bickis, 1956; Bertalanffy, Masin and Masin, 1956; Bertalanffy, Masin, Masin and Kaplan, 1957, 1958; L. v. Bertalanffy, 1959; F. D. Bertalanffy, 1960 I—V). The following discussion concerns the principle of the stain, its technique, and its advantages and disadvantages, compared with those of the Papanicolaou stain on the basis of our own experiences (Bontke, Kern and Schümmelfeder, 1960; Schümmelfeder, Bontke and Kern, 1960; Kern, Schümmelfeder and Kern-Bontke, 1962; Schümmelfeder, 1962).

The fluorescent appearance of fixed cells stained with acridine orange depends on physicochemical properties of the cell and on the particular staining conditions. The difference in the polymerization of RNA and DNA causes the RNA to fluoresce red and the DNA yellow-green within a pH range of 4 to 7 in staining solutions of acridine orange of low concentrations. The red fluorescence disappears upon treatment with ribonuclease, thus proving specificity of the stain for RNA.

DNA can be depolymerized with hydrochloric acid and the green fluorescence thus changed into red, a proof of specificity for the DNA.

Intracellular and extracellular mucopolysaccharides also exhibit red fluorescence and may easily be differentiated by checking with the ribonuclease control, as mentioned above. The staining mechanism is, therefore, much clearer with the acridine orange fluorochrome staining than with the Papanicolaou stain.

BERTALANFFY used the properties of this stain:

1. to achieve good definition of the nucleus and cytoplasm in cytologic smears with a single staining procedure, and

2. to demonstrate selectively the "cancerous cells", which usually are rich in RNA.

This latter idea is indeed attractive and it has often been tried in experiments with numerous stains, histochemical reactions, and enzymatic studies. The results of these experiments have never been satisfactory, however, because the metabolism of malignant cells does not differ essentially from that of benign but altered cells (as in regeneration, inflammation).

STOPPELLI (1960), ELEVITCH and BRUNSON (1961) and SUSSMAN (1961) confirmed BERTALANFFY'S statements. In contrast, FLEGEL (1953/54), UMICKER, PICKLE and WAITE (1959), DART and TURNER (1959), TÖRNBERG, WESTIN and NORLANDER (1960), HOLLAND and ACKERMANN (1961), HOPMAN (1961), HUNTER and BROWN (1961), ANDERSON and GUNN (1962), DUBRAUSZKY and JAEGER (1962) pointed out that a specific selection of "cancerous cells" through red fluorescence was not feasible. A selective demonstration of malignant cells could scarcely be expected to succeed, in consideration of theoretical and practical studies of acridine orange fluorochrome-staining by SCHÜMMELFEDER (1948, 1949, 1950, 1958 I, II), SCHÜMMELFEDER, EBSCHNER and KROGH (1957), SCHÜMMELFEDER, KROGH and EBSCHNER (1958) and others.

We have however, undertaken, a comparative investigation of the acridine orange stain, because the Papanicolaou stain is rather time-consuming and cumbersome and fails to label as such the "cancerous cell", which must be identified on the basis of its structure.

The Process of Staining:

1. Fixation of the moist smears in ether-alcohol (1:1).
2. Descending isopropyl alcohol sequence (80—70—50%).
3. Five minutes 1% acetic acid, renew frequently.
4. Rinse in distilled water.
5. Three minutes 0.01% acridine orange solution in McIlvaine buffer, pH 5.0 (acridine orange Merck).
6. One minute McIlvaine buffer, pH 5.0. The slides are mounted in this buffer, and coverslips applied.

The slides must be examined immediately with the fluorescence microscope in a dark room since the staining does not persist. If preparations are desired for later reference, permanent mounting-media may be used; the slides lose (SCHÜMMELFEDER, KROGH and EBSCHNER, 1958), their fluorescence, however, after several months. Restaining is possible.

For purposes of comparison with the Papanicolaou stain, color photographs were made of fluorescent slides, the cover glasses removed, and the slides taken through the ascending alcohol sequence in ether-alcohol, dissolving the acridine orange completely. The subsequent Papanicolaou stain of the same slide was not impaired. Again, color photographs were taken of the same areas. In this manner, we have examined 1000 smears from 500 patients, among them 40 positive smears, in an attempt to achieve an objective comparison of the two stains.

Since the structure of the cells and their affinity for the Papanicolaou stain were thoroughly described in the preceding chapter, a table presenting a summary of the results is given rather than a description (Table 9).

As seen in this table, the desire to find a selective red staining of malignant cells was not fulfilled. Many cellular elements and microorganisms in the normal smear fluoresce red; conversely, not all pathologic cells fluoresce red. Furthermore, the results are complicated by autolysis and heterolysis. The same morphologic knowledge must be applied to the examination of the smears stained with acridine orange as with the Papanicolaou stain. Because of their red fluorescence a preselection of cells by untrained personnel or even by automatic counters is not possible.

Table 9. *Cytoplasmic affinity of cells and microorganisms in the cytologic smear for acridine orange fluorochrome staining compared with the Papanicolaou stain*

Cell type	Acridine orange fluorochrome stain	Papanicolaou stain
Superficial cells	None or a light green pattern	eosinophilic and basophilic
Intermediate cells	yellow-green to light orange-red	basophilic
Deep cells	orange-red	basophilic
Columnar cells	bright red	basophilic
Endometrial cells	orange-red	basophilic
Histiocytic elements	orange red or deep red-granular	pale basophilic
Leukocytes (neutrophils)	none — or a light green pattern	pale basophilic
Erythrocytes	none — or green-brown shadows	eosinophilic
Pseudodyskaryoses	like normal cells, according to the layer	like normal cells, according to layer
Dyskaryoses in superficial cells	light green to light orange	eosinophilic
Dyskaryoses in intermediate cells	light orange to red	eosinophilic or basophilic
Dyskaryoses in deep cells	orange-red	basophilic
Uniform atypical cells	brilliant orange or red	pale basophilic
Polymorphic atypical cells	light green to red (all variations)	basophilic, sometimes eosinophilic
Cells altered by autolysis and heterolysis (normal and malignant)	light orange to green	pale basophilic
Döderlein's bacilli, cocci, fungi	deep red	basophilic
Trichomonads	orange-red	smudgy pale gray to pale blue

Acridine orange fluorochrome staining saves time and produces extremely well-stained smears that are always technically successful. Considering the morphologic criteria, results equal to those of the Papanicolaou stain are achieved. The important definition of the nucleus with its varying degrees of hyperchromasia also is clearly achieved with the acridine orange stain through varying grades of a yellow-green fluorescence. We have not, in spite of these good features, decided to switch to acridine orange staining because:

1. The purchase of several sets of fluorescence equipment is necessary.

2. The slides must be examined immediately in a dark room. This time schedule imposes difficulties for a clinical service; work in the dark causes considerable fatigue.

3. The preparation of permanent slides for later study nullifies any gain in time.

Summing up, we can make the following statement about acridine orange fluorochrome staining of the cytologic smear:

It is a rapid stain producing beautiful colors. It does not achieve a selective differentiation of malignant cells. With a knowledge of morphology, its results are comparable to those of the Papanicolaou stain. Its application depends on fluorescence equipment. If the customary technique is applied, no permanent slides result and work in the dark room is necessary.

Modified Classification of Papanicolaou

Having examined the cytologic slides and, perhaps, detected pathologic cellular types, the investigator makes a diagnosis according to the groups designated by PAPANICOLAOU. This classification uses the diagnoses negative, suspicious, and positive. *Positive* means pathologic cellular types, hence dyskaryoses of all layers; uniform and polymorphic atypical cells. We reserve the designation *suspicious* for those slides in which there are pseudodyskaryoses or cells that cannot with certainty be classified as benign or malignant. If a slide is marked *negative*, none of the pathologic cells has been found.

We use PAPANICOLAOU'S classification by groups as follows:

Table 10

Group	Evaluation	Cytologic picture
I	negative	Only normal epithelia. No admixture of leukocytes and microorganisms. No pathologic cells
II	negative	More or less substantial admixture of leukocytes and microorganisms together with normal epithelia. No pathologic cellular types
II w[a]	negative	Very substantial admixtures of leukocytes and microorganisms, sometimes signs of inflammation in epithelial cells or atrophy. Also, sometimes obviously faulty smear technique. Smear should be repeated, if feasible, after cleansing treatment (see methodology)
III	suspicious	Pseudodyskaryoses in the smear, or nuclear and cellular changes that cannot be evaluated with certainty. The patient must be kept under observation until a definitive diagnosis can be made. Cleansing treatment
IV	positive	Pathologic cellular types in the smear. Histologic clarification is necessary
V	positive	Great numbers of pathologic cellular types in the smear. Histologic clarification is necessary

[a] Modification used by us.

The clinician is notified of the resulting group and decides on this basis upon his further clinical steps, as described in the chapter on Documentation (see p. 38).

The designation Group I is almost never used by us, because a smear without leukocytes and microorganisms is rare. We mention this group for the sake of completeness.

Any finding that remains equivocal represents a burden for the physician, because the examination must be repeated and the patient may have to be hospitalized. If the suspicion that had been raised proves unfounded, the physician and patient often retain an aversion toward "unnecessary" examinations. Too frequent a use of the diagnosis "suspicious" (Group III) is therefore held against the method and impairs its value. The physician, furthermore, often responds to the label "suspicious" with the feeling that something has to be done. We are, therefore, extremely cautious in using the diagnosis Group III. This diagnosis was made in 1.1% of 13,674 tabulated cases that were examined cytologically.

We make ample use, however, of the Group II W. The slide was labeled II W in 11.1% of 13,674 cases. This diagnosis is usually combined with the request for a cleansing treatment. Many slides classified as Group III by others would appear in our Group II W. It may be a psychological trick, but it is very effective if we consider what has been said above. Marsan, Lecoq and Sicard expressed the same view in 1960. Hall and Rosen warned in 1960 not to use Group III too often, in order to protect the cytologist from liability and criticism.

Groups IV and V are unequivocally positive and must *always* be confirmed histologically. For the method of confirmation, see p. 91 and 163. It should be emphasized at this point that the difference between IV and V is purely quantitative, not qualitative, and that, therefore, the grouping does not permit any conclusion regarding the kind of histologic change.

There remains one group of smears that we do not diagnose because they do not, for various reasons, seem to lend themselves to adequate evaluation. These smears, too, should be repeated. A column "cannot be evaluated" appears in the balance sheet, nevertheless, because ambulatory patients often do not appear for a second examination and must, therefore, be carried as having been examined cytologically with no result that could be evaluated. Slides that dried out, faulty stains (usually because of faulty fixation), and too little material on the smear were carried as "not possible to evaluate".

Summing up, the clinician asks for a repetition of the smear in Group II W, usually after cleansing or hormonal therapy. For Group III, three or four smears are first repeated on different days of the cycle, before dismissal of the patient for a quarterly check-up, if the smear indicates a dysplastic epithelium.

Sufficient histological confirmation must be made in Groups IV and V by the usual means if a carcinoma is suspected; conization is employed if there is no clinical, colposcopic and cytologic (see prediction, p. 91) suspicion of a carcinoma.

This scale of diagnostic methods has been consistently maintained at the women's clinic of the University of Cologne. For special reasons deviations from this scheme were very occasionally made.

Some people may find this intensive cytologic search unusual, because it requires much time and because the goal occasionally could be attained more quickly by histologic methods. We prefer, however, highly sensitive cytology to small biopsy specimens, which do not offer greater certainty; we remove biopsy specimens smaller than a cone only in exceptional cases, except to verify a cervical carcinoma.

What Produces Incorrect Diagnoses in Cytology?

Sources of Mistakes

After having discussed in detail the methods and diagnosis of characteristic cytologic changes, we may enumerate briefly once more the origin of possible mistakes and their corrections:

1. Faulty smear technique.
2. Bacterial contamination (cocci, trichomonads).
3. Faulty stain; nuclear stain too pale or too intense.
4. Menopausal pictures.
5. Admixture of blood too great.
6. Inflammatory or autolytic disintegration of the neoplastic surfaces in cervical carcinoma too severe.
7. Rare tumors with a minimal tendency to shed.
8. Growth of abnormal epithelium primarily downwards into the stroma, with little change in the overlying and superficial epithelial layers.

How May These Eight Sources of Mistakes, Respectively, be Eliminated or at least Limited?

1. Accurate contact smear.
2. Second smear after cleansing treatment.
3. Microscopic control of the nuclear stain before staining the cytoplasm on the slide.
4. Build up the epithelium with estrogens.
5. Wait a few days before repeating the smear, if bleeding follows injury of a friable epithelium of the portio. Hormones may be used to stop intrauterine bleeding before repeating the smear.
6. These are cases of clinically recognizable carcinomas. Cytology was the wrong choice in these cases.

7. and 8. Clear failure of cytology.

Prediction of the Histologic Change from the Cytologic Smear

It was Papanicolaou who in 1949 (I and II) pointed out one can conclude from the occurrence of a dyskaryosis (he referred especially to deep dyskaryosis) that a carcinoma in situ is present. Similar observations were made by Glatthaar (1948, 1950), Ayre (1949, 1959), Nieburgs and Pund (1949), Wied (1950,

1956), SCAPIER, DAY and DURFEE (1952), REAGAN (1952), KOSS and DURFEE (1955, 1957), BLUMENTHAL and HECHT (1956), WIED and DARGAN (1957), GRAHAM (1957 I and II), DE BRUX (1957), CUYLER (1957), TERZANO (1957), ZINSER (1957), WIED and DEL SOL (1958), v. HAAM (1958), COUTIFARIS and COUTIFARIS (1959), BOSCHANN (1960), CITTI (1961), DE BRUX, DUPRÉ-FROMENT, CAMPOS and HOPMAN (1961), DE BRUX, DUPRÉ-FROMENT, GRAHAM, v. HAAM and SIEGLER (1961), and WIED, LEGORRETA, MOHR and RAUZY (1962).

Efforts to reach conclusions regarding the type of histologic change from the presence of single cells met with the greatest skepticism and rejection, especially on the part of anatomical pathologists who are accustomed to arrive at their diagnoses on the basis of the examination of tissue. Accordingly, the authors mentioned above expressed themselves with great caution by merely indicating that dyskaryoses were often shed by carcinomas in situ. This fact, it is generally emphasized, does not allow a prediction of the histologic diagnosis, however. It is often pointed out that inflammations, especially in trichomoniasis, may cause nuclear changes similar to those produced by dyskaryoses, rendering certain prediction impossible (CRAMER, 1951; SCAPIER, DAY and DURFEE, 1952; MACKENZIE, 1955; TERZANO, 1957; NYKLIČEK, 1960).

Others reject entirely such a specified cytology. ANDERSON in 1957 expressed very vigorously that "hairsplitting" of this kind would only discredit cytology, because diagnoses of this sort undoubtedly were bound to create many misinterpretations. LAPID and GOLDBERGER (1951), ROTH (1953), STOLL, MARTIN and GAULRAPP (1954), SCHÜLLER (1957), WACHTEL (1961) and others believed it was impossible to differentiate between invasive cancers and carcinoma in situ on the basis of the cytologic smear. *Acta cytologica* sponsored a symposium published in 1961 (I and II), to consider whether a prediction from the cytologic smear was possible, as judged on the basis of the histologic change. Of some 20 participants, about three-fourths expressed affirmative opinions, stating they considered it possible to draw conclusions about histology from cytology. They warned, nevertheless, that histologic confirmation could not be omitted.

PAPANICOLAOU recognized the possibilities offered by prospective cytodiagnosis, stating in 1952 and 1957 (see p. 33) that the various stages of development of malignant epithelial atypias of the cervix uteri could be traced only by means of cytology. What he had in mind was the observation of the development of an invasive cancer from a carcinoma in situ or its involution. According to PAPANICOLAOU, any removal of tissue for histologic diagnosis involved the danger of totally removing the lesion, thus rendering impossible any further statement about its biologic potential. He indicated also that small biopsies could miss even the most serious lesion; hence with this method of tracing stages of development gross error could also occur.

The success of cytodiagnosis, and especially that of prospective cytology, depends on the cooperation of clinician and pathologist. The clinician will frequently remove tissue from the wrong location if he is not well-acquainted with the extent and location of early changes. Not all pathologists have yet an exact knowledge of the various forms of early stages. Any shortcomings of this kind are bound to result in failures of cytology.

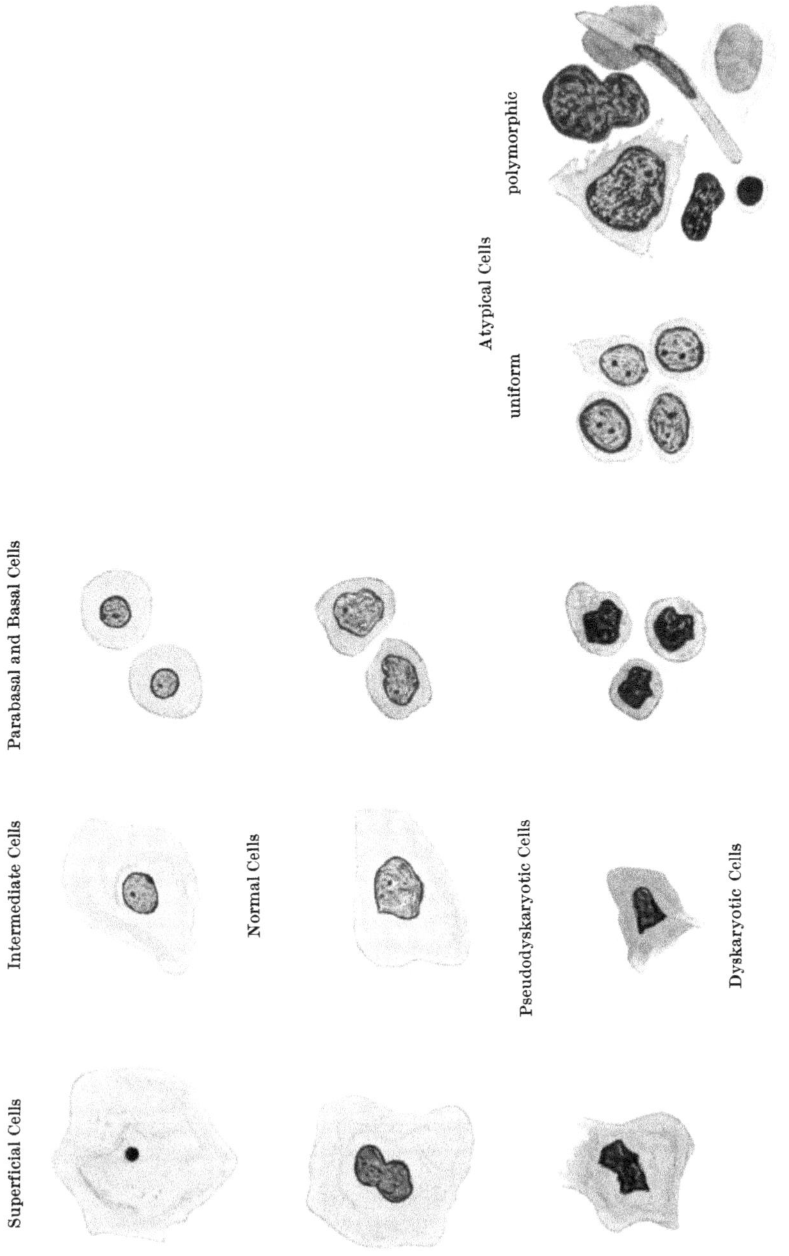

Fig. 46. Partly schematic comparison of the pathologic cellular types with normal cells. Aquarelle. The cells were drawn from colored photomicrographs (KERN, 1962)

For many years we have fortunately been able to clarify cytologic findings in the best possible way, clinically as well as histologically, through teamwork. This cooperation has enabled us to put our impressions of the possibilities of predicting histologic changes from the cytologic smear on an objective basis.

The occurrence of dyskaryosis with the subsequent diagnosis of carcinoma in situ came into focus during our collaboration with ZINSER. Our observations were

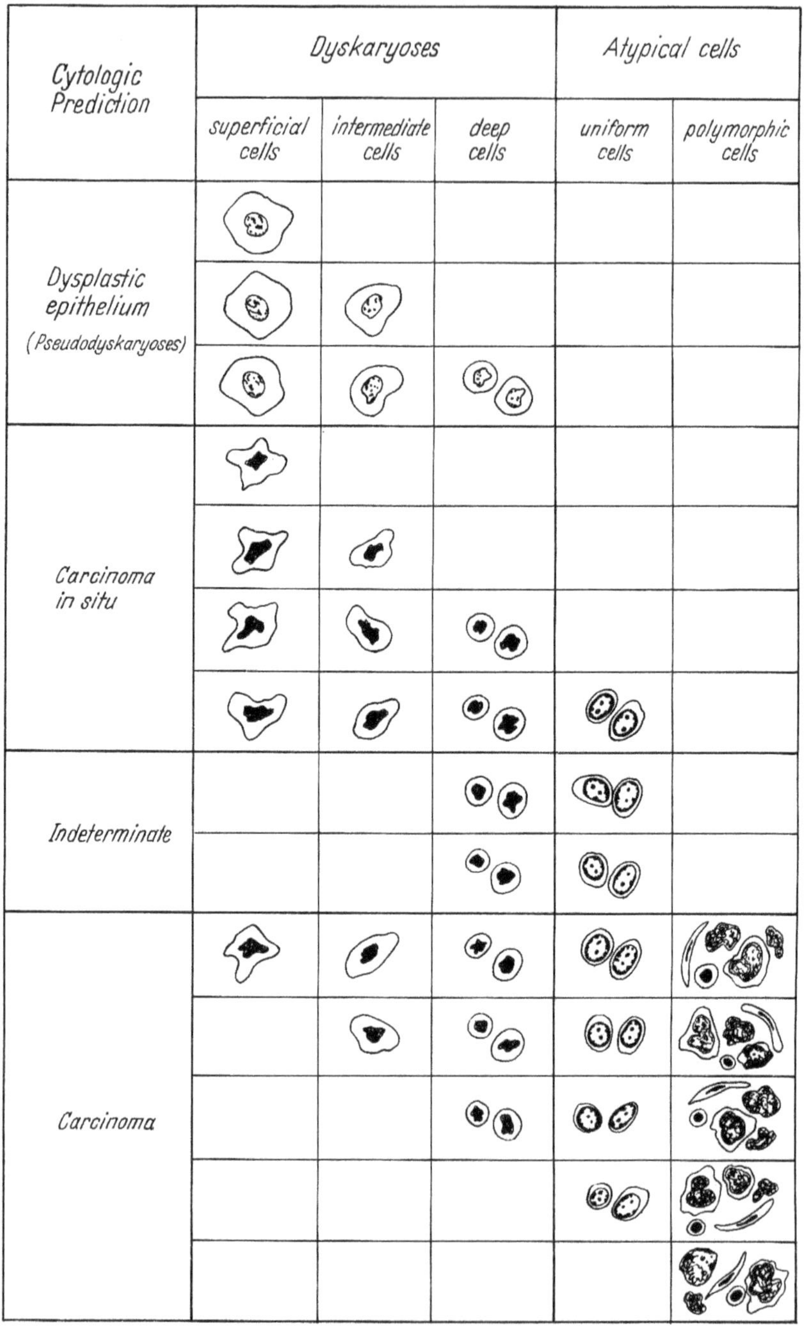

Fig. 47. Partly schematic representation of cellular types in the cytologic smear, from which a prediction can be made about the histologic change (KERN, 1962)

in accord with those in the literature previously mentioned. The following working hypothesis was established in the course of an objective investigation of this phenomenon (KERN, 1959, 1962 I, II) (Figs. 46, 47):

1. A carcinoma in situ is indicated if dyskaryoses of all cellular layers are found in the cytologic smear alone or together with uniform atypical cells.

2. A prospective cytodiagnosis is not possible if, in the smear, only deep dyskaryoses and uniform atypical cells are found together, or if the latter are found alone. The smear can only be labeled "positive".

3. An invasive carcinoma is indicated if polymorphic atypical cells appear either alone or together with dyskaryoses and uniform atypical cells.

This working hypothesis has been tested empirically by comparing the cytologic prospective diagnosis with the histologic diagnosis. For this study 318 cases were available for which an optimal histologic verification had been achieved.

Table 11 (KERN, 1962)

Cytologic prediction	Number of cases	% accuracy	
Carcinoma	154	92.2	87.3
Indeterminate	43	—	
Carcinoma in situ	121	80.99	

According to our definition, optimal verification consists in a conization of the cervix uteri with subsequent multiple sections through the cervix, affording an unequivocal histologic statement of the type and extent of the lesion. There was no case in which a diagnosis would have been reached on the basis of a biopsy. The confirmation of the diagnosis through small biopsies or cervical curettage was sufficient in cases of clinical carcinoma (see OBER and BONTKE, 1959; OBER and BÖTZELEN, 1959).

The results of this study were published in 1959 and 1962 (I and II). They are represented here in sufficient detail to permit understanding of the subsequent discussion.

A prediction could be made from the smear in 86.48%, or 275 times. A combination of cells that made prediction impossible, as mentioned previously, was found in 13.52%, or 43 times. The accuracy of the cytologic prospective diagnoses was 87.3%.

The results are summarized in Table 11.

Prediction of Carcinoma in Situ with Delimitation of the Dysplastic Epithelium from the Cytologic Smear

Table 12 and Fig. 48 show the results of 121 cases diagnosed as carcinoma in situ from the cytologic smear. This prognosis was 80.99% accurate (98 correct and 23 wrong).

There are two possible kinds of error: the change to be expected can be more serious than had been assumed (cancer), or less serious (epidermidalization, metaplasia, dysplastic epithelium).

As Table 12 shows, the mistake of predicting a markedly atypical epithelium rather than an advanced lesion as actually found is quite infrequent (2.48%). Two cases of invasive carcinoma had extensive margins of carcinoma in situ which were the cause of the wrong diagnoses.

More significant was the error of predicting carcinoma in situ when only dysplastic epithelium (13 cases) or epidermidalization (7 cases) was found (a total of 16.53%). The prospective diagnoses among these diagnostic errors ("incorrectly positive") were made on the basis of dyskaryotic nuclear changes. Detection of the mistakes led us to the discovery that these nuclear changes were different from the true dyskaryoses and they have since been called "pseudodyskaryoses". They are described under the heading "Appearance of the Pathologic Cell" (see p. 70). We now group the pseudodyskaryoses with dysplastic epithelium, which

Table 12 (Kern, 1962)

Cytologic prediction: carcinoma in situ	Histologic diagnosis	Number of cases	%
Incorrect	Ascending epidermidalization	7	16.53
	Dysplastic epithelium	13	
Correct	Borderline case, approaching carcinoma in situ	8	80.99
	Carcinoma in situ, simple replacing growth and bulky outgrowth, according to Hamperl	86	
	Early stromal invasion	4	
False	Microcarcinoma	1	2.48
	Invasive carcinoma	2	
	Total	121	100.00

is thought to require mere cytologic observation without therapy. Histologically, these cases are epithelial lesions, for instance basal hyperactivity, epidermidalization accompanied by many mitoses or metaplasia with many mitoses, and dysplastic epithelium (Simm, 1959; Okagaki, Lerch, Younge, McKay and Kevorkian, 1962; Nieburgs, Reisman and Pacheco, 1963). The prospective significance of this change is not clear. Some authors consider it the manifestation of chronic inflammation and, hence, reversible; others suspect it to be a precursor of carcinoma in situ.

The accuracy can be improved in this group if the dysplastic epithelia are eliminated as a cause of incorrect prospective diagnosis of carcinoma in situ. The clinical consequence of the prospective diagnosis of carcinoma in situ made from cytologic smears implies to us conization of the cervix uteri without performing small biopsies. Histologic diagnosis and therapy are begun when the conization is performed.

The reasonably high accuracy of diagnosis of carcinoma in situ suggests a way of elucidating the pathogenesis of cervical carcinoma. It is generally assumed that cervical carcinoma develops from carcinoma in situ. The difference in age between the early stages and invasive carcinoma amounts to an average of 10 years. Increasing differences of age also exist within the groups of carcinoma in situ

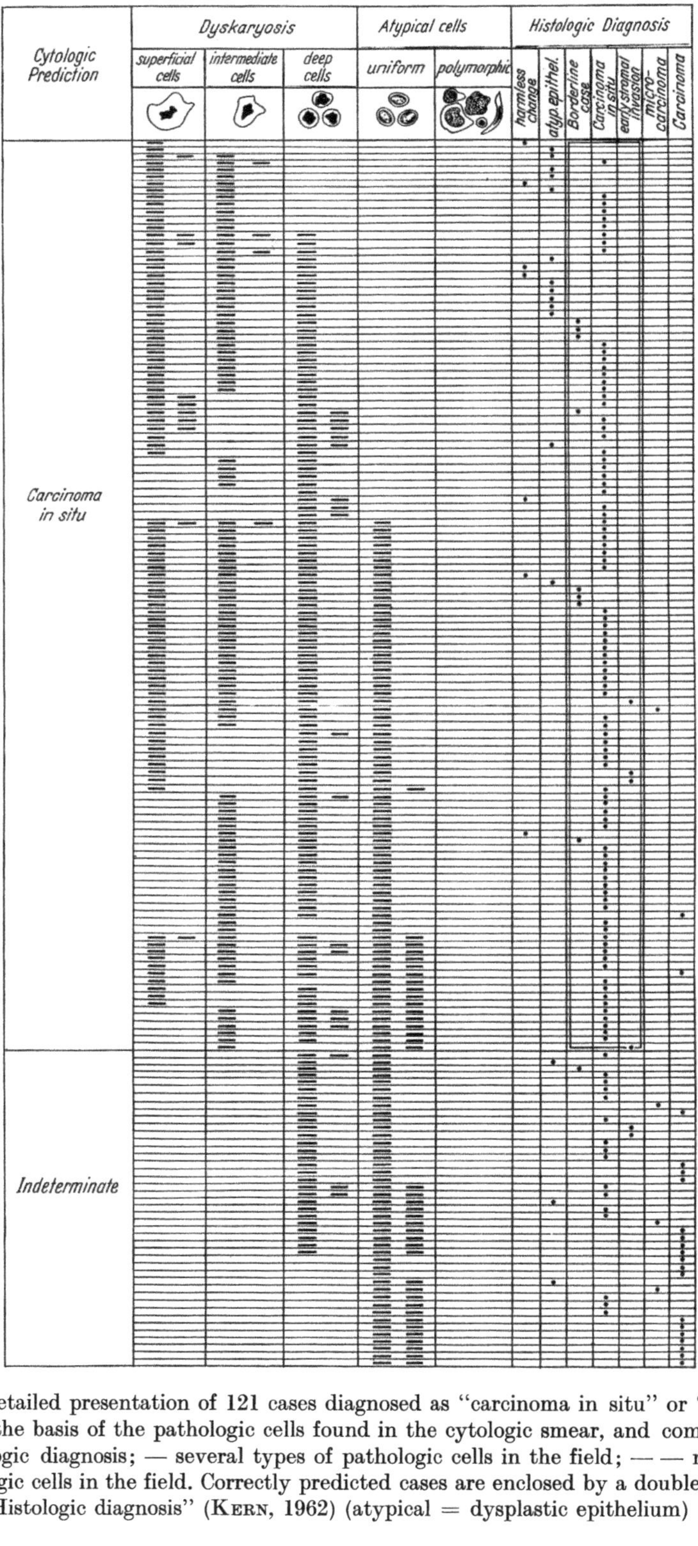

Fig. 48. Detailed presentation of 121 cases diagnosed as "carcinoma in situ" or "indeterminate" on the basis of the pathologic cells found in the cytologic smear, and compared with the histologic diagnosis; — several types of pathologic cells in the field; — — many types of pathologic cells in the field. Correctly predicted cases are enclosed by a double line in the column "Histologic diagnosis" (KERN, 1962) (atypical = dysplastic epithelium)

established by HAMPERL, which represent morphologically progressive stages of development. No cases, however, have been available that would have provided the opportunity to verify this development in any one patient. The possibility of regression of carcinoma in situ also has been discussed, but proof is lacking because there are fundamental objections to the removal of tissue for the purpose of elucidating these problems.

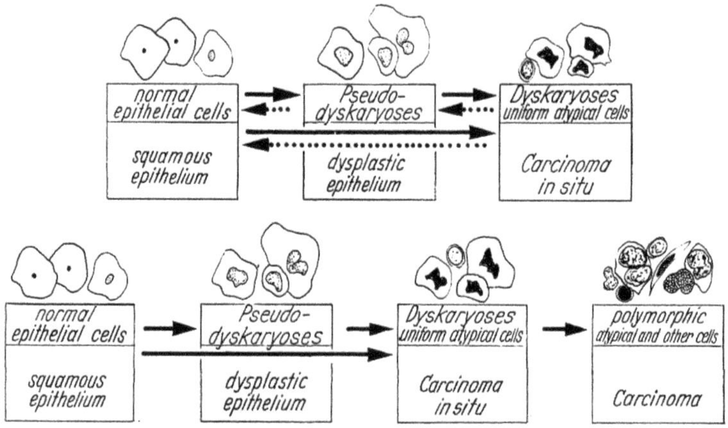

Fig. 49. Cytologic possibilities for depicting the progression or regression of epithelial atypias in the cervix from the changes in certain types of pathologic cells. The black arrow indicates the progression, and the dotted arrow the possibilities of regression

The investigation of the following problems should be feasible through correlation of the individual cellular types and the histologic picture (Fig. 49):

1. Is the dysplastic epithelium capable of regression?

2. Does carcinoma in situ develop from dysplastic epithelium? How long does this development take?

3. Is carcinoma in situ capable of regression?

4. Does invasive cancer develop from carcinoma in situ? How long does this development take?

The investigation of problems No. 1 and No. 2 is feasible without endangering the patient but that of No. 3 and No. 4 is not. Who could calmly stand by and watch the development of a true cancer from a precancerous change? We do not, however, consider it impossible to find an answer to this question, because time and again patients with positive cytologic smears indicating carcinoma in situ avoid treatment for years before they are observed again (HELD, 1957).

Cytologic Smears from which no Histologic Prediction is Possible (Indeterminate)

Among the cytologic prospective diagnoses of "carcinoma in situ" and "carcinoma", there remains a group of smears that do not seem to permit this kind of diagnosis. These are smears in which deep dyskaryoses appear, alone or together with uniform atypical cells. This condition occured in 43 (13.5%) out of 318 cases. Although the slide was classed as positive (Group IV or V according to PAPANICOLAOU), a decision regarding the kind of change could not be made. The composition of the cytologic variations is given in Table 13 in correlation with the histologic diagnoses. It follows that a carcinoma may be expected with reasonable certainty if uniform atypical cells are present. An objection to this group is, of course, its small number. Clinically, these smears call for conization once invasive carcinoma has been excluded.

Table 13 (KERN, 1962)

Histologic diagnosis	Cellular types in the smear	
	Dyskaryoses of deep cells and uniform atypical cells	Uniform atypical cells
Dysplastic epithelium	2	1
Borderline case, approaching carcinoma in situ	1	—
Carcinoma in situ	13	3
Early stromal invasion	2	—
Microcarcinoma	2	1
Invasive carcinoma	8	10
Total	28	15

Prediction of Carcinoma from the Cytologic Smear

Table 14 and Fig. 50 show 154 cases in which the diagnosis "invasive carcinoma" was reached on the basis of the cytologic smear without knowledge of the clinical finding. The presence of polymorphic atypical cells formed the basis for the diagnosis. Comparison with the results of studies of the surgical specimens showed that the diagnosis was correct in 142 cases, or 92.2%. Not a single case designated "false positive" appeared in that group; that is, not one case included a lesion less severe than carcinoma in situ. The mistakes (12 cases) consist of 7 carcinomas in situ of Group I and II according to HAMPERL (simple replacing growth and bulky outgrowth) and of 5 cases of early stromal invasion.

Table 14 (KERN, 1962)

Cytologic prediction carcinoma	Histologic diagnosis	Number of cases	%
Incorrect	Carcinoma in situ (simple replacing growth, bulky outgrowth according to HAMPERL)	7	7.8
	Early stromal invasion	5	
Correct	Microcarcinoma	11	92.2
	Invasive carcinoma	131	
Total		154	100.0

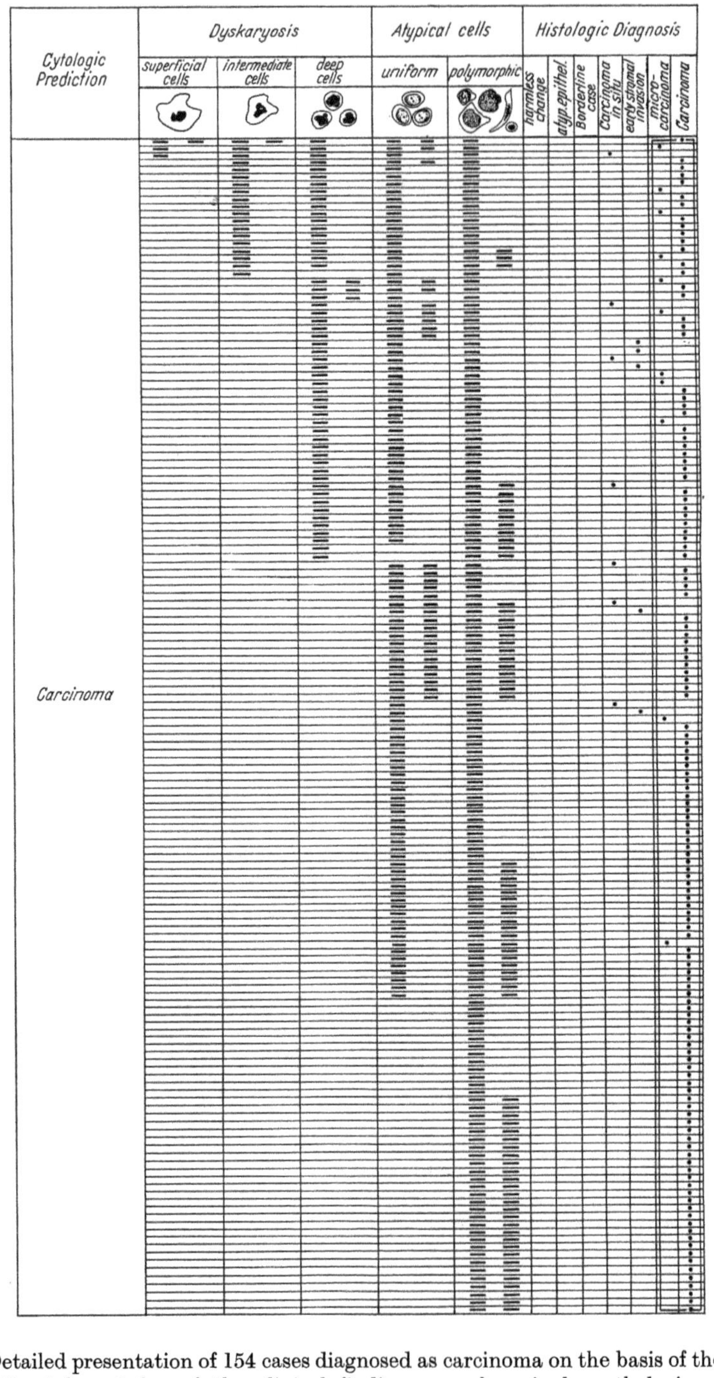

Fig. 50. Detailed presentation of 154 cases diagnosed as carcinoma on the basis of the cytologic smear, without knowledge of the clinical finding; — a few single pathologic cells in the field; — — many pathologic cells in the field. Cytologically correctly predicted cases are indicated by a double line in the column "Histologic diagnosis" (KERN, 1962) (atypical = dysplastic epithelium)

The accuracy of 92.2% achieved for the prediction of carcinoma from the cytologic smear is very high for a biological method. Invasive cancer may, therefore, with reasonable certainty be assumed to occur whenever polymorphic atypical cells are found.

This finding has more than theoretical significance. It is true that in 90% of all invasive cancers a tentative diagnosis may be reached through inspection and palpation, without cytology. The problem, however, is different when clinically questionable carcinomas are concerned, carcinomas designated "histologically detected cancers" by OBER, KAUFMANN and HAMPERL (1961).

In view of the great difference between the treatment for cancers that cannot be detected clinically and that for carcinoma in situ, knowledge of the type of change present should be as precise as possible before therapy starts. In our institution, every smear indicating carcinoma in situ is diagnosed by conization and treated simultaneously in sexually mature women. It is, therefore, very important to know whether a carcinoma is present. We try to verify the diagnosis of cancer through a careful cervical curettage if it is indicated by the cytologic smear. Extremely small endophytic growths are found as a rule; they would have been noticed clinically had the direction of their growth been outward. This course of action makes it possible, if a clinically occult cancer is present, to avoid conization, a procedure known to create difficulties in subsequent definitive operations for cancer. Fig. 51 shows the histologic findings in 116 conizations. The 17 invasive carcinomas found in the cone come from the group of indeterminate smears.

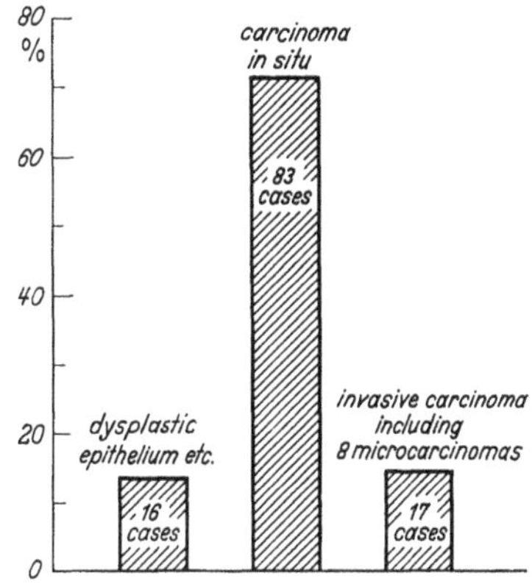

Fig. 51. Histologic finding in multiple survey sections from 116 conizations of the cervix (KERN, 1962)

A prospective diagnosis based upon the cytologic smear can thus be made with relatively high accuracy for the epithelial atypias of the cervix if the specimen has been gently removed, and the surgical verification and histologic preparation have been optimal. Disregard of these conditions will lead to considerable frustration. All of our results have been reached through such cooperation.

The harmony of this interplay between clinical practice - cytology - histology depends on the use of instruments that may easily get out of tune. The results of cytology deteriorate if the clinician is careless in removing secretions from the vagina, and he loses confidence. At the same time, he loses his willingness to expose the patient to major diagnostic techniques, such as conization, because of uncertain cytology. The clinician begins "snipping" away at the portio in a more or less expert manner; the small biopsy specimens obtained in turn limit histological examination, thus discrediting even more the allegedly bad cytology. In this vicious cycle the blame for misinterpretation usually remains with the cytologic

diagnosis, even though its causes often are to be found in the technique of biopsy. Since cytologic diagnoses may approach in accuracy those reached by histologic studies, the importance of carefully removing secretions for smears should be self-evident.

The following procedure is appropriate if removal, surgical verification, and preparation of the material are optimal:

1. When pseudodyskaryoses are present in the cytologic smear, it is classified in PAPANICOLAOU'S Group III, indicating dysplastic epithelium. Therapeutic intervention is not necessary but a cytologic check-up is required at regular intervals (every 3 months).
2. With dyskaryoses alone or together with uniform atypical cells, the smear is classified in PAPANICOLAOU'S Groups IV or V and indicates carcinoma in situ. A conization is performed and the cone is histologically prepared in multiple survey sections.
3. If the cytologic smear is positive but the prospective diagnosis is indeterminate, it is classified in PAPANICOLAOU'S Group IV or V. If a carcinoma in all probability can be excluded, a conization is performed.
4. If the cytologic smear contains polymorphic atypical cells alone or with other pathologic cellular types, it is classified in PAPANICOLAOU'S Group IV or V and indicates invasive carcinoma. The diagnosis of cancer must be verified histologically through removal of small specimens of tissue (cervical curettage, biopsy of cervical fragments), and the patient must undergo the usual treatment for cancer. If cancer cannot be demonstrated unequivocally, conization should also be performed in such cases.

General Review of the Cytologically Examined Material

The cytologic material collected during $4^1/_2$ years is presented below; first, a few general aspects (age, menstrual phase and number of deliveries) will be correlated with PAPANICOLAOU'S groups.

There were 22,249 cytologic examinations performed on 13,674 patients from January 1, 1957 through June 30, 1961, entailing the microscopic inspection of 44,498 slides.

The number of examinations has increased every year since 1957, and by 1960 had almost doubled.

The evaluation has been based on the number of patients examined (13,674), not on smears taken. Any patient examined with several smears was classified under the "most serious" diagnosis; hence a patient with smears evaluated as IIW, II, II, respectively, was listed in the column headed "IIW"; or a patient with smears evaluated as IIW, III, III, IV was listed in the column "IV/V".

The diagnosis in relation to the total number of cases is presented in Fig. 52. In more than 80% of the patients no variety of epithelial atypia was noted. In 11% the smears were repeated after cleansing treatments, but they showed no further indication of epithelial atypia. This percentage is an indication of the frequency of admixtures in vaginal secretions that require treatment. Group III is very low — 1.1%, accounted for by our concept of interpretation as previously explained. The positive smears in Groups IV and V are characterized by the high rate of 4%. It comprises, in addition to the cytologically detected, clinically occult epithelial diseases of the portio, clinical cancers that had been examined cytologically during first years covered by the report. The smears of clinical carcinomas were used mainly for the analysis of cellular types (see prediction). The smears from 418 patients (3.1%) could not be evaluated. An improved smear technique substantially reduced the number of smears that could not be evaluated each year.

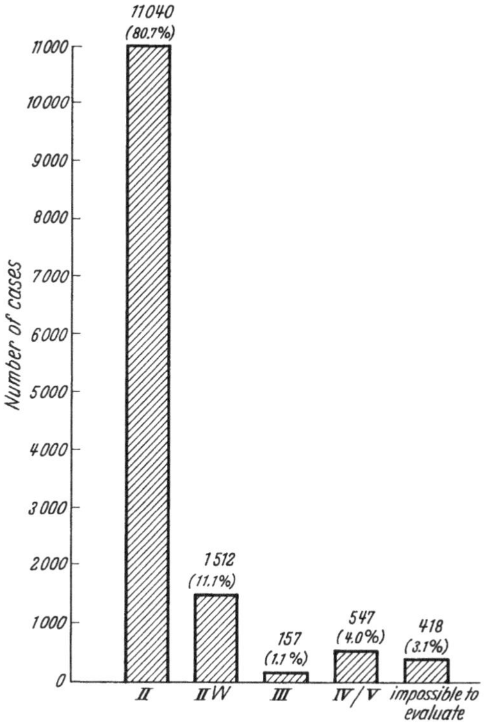

Fig. 52. Results of the cytologic examination of 13674 cases according to PAPANICOLAOU'S groups (KERN, RISSMANN and HUND, 1964)

It is customary to attempt a comparison of one's own results with those of other investigators. A direct comparison is unfortunately not possible in most cases because of differences in methods and in the interpretation of cytologic smears.

CUYLER, KAUFMANN, CARTER, ROSS, THOMAS and PALUMBO reported in 1951 on 51,022 smears taken from 15,217 women, with these results: Papanicolaou Class I: 12.3%; II: 80.4%; III: 3.6%; IV: 0.9%; V: 2.6%; and not evaluable: 1.1%[1].

STOLL, RIEHM and BACH in 1955 obtained the following results among 5,619 women: Papanicolaou Class I and II in 88.6%; III in 7.6%; and IV and V in 3.8% of all cases.

[1] The total percentage is 100.9; figures taken from the original paper.

KAISER, BOUSER, INGRAHAM and HILBERG reported in 1960 on the overwhelming total of 608,200 cytologically examined women. Their results were: negative, 95.2% ; atypical, 3.0% ; suspicious, 0.7% ; positive, 0.2% ; unsatisfactory, 0.9%. "Atypical" seems to be equivalent to our Group III, and "suspicious" to our Group IV.

SOULE and DAHLIN (1960) found 2.5% to 3% of smears that could not be evaluated in a total of 139,503.

JAEGER and ERDENEN (1961) diagnosed 2.6% as Group III and 1.4% as Groups IV and V out of 21,520 smears taken in their clinic. Of the slides sent in, 3% could not be evaluated, as against only 1.5% of their clinical material.

Table 15. *Distribution of cytologic findings in 13,256 patients according to age groups.* (KERN, RISSMANN and HUND, 1964)

Age Groups Years	Cytologic Result Normal II/IIW	Suspicious/Positive III/IV/V
0—19	309	4
20—29	2,136	51
30—39	3,340	198
40—49	3,263	196
50—59	2,403	153
60—69	821	67
70—79	255	32
80 and over	25	3
Total	12,552	704
Average age	42.1 years	46.2 years
Confidence limits for $t = 3$	41.7—42.5 years	44.7—47.7 years

The group of smears that could not be evaluated had to be excluded in further calculations, leaving 13,256 cytologically examined and diagnosed patients with complete files.

Table 15 shows the distribution by age-groups of the patients examined and their respective cytologic findings.

Using the Chi square test, the accuracy of difference between the age distribution of the normal cytologic findings (II, IIW) and that of the suspicious and positive findings (III—IV, V) was 99% (Chi square = 82 for $n = 7$).

A possible correlation of the suspicious and positive cytologic findings with the menstrual status of the groups of patients examined was investigated. Women in the menopause have the highest rate of cytologically positive smears (6.2%), about 1% higher than that of younger sexually mature patients, but the difference cannot be ascertained statistically (Chi square test).

The correlation of the suspicious and positive findings with the number of births of the women examined is represented in Fig. 53. The deviation of the distribution of the number of births among patients with normal cytologic findings from that of those with suspicious and positive findings has been ascertained (Chi square = 116 for $n=5$). The percentage proportion of the suspicious and positive findings in the total material rises as the number of births increases (3.1%, 5.1%, 5.4%, 7.1%, 8.3% and 12.1%). It can be found by dispersion analysis that a straight line of regression is barely admissible, $y=(3.13+1.45x)\%$. The coefficient has been well ascertained to be not equal to zero.

This presentation emphasizes the importance of the examination by cytologic smear in a woman who has had many children.

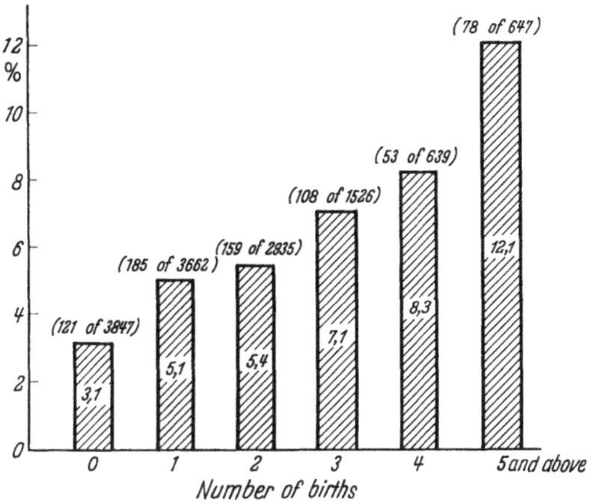

Fig. 53. Percentage increase of cytologically suspicious and positive findings in relation to the increasing parity of the patients

Accuracy of Cytodiagnosis in Our Material

All positive findings require histologic verification, either to confirm or refute them. The value of any method of early diagnosis, therefore, depends largely on histology.

Of the 13,674 patients examined cytologically tissue was removed from 2,281 and studied histologically. Very strict criteria were applied in the comparison with cytology to provide unequivocal confirmation or refutation of the cytologic diagnosis. The number of cases compared was 1,106. Table 16 presents a survey of the composition and histologic method of studying this material. (The complete histologic findings were available in another 35 cases, but the cytologic findings could not be evaluated.)

The group of cases not optimally comparable consisted of those in which tissue was removed by 1,089 curettages of cervix and corpus, by polypectomy by a few biopsies (none of these cases showed any indication of malignancy) and from 51 genital carcinomas unrelated to the cervix or corpus.

Table 17 presents a survey of the relations between cytologic findings and histologic diagnoses. In this table only those cases are considered in which an unequivocal diagnosis was made on the basis of the histologic evaluation.

The corpus carcinomas are excluded from the following discussion since their detection is not the purpose of cytology. In addition, the figures shown in Table 17 demonstrate how unsuitable our smear technique is for this type of carcinoma.

Tables 17 and 18 show the cytologic results for 999 portios. They invite a challenge to test the accuracy of cytology. A certain percentage of cytologic findings was "false positive", that is, the suspicious cytologic diagnosis could not be confirmed through histologic examination. Surgical intervention, therefore, would not in retrospect have been necessary in these patients (1.5%). Another percentage of the cytologic findings was "false negative", consisting of incidental epithelial lesions detected histologically (1.2%). They are early cases (the women were operated on for other indications) and "false negative" clinical cancers. A group of suspicious findings remains (3.6%). Calculation of the cytologic accuracy according to customary methods shows agreement with the histologic diagnosis in 93.7%, a suspicious result in 3.6%, and an incorrect result in 2.7% of cases. The question whether this accuracy of 93.7% could be fallacious will be discussed later.

Table 16. *How did the histologic diagnosis evolve?* (Kern, Rissmann and Hund, 1964)

Histologic diagnosis	Removal of tissue	Histologic preparation	Number of cases
Benign lesions of the portio: ascending epidermidalization, metaplasia, etc.	Hysterectomy, amputation of the portio or conization	Multiple transections through cervix	615
Early cases of cervical carcinoma	Conization of the portio, hysterectomy	Multiple transections through cervix	205
Cervical carcinomas	Multiple biopsies Cervical curettage	Customary histologic preparation confirming the diagnosis	206
	If treated surgically: surgical specimen	Multiple transections through cervix	
Carcinoma of the corpus	Curettage of corpus	Customary histologic preparation confirming the diagnosis	80
Total			1,106

Table 17. *Histologic diagnosis compared with the cytologic finding.* (Kern, Rissmann and Hund, 1964)

Histologic diagnosis	Cytologic diagnosis				
	II	IIW	III	IV/V	Total
Benign lesions of the portio	454	129	17	15	615
Early cases (without dysplastic epithelium)	3	1	12	162	178
Cervical carcinomas	2	6	7	191	206
Total					999
Corpus carcinomas	26	24	15	15	80

We have pursued the "false negative" and "false positive" findings and present them in Tables 19—21.

BONNEY's plastic procedure was performed on two patients (cases No.1 and 2) with cytologically "false negative" carcinomas in situ because of large ectropions

Table 18. *Incorrect results of cytology, as compared with histology.* (KERN, RISSMANN and HUND, 1964)

Histology	False negative cytologic finding	Suspicious cytologic finding	False positive cytologic finding	Total of all cases
Benign lesions of the portio	—	17 (2.8%)	15 (2.4%)	615 (100%)
Early cases (without dysplastic epithelium)	4 (2.25%)	12 (6.75%)	—	178 (100%)
Cervical carcinomas	8 (3.9%)	7 (3.4%)	—	206 (100%)
Total	12 (1.2%)	36 (3.6%)	15 (1.5%)	999 (100%)

Table 19. *Cytologically "false negative" carcinomas in situ.* (KERN, RISSMANN and HUND, 1964)

Cur. No.	Indication	Cytologic findings	Cytologic result on check-up and error	
1	Plastic surgery (Bonney) for ectropion with profuse discharge	1. II 2. too little material 3. too little material	1. II 2. too little material 3. too little material	Faulty smear technique
2	Bonney for ectropion with profuse secretion	1. II	1. II	Smear markedly contaminated, faulty smear technique
3	Hysterectomy for descensus	1. II 2. II 3. II	1. II 2. IV 3. III	Error of the investigator and faulty smear technique
4	Hysterectomy for descensus	1. IIW 2. IIW 3. II 4. II	1. IIW 2. IV 3. IV 4. IV	Error of the investigator

with discharge resistant to therapy. A faulty smear technique (no contact smear), possibly because of the profuse mucous secretion, seems to have caused the failure in both cases. The uterus was removed in two other patients (cases No. 3 and 4) because of prolapse. One of these patients had a minute region of markedly atypical epithelium of the endocervix; the other patient had an extensive endocervical carcinoma in situ. In both instances, reinspection of the cytological smears proved the cytologist to have been in error. These four cases had been diagnosed in the years 1957 and 1958.

Cytologic smears made after surgical operations on the cervix (biopsy, curettage, electrocoagulation) were examined in four cases of cytologically unrecognized cervical carcinomas. One case represented a recurrence of tumor after intensive radiation therapy; another was a histologic rarity, an invasive tumor of the portio exhibiting extreme keratinization and not fitting into any histologic classification.

Cytology as a method failed twice (Table 20).

Table 20. *Cytologically "false negative" cervical carcinomas.* (Kern, Rissmann and Hund, 1964)

No.	Clinical Diagnosis	Cytology	Attempted explanation
1	Electrocoagulation after biopsy (extramural)	II	considerable nonspecific shedding after electrocoagulation
2	Condition after biopsy (extramural)	II W	profuse discharge from the granulation tissue of the biopsy wound
3	Condition after biopsy (extramural)	II W	profuse nonspecific discharge from the wound
4	Condition after curettage	II W	nonspecific discharge from the site of curettage
5	Recurrence in vagina after Wertheim and irradiation	II W	much detritus (reaction to irradiation)
6	Histologically exceptional case. Differential diagnosis: papilloma or markedly keratinizing squamous epithelial carcinoma	II W	extreme keratinization explains the cytologically negative diagnosis
7	Long misdiagnosed clinically as an adnexal tumor, high endocervical	II	incorrect smear technique (not from the endocervix)
8	Exophyte	II W	mistaken cytologic diagnosis

The "false positive" cases are presented in Table 21.

The operations performed on 15 "false positive" patients were seven hysterectomies, one excision of a cervical stump, and seven conizations. Other clinical indications were the cause of surgical intervention in eight cases in which the cytologic finding was only incidental.

A severe cervicitis was found in nine cases; consequently, an important cause of discharge was eliminated by the operation. Hyperactivity of the basal epithelium was prominent in six cases, in two of which epithelial artifacts may have been the reason for an interpretation that was not entirely satisfactory from the cytologist's point of view. Graham and McGraw (1950) and Milligan, Carrow and Eggers (1959) reported similar observations.

The *dysplastic epithelium* represents a special case, cytologically as well as histologically. The histologic diagnosis of dysplastic epithelium has not been accurately defined. Its scope may extend from disturbance of the basal cells to

Table 21. *Fifteen cytologically "false positive" results.* (KERN. RISSMANN and HUND, 1964)

No.	Indication and kind of operation	Histologic diagnosis
1	Uterine leiomyoma, size of a man's fist, with adnexal tumor. Cytologic Group IV. Hysterectomy with removal of both adnexa	1359/57; ascending epidermidalization, metaplasia of the endocervix
2	Ovarian tumor on the right. Cytologic Group IV. Hysterectomy with removal of adnexa	957/57; papillary ovarian tumor Peculiar squamous epithelial metaplasia of the endocervix
3	Cytologic Group IV. Conization	203/58; metaplasia, cervicitis
4	Vaginal prolapse. Cytologic Group IV. Anterior and posterior plastic surgery with conization	52/58; ascending epidermidalization
5	Climacteric hemorrhagic disorder. Cytologic Group IV. Hysterectomy	224/59; ascending epidermidalization, metaplasia of the endocervix
6	Adnexal tumors on both sides. Cytologic Group IV. Hysterectomy with removal of adnexa	1085/59; ascending epidermidalization severe cervicitis, endometriosis
7	Intermenstrual bleeding. Cytologic Group IV. Conization	911/59; severe cervicitis, metaplasia of the squamous epithelium of the endocervix, epithelial artifacts
8	Discharge resistant to therapy. Cytologic Group IV, conization	357/59; severe cervicitis, ectropion
9	Cytologic Group IV, vaginal hysterectomy	367/59; ascending epidermidalization
10	Cytologic Group IV, conization	423/59; severe cervicitis, basal disturbance in process of epidermidalization around the external cervical os
11	Cytologic Group IV, conization	972/59; cervicitis, basal disturbance in metaplastic epithelium
12	Cytologic Group IV, cervical stump, excision of the stump	782/59; widespread leukoplakia of the portio. Basal disturbance in epidermidalization
13	Descensus, cytologic Group IV, vaginal hysterectomy	104/60; cervicitis, epithelial artifacts in area of external cervical os
14	Adnexal tumors on both sides, cytologic Group IV, hysterectomy with removal of adnexa	559/60; endometriosis, ovarian carcinoma, cervicitis, basal disturbance in metaplasia
15	Severe discharge during last 4 years, extensive laceration: cytologic Group IV, plastic surgery on the portio	252/61; severe cervicitis, processes of epidermidalization

squamous epithelium with an abundance of mitoses to manifestations that cannot, without difficulty, be differentiated from the "simple replacing growth" (in HAMPERL's terminology) of carcinoma in situ. Some of the cases designated "metaplasia" in Table 21 could, for instance, be considered dysplastic epithelium as well. Credit is due, on the other hand, to the histologic evaluation of 18 dysplastic epithelia classified under IV and V and not included in this tabulation because of the special categorization of the pseudodyskaryoses. It is since that time that we keep cases of this kind under cytologic observation. Seven dysplastic epithelia were not cytologically suspicious. The question whether the degree of atypia in these cytologic smears was perhaps adequate for a suspicious or positive diagnosis remains open. A review of the histologically confirmed early cases and cervical carcinomas that were diagnosed "Groups IV and V" cytologically shows that the great majority had been positive in the first smear (Table 22), but an evaluation of the method from the first smear would produce a less favorable result.

Table 22 (Kern, Rissmann and Hund, 1964)

1. Smear	III, IV, V	IIW	II	Total
Early cases	141 (87.1%)	14 (8.6%)	7 (4.3%)	162 (100%)
Cervical carcinomas	183 (95.8%)	4 (2.1%)	4 (2.1%)	191 (100%)

Navratil gave extensive consideration to the methods of calculation of the cytologic accuracy in the Handbuch of Seitz-Amreich, Vol. 4/1, 1955, and tabulated a large number of reported accuracies. He quotes 22 authors who had reported on the accuracy of their cytologic studies. The range is between 80% and 99.26%, with 17 reports above 90%. Further data on cytologic accuracy have been published after Navratil's article in the Handbuch.

Author	Accuracy of cytodiagnosis %
Walz (1955)	86.7
Igel and Müller (1956)	93.15
Klein, Kofler and Kremer (1957)	93.7
Janisch and Kremer (1959)	93.4
Navratil, Bajardi and Burghardt (1959)	92.5
Deimel (1960)	92.99

One of the principles followed in calculating the accuracy is described as follows: A known number of histologically verified cases is used as 100% in the calculation of the percentage of the cytologic false positive and false negative results. The % accuracy is:

100% — (% false negative + % false positive) = % accuracy.

The suspicious findings (Group III) were classified as positive by Navratil. We let this group stand by itself, thus calculating:

100% — (% false negative + false positive + % suspicious) = % accuracy
100% — (1.2% + 1.5% + 3.6%) = 93.7% (Table 18).

Evaluation of the accuracy on the basis of the first smear has been recommended. Using this method, our calculation would give this result (Tables 18 and 22):

100% — (% false negative + % false positive + % suspicious) = % accuracy
100% — (4.1% + 1.5% + 3.6%) = 90.8%.

We would have to use 41 false negatives rather than 12, and the accuracy thus falls to 90.8%. Limitation of the method to the first smear, however, should not be too strongly emphasized for smears from clinic patients; material sent to the clinic, however, might well be restricted to only one smear. KIMMELSTIEL, BOS and NOLEN (1958) emphasized the increase of accuracy through repeated cytologic examination. STOLL, BACH and RIEHM (1955) found 10.04% of 229 cervical carcinomas *not* in the *first* smear.

False negative and false positive results have been reported repeatedly, but it is difficult to make comparisons, because the raw data vary greatly. Authors who have studied these problems intensively are: NIEBURGS and PUND (1950), HELD, SCHREINER and OEHLER (1954), FENNELL and GRAHAM (1955), STÜPER (1955), MORICARD (1955), SIEGEL (1955), LUKSCH and SEBEK (1957), JENNINGS, DALE, NELSON, BRINES and WILSON (1959), MUSSEY and SOULE (1959), LEVRIER and CATOR (1960), ZINSER, MEISSNER and BÖTZELEN (1963), and ULM, BACHER, JANISCH, KOFLER and KREMER (1963).

One more thought about the method used to calculate the cytologic accuracy should be mentioned: excluding clinical cancers from this consideration, cytology has been applied to the search for the early stages of cervical carcinoma. The number of early cases found during 5 years in 13,050 (13,256—206 carcinomas = 13,050) suitable cytologic examinations amounted to 174, or 1.3%. Four cytologically false negative carcinomas in situ were found accidentally during the same period in 619 uteri (615 benign lesions of the portio and four false negative carcinomas in situ) removed for various clinical reasons. Could it be assumed that the number of carcinomas in situ accidentally detected by us might have been greatly increased if the cervix or uterus had been removed from *all* patients examined cytologically, and if histologic specimens had been evaluated with multiple transections of the cervix?

The following calculations would have pertained:

cytologically examined	13,050 women
found	— 174 carcinomas in situ
histologically verified	— 619 cervices
histologically not verified	12,257 cases.

In 619 uteri four cytologically "false negative" carcinomas in situ were accidentally detected. With a 95% accuracy in diagnosis, one should expect to find between 27 and 170 unsuspected carcinomas in situ in 12,257 uteri. These figures mean that 174 early cases would have been found during the reported period, and 27 to 170 would have been overlooked, assuming a frequency of 1.6 to 2.7% of early cases. Applying these figures, the accuracy increases to 99% if the basic figure of 13,050 cases is used, even though the number of cytologically "false negative" findings has increased substantially.

This method of calculation results in a distorted picture. The essential fact remains that during the period reported 178 were found, and possibly 27 to 170 overlooked out of 13,050. This figure is even more significant in view of our prevalence rate for early stages (1.3%), which is rather high. The thought that despite all efforts perhaps 13—50% of possible carcinomas in situ remain unrecognized continues to cause anxiety.

These considerations certainly provide a reason for emphatic repetition of the request that every woman submit once a year to a cytologic examination after the age of 30, because the cases that had been overlooked may be recognized on reexamination, especially since the time required for an early case to develop into a clinical cancer is estimated to be 5—10 years. We can only guess why these cases are overlooked in cytology, since it is impossible to check an error, perhaps of the examiner, by reviewing all 22,249 cytologic smears. Both the method and the examiner probably contribute to the error.

Colposcopy

Historical Introduction

The father of colposcopy was HANS HINSELMANN who was born in Neumünster, Holstein, in 1884. He received his training in Kiel, completing it in 1908. After a relatively short period of work in Dresden, Heidelberg, Kiel, Jena, and Giessen, he spent 13 years working under v. FRANQUÉ in Bonn. In 1925 he became medical director of the Department of Obstetrics and Gynecology of the General Hospital in Hamburg-Altona.

At about that time he worked on the article "Etiology, Symptomatology and Methods of Diagnosis of the Carcinoma of the Uterus" in the Manual of VEIT-STOECKEL (1930). In directing his attention particularly to the detection of the small and earliest carcinomas of the portio, he conceived the simple but ingenious idea of looking at the surface of the portio through a magnifying glass. The device for binocular inspection through a magnifying glass utilizing intense focused light was called a "colposcope" by its inventor. It led to a new line of research, "colposcopy", which aroused the greatest interest during the subsequent decades. The surface of the portio can be studied in detail with the colposcope, which is capable of tenfold to fortyfold magnification, according to its optical system. Various kinds of epithelium can be differentiated that cannot be distinguished with the naked eye. HINSELMANN thus laid the foundation in Germany for the early diagnosis of cervical carcinoma, for it was through colposcopy that many superficial carcinomas were detected that had been recognized only as incidental findings in surgical specimens. The founder of this method continued reporting on his experience in many monographs to the end of his life. The central subject was the early detection of carcinoma of the portio (1930—1959). HINSELMANN died in Hamburg in 1959. His terminology is that of a clinically oriented investigator, and there is no analogy to it in pathological anatomy. Most of his terminology originated from visual impressions and is still in use. The difficulties encountered in translating his terminology as well as those in handling the cumbersome earliest colposcopes seem to be reasons why colposcopy has scarcely been accepted in Anglo-Saxon countries. The terminology was criticized by NOVAK (1955) after a lecture given by SCHEFFEY, LANG and TARTARIAN, who spoke on colposcopic examinations in America. Other reports, too, produced little response (SCHEFFEY, BOLTEN and LANG, 1955; LANG and RAKOFF, 1956; LANG, RAKOFF and TARTARIAN, 1957; SCHMITT, 1956, 1959; LANG, 1958 I, II; OLSON and NICHOLS, 1961; LANG, 1962). German gynecologists, however, took up the method enthusiastically, and colposcopic reports appeared in countless numbers. The knowledge gained through colposcopy has been compiled in monographs, some with excellent illustrations, by WESPI (1946), MESTWERDT (1953), GLATTHAAR (1955), CRAMER (1956,

1962), LIMBURG (1956), GANSE (1958), BRET and COUPEZ (1960), and MESTWERDT and WESPI (1961).

Colposcopic pictures were, at first, reproduced through drawings and aquarelles, but these methods were soon replaced by photography, utilizing equipment directly combined with the colposcope. Colpophotography was developed mainly by WESPI (1951, 1958), GANSE (1953), MENKEN (1954), WESPI and LOTMAR (1954), LITTMANN and WALZ (1955), SCHMITT (1955, 1956), KORTE (1957) and KRÜGER (1957). It is important for objective documentation of the condition on the surface of the portio and is an ideal means of tracing and comparing the findings as they change in the course of time.

HINSELMANN recommended, in addition to the study of the normal portio through the magnifying glass, treatment of the region with certain reagents to improve optical contrast. He called this method "extended colposcopy" (1933).

Several authors tried to overcome the limitation to the surface of the portio of the area examined with the colposcope (MENKEN, 1955; EISEN, 1955) by developing a method for inspection of the cervical canal with dilators. This method has not found general use; it does not permit observation of the upper sections of the cervical canal.

The latest development of colposcopy was introduced with the use of substantially greater magnification, similar to that of incident light microscopy. The *colpomicroscopy* of ANTOINE, GRABNER and GRÜNBERGER (1953) and ANTOINE and GRÜNBERGER (1956) uses a 240-fold magnification that makes single cells on the surface of the portio visible. This method is not simple technically, for the optical system must be placed practically on the surface of the portio, and the field of vision is less than 1 mm square, thus rendering orientation difficult. Colpomicroscopy seems, nevertheless, to extend substantially the scope of colposcopy, particularly with regard to the correlation of colposcopic and histologic specimens (GRÜNBERGER and BRANDL, 1954; WALZ, 1958; ANTOINE, BRANDL, GRÜNBERGER, KOFLER, KREMER and WALZ, 1961; BANGEN, FOCKEN and FRANZ, 1961).

Methods of Colposcopy

The following section presents the colposcopic methods in use at the Gynecological Clinic of the University of Cologne, in order to explain how the findings and the knowledge derived from them were reached.

Simple Colposcopy

Any patient (with the exception of virgins) who is not bleeding may be examined colposcopically, if the surface of her portio can be positioned in the field of vision.

The patient is placed in the proper position on the gynecological table and her vagina is held open with SIMS specula. The posterior blade of the speculum is directed towards the perineum and the anterior blade towards the bladder after passing through the introitus. The two blades point in opposite directions to avoid all possible contact with the surface of the portio, since the epithelium may be injured, causing hemorrhage and thus disturbing the field of observation.

The blades should be dry upon insertion, neither lubricated nor moistened, to avoid any detrimental effect on the cytologic smear, which is taken first.

If both blades are well positioned within the anterior and posterior fornices, the surface of the portio may be manipulated, through varying degrees of separation of the fornices, into a position as nearly as possible vertical to the observer's line of vision. The separated blades are especially useful if the portio cannot be moved easily because of adhesions, tumors, or abnormal positions of the uterus, for example.

An assistant then holds the upper blade; secretions are carefully removed from the surface of the portio and colposcopic examination is performed at a magnification of 10 to 20 times. Magnification of 40 times is not ordinarily employed in routine colposcopy. The whole surface is scanned clockwise.

By distending the vaginal vault, the lowest portion of the cervical canal can be examined through an external os if it is transversely lacerated or "fishmouth" in shape. This procedure is not feasible if the external os is just a dimple. We do not use special dilators for inspection of the cervical canal. It may be possible, at times, to extend the field of observation but in most cases it cannot be done satisfactorily. Observation becomes difficult, furthermore, because of the tangential examination of the cervical canal.

Several models have been developed by various manufacturers since HINSELMANN'S first colposcope. All of them are well suited to their purpose. Portable colposcopes mounted on the examining table are very useful in practice, whereas other kinds with individual, usually not easily movable stands often block access to the table. Our experience with MÖLLER'S colposcope for routine colposcopy has been good.

Extended Colposcopy

Simple colposcopic examination is immediately followed by treatment of the portio with reagents.

Acetic Acid Test. The surface of the portio is gently swabbed with an applicator dipped in 3% acetic acid, which causes precipitation of the mucus as well as a superficial blanching. Better contrast and three-dimensional impressions are obtained in this manner, against the background of the surface of the portio (Fig. 54). An applicator of the kind used for the cytologic smear is dipped in acetic acid and inserted into the cervical canal in an attempt to remove any vitreous, sticky mucus that may have remained there. The purpose is to permit an impression of the visible part of the lower cervical canal. The effect appears in about 3 seconds and lasts about 10 seconds. The change in the epithelium and the vessels resulting from the effect of the acetic acid should be observed with the colposcope. At the start, the epithelium appears increasingly white and the vessels become narrow. As the effect decreases, the epithelium regains its red color, the supply of blood increases, and the vessels dilate (GANSE, 1959). The vessels should be observed particularly during the decline of the acetic acid effect, preferably through a green filter.

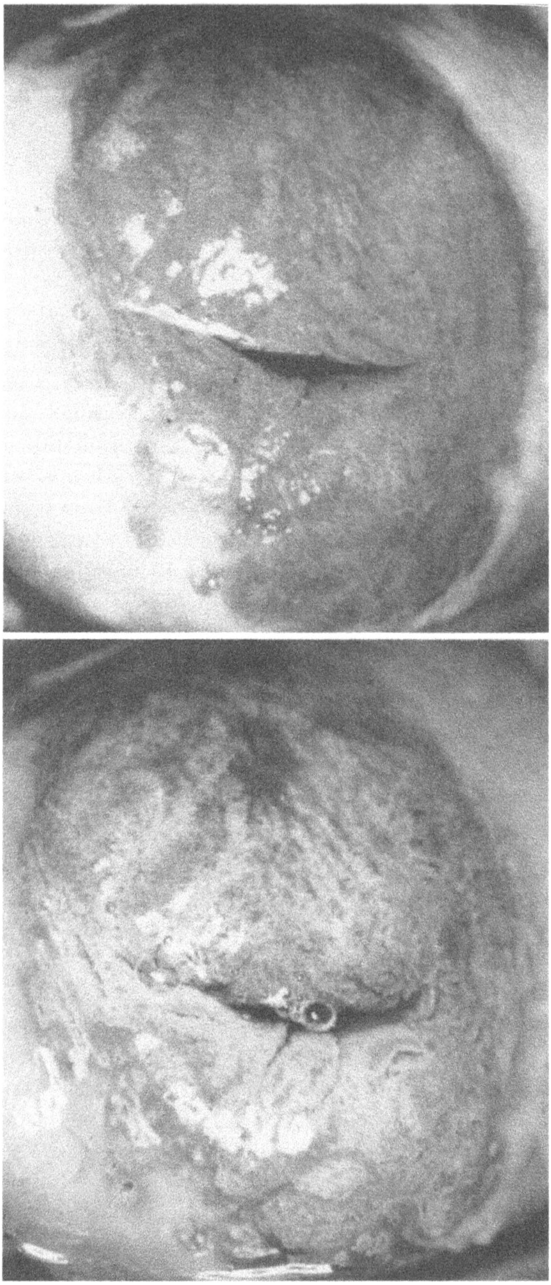

Fig. 54. Effect of 3% acetic acid on the colposcopic picture of an ectopy. The two pictures show the findings before and immediately after application

We perform the acetic acid test routinely during colposcopic examination. The effect of the acetic acid lasts just long enough for an examination of all details of the surface of the portio. The acetic acid test may be repeated several times in succession without impairing its effect, as described above. A cytologic smear can be obtained in exceptional cases even after application of acetic acid without destroying its value for diagnosis, if a few minutes are allowed for the effect of the acetic acid to disappear.

A similar effect may be obtained with lactic acid, but it takes longer to appear and to disappear. Much more time is therefore needed to observe the increasing and decreasing effects (MADEJ, 1962).

Schiller's iodine test. The vital staining of glycogen in squamous epithelium of the surface of the portio was adopted from SCHILLER by HINSELMANN as an addition to the examination by colposcopy. The results of this test may indeed be followed particularly well with the colposcope. We consider Schiller's iodine test especially important and shall therefore discuss it in detail beginning on page **142**. The test is performed regularly at the completion of the colposcopic examination. The duration of the intense brown staining of squamous epithelium varies from test to test and it must be remembered, therefore, that a colposcopic examination can often be repeated only after 1 to 3 days. A cytologic examination should not be performed after an iodine test (SMOLKA and BERIĆ, 1958; BERIĆ and SMOLKA, 1958).

Demonstration of Vessels. The vasculature of the surface of the portio is an essential criterion for judging benign, suspicious, or positive colposcopic findings, as has been emphasized by HINSELMANN.

The vessels appear red in a normal colposcopic examination, against a more or less reddish background. Some blanching may be produced by constriction of the vessels; on the other hand, congestion from venous obstruction may result if the fornices are too greatly dilated, especially by duckbill specula.

Improvement of contrast for demonstration of vessels can be achieved with the acetic acid test, and even more satisfactorily with a green filter. Such a filter is routinely attached to all colposcopes and needs simply to be brought into the path of light.

The vessels appear dark green against a light green background. The pictures are remarkably clear, especially for observation of the smallest vessels, and are better than if normal light were used.

MAJEWSKI (1960) suggested the use of a solution of Arterenol for improved vascular colposcopy. We are not familiar with it.

Numerous other chemicals suggested for use in extended colposcopy have not been tried out by us [$^1/_2$% salicylic alcohol, 3 to 10% silver nitrate solution, Albothyl solution (STOLL and POLLMANN, 1957) and so forth].

The turgor of the tissue may be tested with a blunt probe under colposcopic examination to ascertain the extent to which the tissue may be depressed. This method of observation is more subtle than that utilizing Chrobak's probe.

A second or even third examination at intervals of several days, or in other phases of the cycle, is advisable if colposcopic findings are equivocal, particularly in the large group of regional atypical transformations. Findings sometimes may be clarified on repeated examination (GANSE, 1954, 1958; GLATTHAAR, 1954).

Colpophotography

The photograph of what is seen on colposcopic examination is an unerring and objective documentation of the finding. The observation of colposcopic findings over a long period of time and the possible changes in them can be verified by colpophotography. The histologic picture of a surgical specimen can be most reliably compared with the preoperative colposcopic finding through the use of the photograph (GANSE, 1954; WESPI, 1954).

A detailed colposcopic report, however, cannot be completely replaced by colpophotography. The explanation lies in the nature of the subject. The portio is three-dimensional and its surface is uneven. At certain magnifications the entire surface of the portio cannot be placed in sharp focus, because the depth of field is limited. The mucosa of the portio is always moist and shiny, and may create reflections of light precisely in the area where an important examination is to be performed. Such highlights may be deflected to areas where they cause no difficulty if polarizing filters are employed. Use of these filters in colpophotography is limited, however, since the source of the light used to focus the camera (pilot light) produces reflections different from those produced by the electronic ring flash for photography. The highlights consequently, cannot be deflected in advance to the point where they will cause the least disturbance. Experts, on the other hand, have repeatedly emphasized that the reflections usually do not cause difficulty, but rather contribute to the three-dimensional effect of the picture (WESPI, 1951; GANSE, 1953). The surface of the portio is part of a living organism, and the slightest unconscious movements of the patient, even her pulse and respiration, may throw the area under study out of focus at the precise instant the photograph is taken, especially with high magnifications, if the area is moved beyond the limits of sharpness in depth.

There are basically two different systems of photography: photographic equipment coupled with the colposcope in which the various magnifying glasses of the colposcope are identical with the lenses of the camera, and separate photographic equipment consisting of a teleobjective and bellows. Both have their advantages and disadvantages. The first system combines colposcope and photographic equipment; with the other system, the colposcope must be exchanged for the photographic equipment with teleobjective and refocused. Work with the combined equipment is restricted to the magnification of the colposcope, while the teleobjective permits the use of any desired magnification within the limits determined by the length of the bellows. That feature is of great advantage if color photography is used, because the specifically desired part of the picture may be brought into focus immediately, whereas the enlargement of parts of color diapositives is still scarcely feasible. The enlarged picture of the portio or of a detail may be as large as the negative. This advantage is of lesser importance for black and white photography, because any desired enlargement of parts can be used in making black and white copies.

Technique. We insert COLLIN's self-retaining duckbill speculum for photographic work to maintain the portio as long as necessary in the same position. It may be difficult to bring the portio into focus, especially if it cannot be moved very easily. It is advisable to use a blackened speculum to reduce the reflections on the surface of the portio. Too much dilation must be avoided, lest the vessels at the surface of the portio be constricted. We use the Kolpophot of Ihagee, Dresden, which takes photographs from 1:1 to 1:4. The equipment consists of a camera (Exakta Varex), bellows expansion, and teleobjective.

The light is produced by an annular electronic flash (400 Watt) mounted around the opening of the objective. The diaphragm may be reduced to 32 and 48 to secure the greatest possible depth of focus. We take our photographs exclusively in color, using the Agfa CT 18 reversible diapositive film.

A survey picture of the portio is always taken first during colpophotography, the outline of the portio coinciding with the edges of the picture. Enlargements are made of details in special cases. Two exposures are made with different diaphragm settings for every picture in order to compensate for differences in the intensity of light on the portio. The variations may be caused by differences in the width of the vagina or in the position of the portio (low or high).

Fig. 55. Sketch of the colposcopic finding described in the text as an example

Colpophotography is performed on all patients with findings worthy of note. It is obligatory in all cases in which surgical excision of the cervix is planned.

Wespi (1961) wrote a lengthy chapter on colpophotography with many technical details in the third edition of the Atlas of Mestwerdt-Wespi.

In summary, the procedure in colposcopic examination is as follows:

1. Positioning of the portio with dry, separated blades of the speculum.
2. Careful removal of excess mucus and discharge from the portio.
3. Cytologic smears taken from the surface of the portio and the cervical canal.
4. Brief inspection of the entire portio.
5. Acetic acid test.
6. Green filter if advisable.
7. Schiller's Iodine test.

Colposcopy with intended colpophotography:

1.—4. As above.
5. Exchange of specula. The blackened duckbill speculum is lubricated.
6. Acetic acid test and survey photograph.
7. Green filter if advisable.
8. Sectional magnification if needed.
9. Schiller's Iodine test and photograph.

Documentation of the Finding. Every colposcopic finding is put in writing. For this purpose we use the same clinical forms described on page 38. A brief description of the colposcopic picture requires a sketch that is sufficiently realistic. The finding may, for example, be "Mosaic area about 1 cm in diameter on the anterior lip of the cervix around the external os, and extending into the os. On the posterior lip of the cervix a narrow, closed transformation zone with marked vascularity. Mosaic area iodine-negative, sharp edges, transformation zone iodine-light, edges not sharp." The sketch is drawn within the circle printed on the clinical form (Fig. 55).

Following GLATTHAAR's (1955) suggestion, we use a special symbol for every colposcopic finding that deviates from the norm to characterize accurately the findings in the sketches. Figure 56 shows the symbols in use. The cervical os is diagrammed according to the individual case with heavy black lines. Proportions are estimated for the sketch. The accuracy and clearness of the colposcopic finding are improved by this procedure.

The colposcopic findings are written out in full on the status card, and transferred to the punch card in code (see p. 38—44).

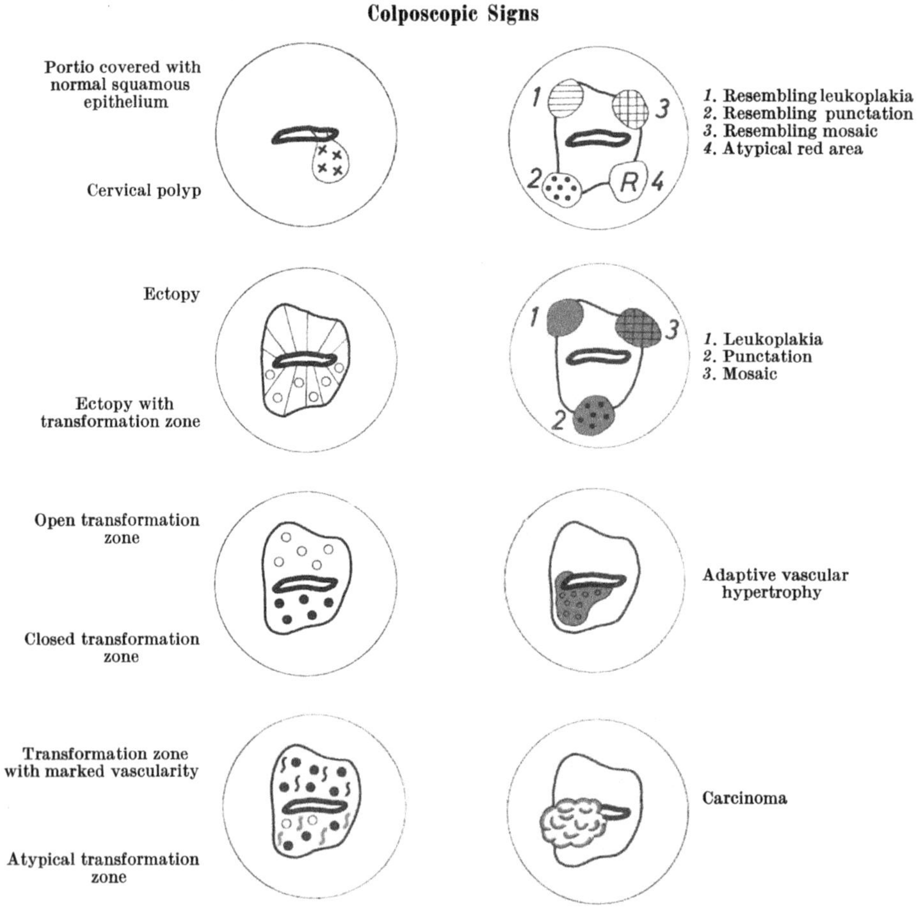

Fig. 56. Colposcopic symbols used for documentation, modified from GLATTHAAR (KERN and BÖTZELEN, 1961)

Normal Colposcopic Findings

Colposcopy is better suited than any other method to tracing *in vivo* the physiologic migrations of cervical epithelium during a woman's life. A presentation of normal colposcopic pictures will therefore be attempted in correlation with the histology of the cervical epithelium (see p. 18—23).

Portio Covered with Normal Squamous Epithelium

The surface of the portio is pale pink and iridescent, resembling mother-of-pearl. At regular intervals slender vessels may be seen that disappear after a short distance. Nowhere are there any signs of epidermidalization. The boundary between squamous and columnar epithelia is within the cervical canal, and therefore invisible. In a few rare cases this boundary may be just visible at the external cervical os, forming a relatively sharp line along which the squamous epithelium abuts the columnar epithelium of the cervical canal.

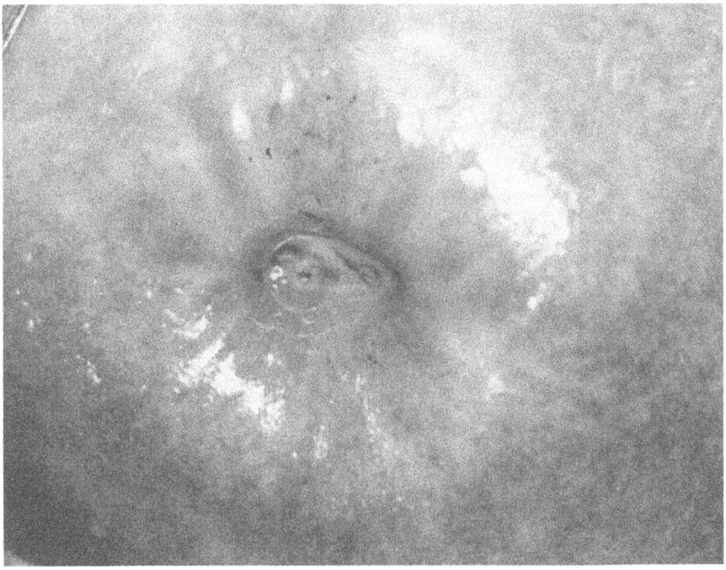

Fig. 57. Portio, covered with normal squamous epithelium, primary with dimple-shaped cervical os. A plug of clear mucus is visible in the os. The entire portio is covered by squamous epithelium. Cervical glands are not visible

If the surface of the portio is covered with smooth squamous epithelium, it is called a "primary portio covered with normal squamous epithelium" (Fig. 57). If all transformations have been removed from the portio through conization, annular biopsy, or electrocoagulation, or if they are, as in older women, no longer visible, the portio is called "secondary, covered with normal squamous epithelium" (Fig. 58).

It is often impossible to differentiate between a primary and a secondary portio, as in cases in which the squamous epithelium is so thick that the cervical glands beneath it cannot be seen.

A portio completely covered with squamous epithelium is relatively rare in sexually mature women, whereas it is found much more frequently in the climacteric period and after the menopause, as a result of the increasing ascending epidermidalization and the change of shape of the cervix in older women. The covering of squamous epithelium is atrophic in senility, consisting of only a few layers of cells (Fig. 13). An extravasation can often be seen in these cases as subepithelial petechial hemorrhages. A patchy vaginitis is not infrequent, even on the surface of the portio, at any age in the presence of vaginal inflammation (HOLTORFF, 1961).

The squamous epithelium is slightly paler after the acetic acid test. Further details can not be discerned on the portio by this test.

Schiller's iodine test often reveals, to the observer's surprise, areas deficient in glycogen, previously unnoticed, on the portio covered with normal squamous epithelium. The test therefore should never be omitted.

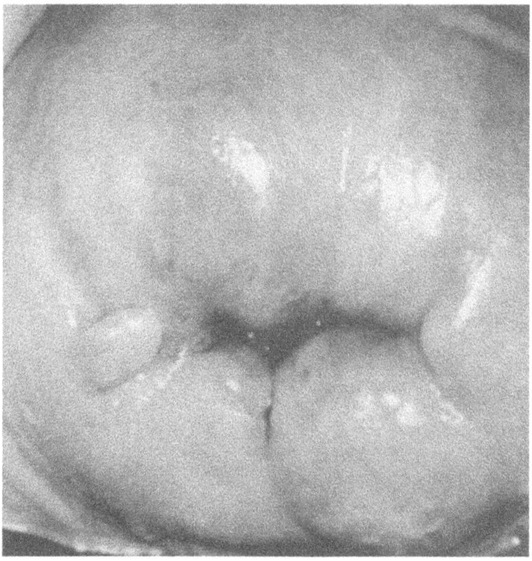

Fig. 58. Secondary portio, covered with normal squamous epithelium. Processes of transformation are no longer visible

The Ectopy

An ectopy is a displacement of the boundary between squamous and columnar epithelia onto the surface of the portio. An ectopy may be concentrically located around the os, spread asymmetrically on both lips of the os, or limited to one cervical lip.

Ectopy is a physiologic condition of the sexually mature woman in whom the cervical os is usually oval or transverse and is largely independent of the changes in pregnancy (Figs. 14, 59).

Certain visible red spots may be called "erosions of the portio" and often treated as such unless the colposcope is used. LIMBURG (1956) emphasized that the greatest number of unnecessary biopsies is performed with such findings.

The structural details of the "red spot", also called "erythroplakia" (NAVRATIL, 1958) can be resolved with the colposcope. Well-vascularized tissue that resembles a bunch of grapes may be seen secreting clear mucus. The resemblance

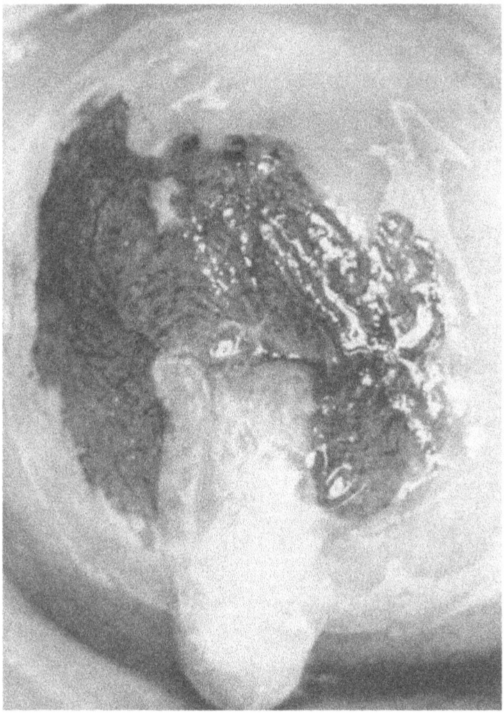

Fig. 59. Circular ectopy with marked secretion of mucus. Change resembling leukoplakia in the squamous epithelium at the periphery

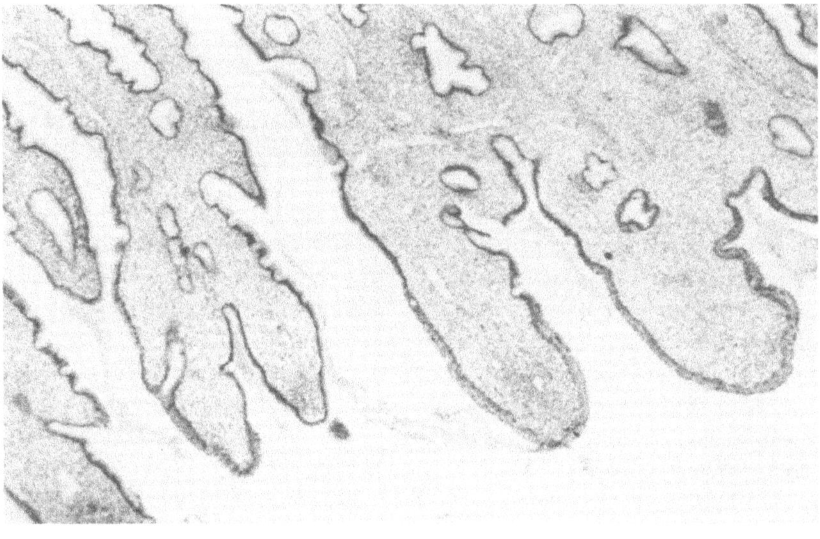

Fig. 60. Histologic section showing why an ectopy resembles a cluster of grapes

to a bunch of grapes is caused by the pattern in which the funnel-shaped ducts of the cervical glands are arranged (Figs. 60, 61).

During pregnancy this grapelike picture grossly may create the impression cf a neoplasm, since the region of the cervical glands exhibits true hypertrophy. This picture can be clarified quickly by means of the colposcope. A vascular loop is frequently found at the tip of the small clusters between the necks of the cervical glands.

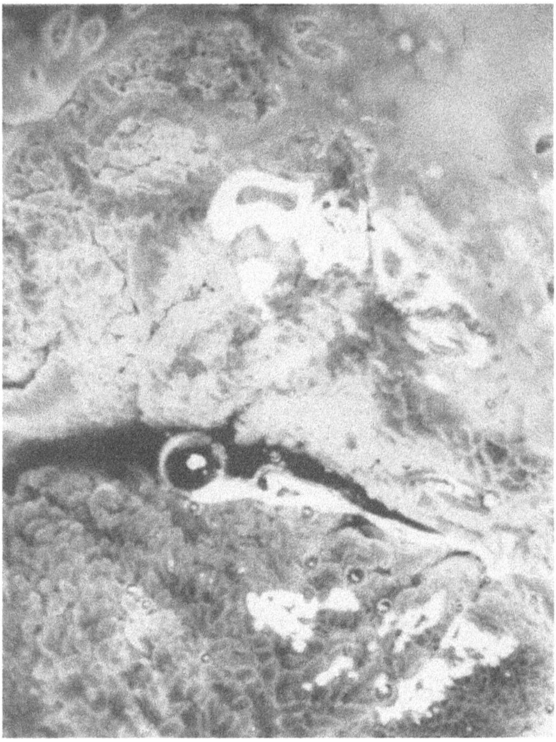

Fig. 61. Ectopy resembling a cluster of grapes after swabbing with acetic acid. An early transformation of the ectopy at the periphery. The squamous epithelium begins to grow over the columnar epithelium from the periphery, leaving behind islands of cervical mucosa. as can be seen in the left upper corner of the picture

An ectopy is quite susceptible to injury and may bleed slightly even when touched with a swab to remove mucus. Colposcopy makes it possible to recognize the innocuous cause of bleeding in these cases; the lesion may be shown to be benign and unnecessary biopsies may be avoided.

When the cervical mucosa appears on the surface of the portio, it becomes a point of reduced resistance (a vulnerable spot and a locus for bacteria). Inflammation often occurs therein, causing the ectopia to appear redder than normal and to secrete mucus with pus.

Acetic Acid Test. A surprisingly clear picture results when the ectopia is carefully swabbed with acetic acid. The tissue becomes pale, and the impression of clusters of grapes appears (Figs. 54, 61).

A thorough inspection can be performed after the acetic acid test, particularly of the boundary between squamous and columnar epithelia. The ectopic columnar epithelium occasionally abuts the squamous epithelium as a sharp line, but more frequently the squamous epithelium can be observed to advance as delicate, pale-white processes into the columnar epithelium.

Iodine Test. The ectopy appears light after application of Lugol's solution because the epithelial invaginations take up the iodine. The outline of the ectopy is usually blurred. The columnar epithelium does not contain glycogen.

Ectopy with Transformation Zone

As mentioned in the chapter on histology, the squamous epithelium has a tendency to grow over the columnar epithelium located on the portio. This process

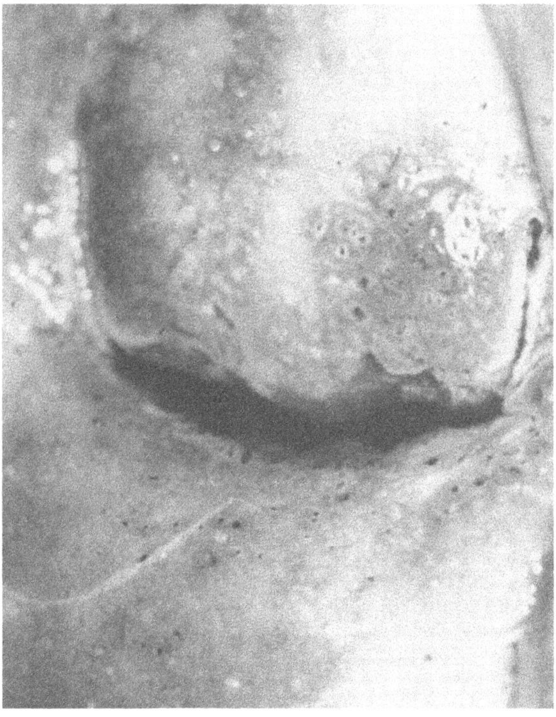

Fig. 62. This surface of a portio is completely covered by squamous epithelium. The necks of the cervical glands have remained open. Cervical glands are beneath the squamous epithelium at the periphery of the surface of the portio. "Open transformation zone"

can be observed very well with the colposcope. The squamous epithelium may grow in a broad front, but more often it forms long tonguelike processes projecting toward the ectopy. Arising from the periphery, these processes may reach the cervical os, leaving at first large islands of cervical epithelium untouched. The slender processes of the squamous epithelium eventually grow wider and surround the ducts of glands, from which clear mucus frequently can be seen to ooze. The advancing tongues of squamous epithelium are quite thin and can be wiped off if roughly swabbed. Bleeding may occur in such cases.

Acetic Acid Test. The picture just described becomes considerably clearer after acetic acid has produced its effect. This condition, therefore, should always be photographed after application of acetic acid (Fig. 61).

Iodine Test. An ectopy with transformation appears light after application of iodine and it has an indistinct margin. Sickle-shaped, iodine-negative areas may appear at the periphery.

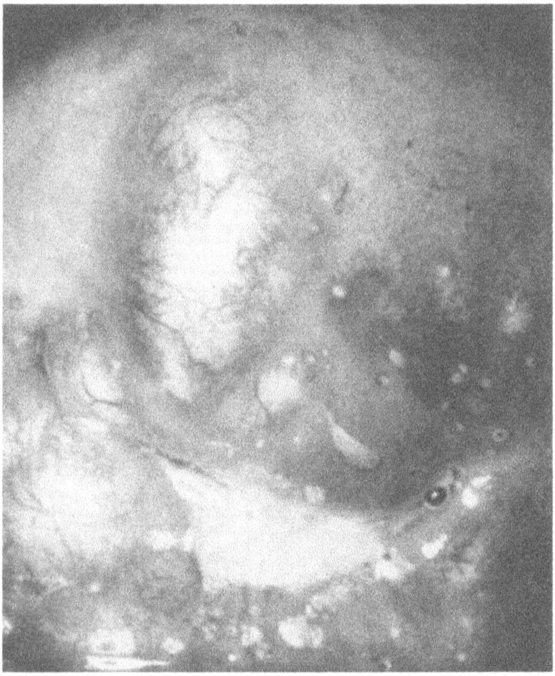

Fig. 63. Partly closed and partly open transformation zone. The Nabothian follicles exhibit especially striking vascularity. Open glandular ducts are visible, mainly near the lower margin of the picture and in the left corner of the os

Open Transformation Zone

The columnar epithelium on the surface of the portio is completely overgrown by squamous epithelium in this colposcopic picture. The necks of the glands are still patent. Accordingly, the portio may appear covered with pale-red squamous epithelium containing pinhead-sized holes at irregular distances from one another. From these holes mucus may occasionally well forth. Differences in thickness produce uneven shades of color in the squamous epithelium. The open transformation zone may occasionally persist for a long time, causing the squamous epithelium to become thicker and whiter. The open transformation zone usually

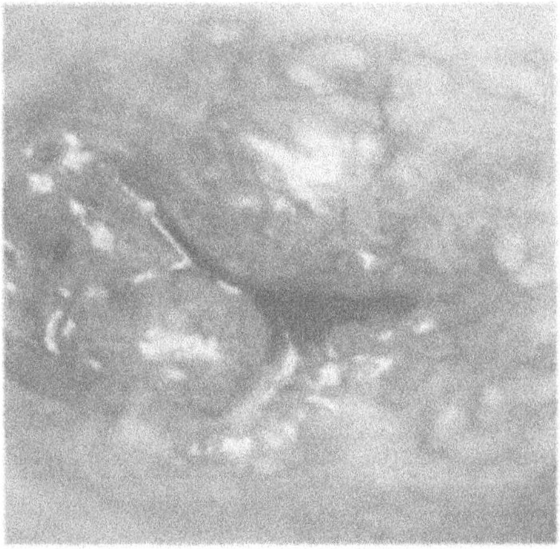

bb. 64

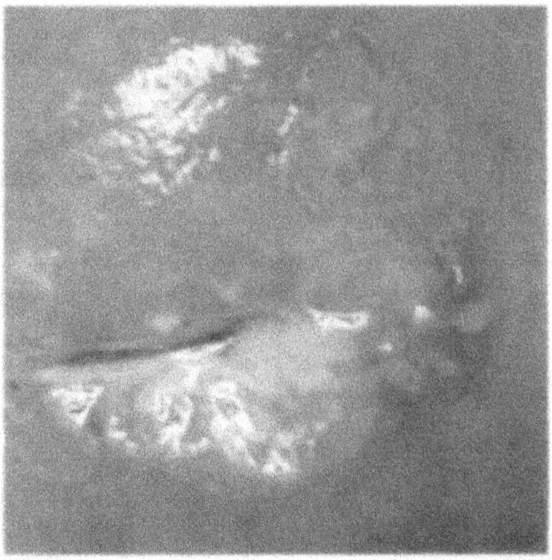

Abb. 71

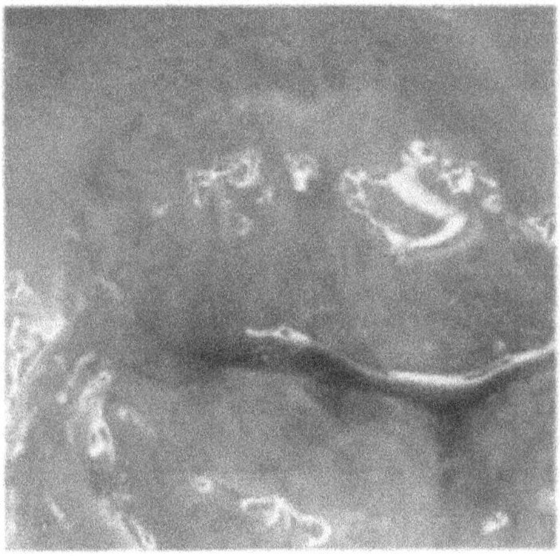

bb. 74

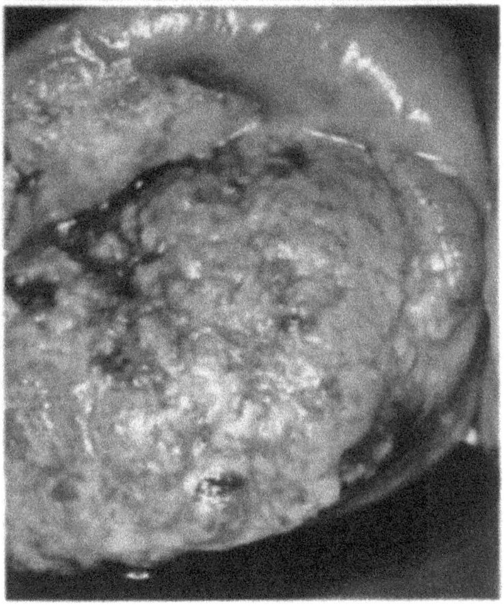

Abb. 77

Fig. 64. Transformation zone with marked vascularity and typical arborescent ramification of vessels

Fig. 71. Finding resembling leukoplakia. Slight circumoral keratinization, especially in the right upper corner of the picture

Fig. 74. Example of an atypical transformation zone. Epidermidalization and vascular pattern give the impression of a disturbance. It is difficult to find a single characteristic picture of the atypical transformation zone because of the great morphologic variation

Fig. 77. Cancer growing mainly outwardly. Photograph taken after application of acetic acid includes no visible vessels. The appearance of vessels indicates a previous epidermidalization.

Acetic Acid Test. The three-dimensional quality of the picture is improved by the action of acetic acid. The glandular openings appear more prominent. In this condition there is also the danger that in cases of fresh epidermidalization the squamous epithelium may be wiped off and bleeding provoked (Figs. 62, 63).

Iodine Test. The outline of the open transformation zone is usually blurred, and iodine-negative or iodine-light. The age of the zone of epidermidalization can probably be deduced from the quantity of glycogen stored.

Closed Transformation Zone

Epidermidalization is completed in a closed transformation zone. Occluded glands may be discerned together with glands that are still open. The glandular ducts after occlusion may be recognized as whitish epithelial bulges. Eventually all glandular ducts are occluded and retention cysts develop rapidly in the cervical glands (Nabothian follicles). Often the squamous epithelium covering the cysts is so thin that the mucus within them appears white. The size of the cysts may vary widely. They are often surrounded by delicate, branching vessels, even if the squamous epithelium outside the Nabothian follicles does not show any vessels (Fig. 63). The closed transformation zone is a transition to the secondary portio covered with normal squamous epithelium, as seen in old women.

Acetic Acid Test. The acetic acid emphasizes particularly the differences in thickness of the squamous epithelium: the thicker it is, the less transparent and, therefore, the whiter it appears after acetic acid.

Iodine Test. The closed transformation zone may exhibit all reactions from iodine-negative to iodine-light to iodine-positive. The glycogen is not apparent in the epithelium involved in epidermidalization before the iodine test is applied. The result, therefore, is frequently surprising. The edges of the iodine-light and iodine-negative spots vary greatly from case to case.

Transformation Zone with Marked Vascularity

This colposcopic picture may be observed in the stages of the open and the closed transformation zones. Vessels of moderately large caliber proliferate into the zone of epidermidalization from the periphery. MESTWERDT (1953) very clearly described this process. Typical of this condition is the arborescent ramification of the vessels, the direction of their growth towards the cervical os, and their diameter, which decreases gradually in the same direction (Fig. 64). The transformation zone with marked vascularity gives the gross impression of a red spot, or an erythroplakia.

Acetic Acid Test. As the epithelium blanches, the vascular pattern becomes clearer. This impression may be enhanced through insertion of a green filter.

Iodine Test. The reaction is the same as in the open and closed transformation zones. The vascular picture can no longer be evaluated after application of the iodine solution.

General Considerations

The portio covered with normal squamous epithelium, the ectopy, and processes of transformation are considered normal, nonsuspicious colposcopic findings. The question whether this is a reliable method for the elimination of nonsuspicious cases in the early diagnosis of cancer requires further investigation (see p. 132, 140).

These pictures of physiologic conditions reflect the epithelial displacement, as demonstrated by OBER (1958) histologically, as well as the change of the cervical shape *in vivo*. ZINSER and KERN (1958) and VÖGE (1960) have used their own material to show that, with regard to correlation with age, the colposcopic investigations were in agreement with the studies of OBER. Colposcopically normal findings were reviewed with the same result (KERN, RISSMANN and HUND, 1964).

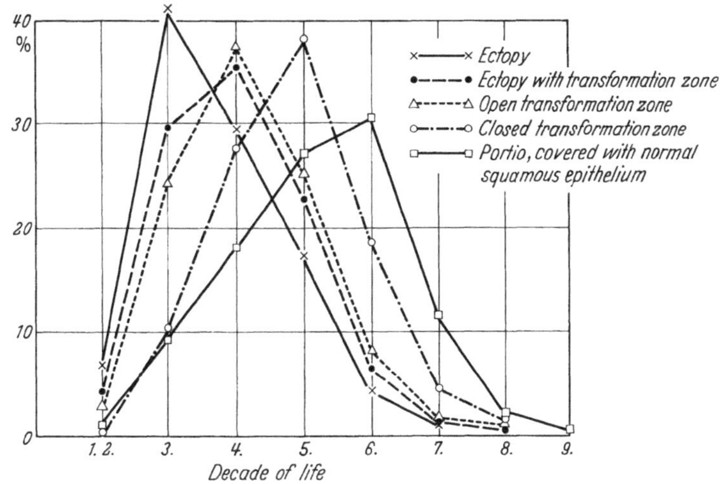

Fig. 65. Age curves in normal colposcopic findings. A definite displacement of the peaks over several decades of life is obvious (KERN, RISSMANN and HUND, 1964).

The statistics of the normal colposcopic findings at various ages are based on 4019 cases. A definite displacement of the peaks of the graphs from the ectopy in the third decade to the portio covered with normal squamous epithelium in the sixth decade of life is found (Fig. 65). Statistical calculation based on the Chi square test showed that the age distribution of the individual colposcopic findings definitely varies (with the exception of the difference between "ectopy" and "ectopy with transformation zone", $\chi^2 = 4.6$ for $n = 6$). Calculation of the average age results in a continuous increase (with confidence limits for $t = 3$): ectopy 32.3 years (30.7—34.0), ectopy with transformation zone 35.3 years (34.1—36.6), open transformation zone 36.8 years (35.0—38.8), closed transformation zone 43.4 years (42.4—44.1) and portio covered with normal squamous epithelium 46.9 years (45.7—48.2).

A study of the same material with regard to the *menstrual status* of the patients resulted in the following correlation. Most patients with a portio covered with normal squamous epithelium are in the menopause. Women with a regular cycle have the largest share of ectopy and recent epidermidalization. This relation is statistically significant.

Another subject of investigation was the relation between the number of births and the colposcopic finding. The Chi square test showed that the distribution of the number of births varied for every colposcopically normal characteristic (with the exception of the difference between "ectopy with transformation zone" and "open transformation zone"). The average number of births (with confidence limits) was: ectopy 1.2 (1.0—1.4), ectopy with transformation zone 1.6 (1.4—1.7), open transformation zone 1.5 (1.3—1.7), closed transformation zone 2.0 (1.8—2.1) and portio covered with normal squamous epithelium 1.3 (1.2—1.4). This result indicates that women with a portio covered with normal squamous epithelium have had substantially fewer children than those with other colposcopic findings.

Pathologic Colposcopic Findings

The pathologic colposcopic findings are divided into two categories: the *suspicious* findings with a suspected malignant epithelial lesion, and the *positive* findings with a clearly demonstrable epithelial atypia.

Suspicious Colposcopic Findings

A whitish thickening of the squamous epithelium with or without certain visible signs in the epithelium is typical of most suspicious colposcopic findings. These findings were called "matrix areas" by HINSELMANN, who considered them the source of a possible cancer.

For the following discussion, we have separated from the distinctive findings of matrix those in which the characteristics of the matrix areas are merely suggested, and we have designated them "matrix-like". GANSE has included findings of this kind in his collection of pictures and indicated the differences in the development of the matrix areas.

GLATTHAAR (1955) pointed out a finding that has since been included among the suspicious colposcopic findings. It concerned atypical vascular patterns or atypical epidermidalizations within the zones of transformation. GLATTHAAR appropriately called this finding an "atypical transformation zone". MESTWERDT's "abnormal transformation zone" is synonymous.

Matrix Areas

Leukoplakia. The longest known matrix area is a whitish, usually somewhat elevated thickening in the squamous epithelium called "leukoplakia". Leukoplakia was known even before the colposcope was introduced. v. FRANQUÉ (1927 and 1930) published several cases in which "a very small carcinoma" was hidden behind this lesion. A designation used even earlier, "sugar-icing carcinoma", described this change rather well. The epithelial thickening appears remarkably clear under the colposcope. There are no special signs visible within this area. Its outline may be sharp or blurred.

The surface of the lesion may be smooth or, occasionally, rough and scaly. The latter condition is called "coarse leukoplakia". The white spots may appear singly or in considerable numbers. Their size may be that of a grain of rice or occasionally as large as the entire portio. Leukoplakia may sometimes be wiped off; at other times it firmly adheres to its base. When wiped off there may appear an area that is called "punctation" or "ground leukoplakia" (Fig. 66) (FRANKEL, 1960; BAJARDI, BRET, COUPEZ, LANG and WALZ, 1961).

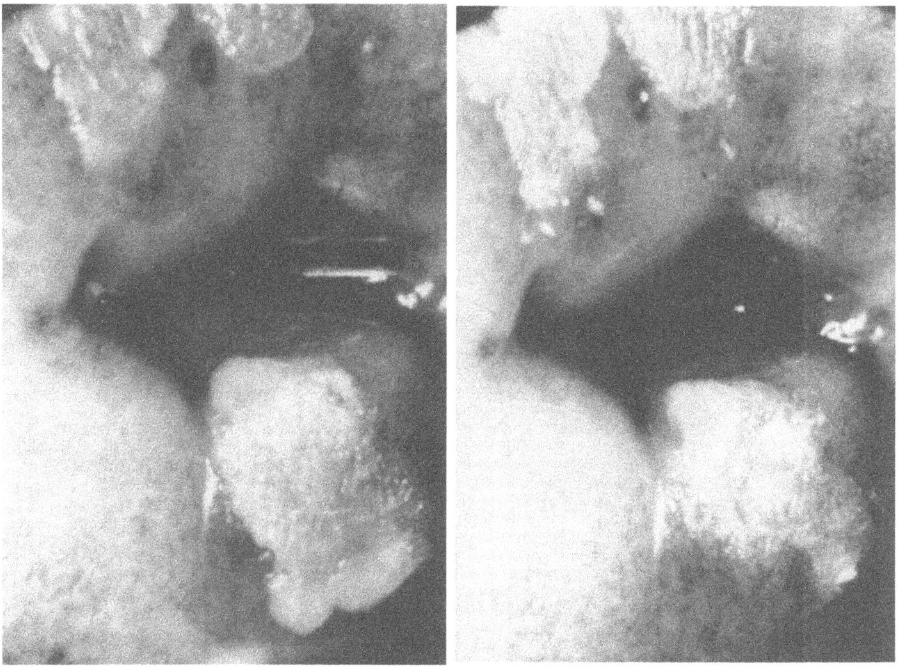

Fig. 66. Leukoplakia of both lips of the os. Left half of the picture before application of acetic acid, right half afterwards. Part of the leukoplakia at the posterior lip could be "wiped off"

Acetic Acid Test. The leukoplakia becomes even clearer and appears in bolder relief after application of acetic acid.

Iodine Test. Leukoplakias usually are sharply outlined and iodine-negative.

Punctation (Ground Leukoplakia). In addition to the lesion that appears when an area of leukoplakia is wiped off, there are similar areas without any thickened overlying epithelium. These were called "ground leukoplakia" by HINSELMANN and "punctation" by the American Society for Colposcopy.

The punctations may be recognized only with a colposcope. They are pale pink, sometimes paler and sometimes redder than their environment. They are usually slightly elevated above the normal squamous epithelium. Typical of punctation areas are dense accumulations of small red spots that under high magnification prove to be many capillary loops near the surface. Spotlike capillary loops generally may be seen in the punctation but not vessels running along the

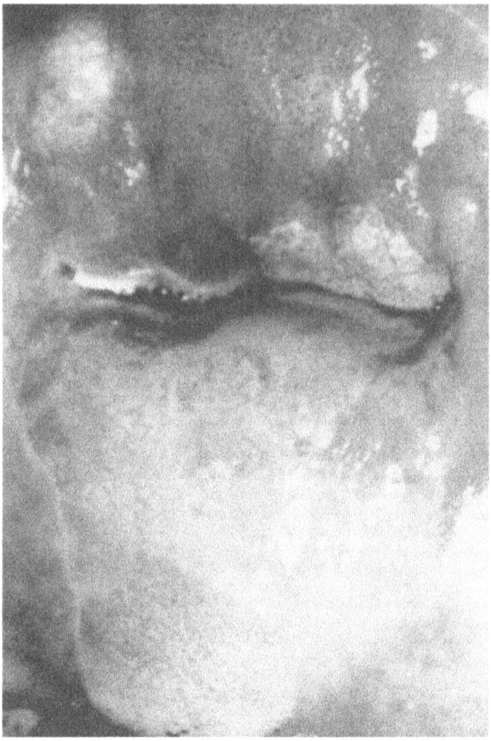

Fig. 67. Relatively large punctation at the anterior and posterior lips of the os

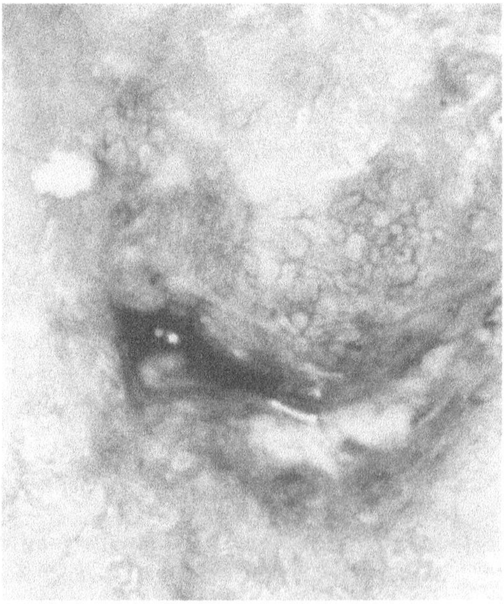

Fig. 68. Mosaic, mainly at the anterior cervical lip

surface. Unlike leukoplakias, punctations usually appear singly. They are small to medium in size (Fig. 67). Large areas are rare on the surface of the portio. The surface of such lesions is usually smooth, but occasionally it is granular. The latter

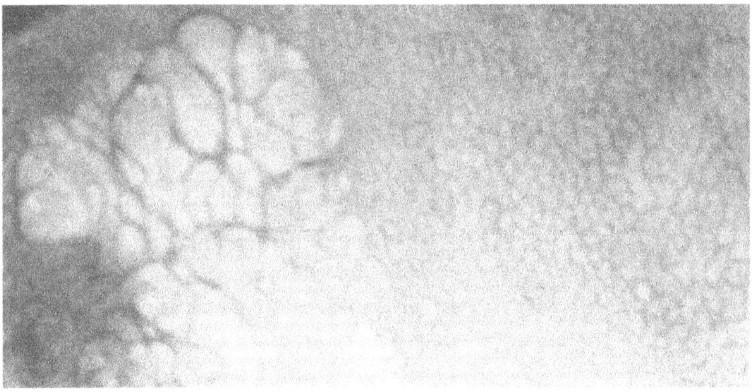

Fig. 69. Mosaic with coarsely and finely meshed patterns. In this example the coarsely meshed mosaic is somewhat elevated

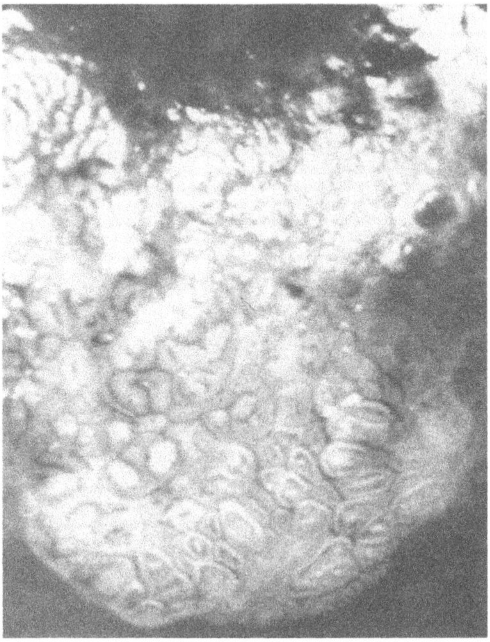

Fig. 70. So-called "trough" pattern of mosaic

condition may be taken for reactive vascular hypertrophy unless attention is paid to the typical vascular pattern. A punctation with papillary elevations is called a "papillary punctation area". The peripheral outline is usually sharp but may occasionally be blurred.

Acetic Acid Test. The punctation assumes a whitish-yellow, often somewhat glassy appearance. The vascular dots become clearer. The punctation becomes paler than its environment.

Iodine Test. Usually iodine-negative with sharp outlines.

Mosaic. The third kind of matrix area is the so-called "mosaic". This also is a more or less marked epithelial thickening crosshatched on its surface with thin red lines that produce a design resembling a mosaic (Fig. 68). These mosaics may have polygonal, honeycomb patterns or flat, converging borders. The mosaic pattern is coarsely or finely meshed (Fig. 69). The epithelium within a single element of the mosaic may be elevated or depressed (Fig. 70). Vessels are sometimes found, often as accumulations of red dots, within the red lines running through the mosaic.

The mosaic results from a peculiar relation of epithelium to vascular stroma that can be demonstrated histologically (MESTWERDT). WESPI (1946) published a very clear picture by means of a moulage. The typical appearance of the vessels was ideally demonstrated by ZINSER by use of a vascular injection technique with surgical specimens (ZINSER, 1960; ZINSER and ROSENBAUER, 1960 I and II; KOŠ, MIKOLÁŠ and LANĚ, 1960). STAFL, LINHARTOVA and DOHNAL (1963) showed the vessels well in histologic sections of mosaics by demonstration of alkaline phosphatase in the vascular endothelium.

Table 23

Matrix areas	Number of cases
Leukoplakia (L)	65
Punctation (P)	54
Mosaic (M)	44
M, P, L	14
M, P	22
M, L	8
L, P	7
Total	214

Mosaics usually do not appear in numbers. Their size varies considerably and their outlines are usually sharp.

Acetic Acid Test. The thickened epithelium becomes whiter upon application of acetic acid, and it appears more distinctly three-dimensional. The entire picture increases in clarity.

Iodine Test. The mosaics are generally iodine-negative with sharp outlines.

It is easy to diagnose matrix areas with the colposcope and impossible to overlook them. They may appear singly or in combinations.

The following single or multiple findings were observed in 214 portios of our own material with matrix areas (Table 23). Among the single findings, leukoplakia is the most frequent; among the multiple findings the mosaic and punctation lead numerically. A matrix area may also, however, be found in combination with other suspicious or positive colposcopic findings, for example with the atypical transformation zone or the IVa area. Matrix areas frequently appear also in the surfaces of the margin around a carcinoma.

Matrix-Like Areas

This is our designation for colposcopic pictures that merely suggest typical matrix areas. They are usually smaller. The meaning of the term "matrix-like areas" is not identical with that of "praematrix", the expression coined by HIN-

SELMANN (1933) in describing a histologic change in the squamous epithelium, approximately within the area of the dysplastic epithelium.

On evaluating colposcopic findings for detection of early cancer, the significance of the "matrix-like areas" does not seem to be equal to that of definite matrices. We therefore felt justified in treating these findings separately. Findings resembling matrices appear singly or in combinations.

The acetic acid test becomes especially important in matrix-like areas, for areas of this kind often become visible only after application of acetic acid, particularly at the time when the effect of the acetic acid subsides.

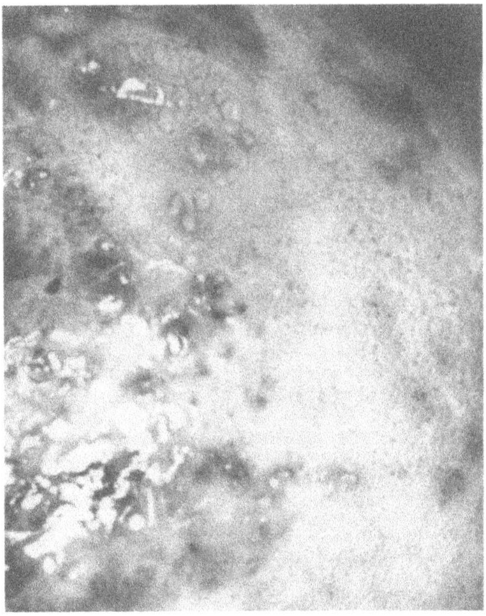

Fig. 72

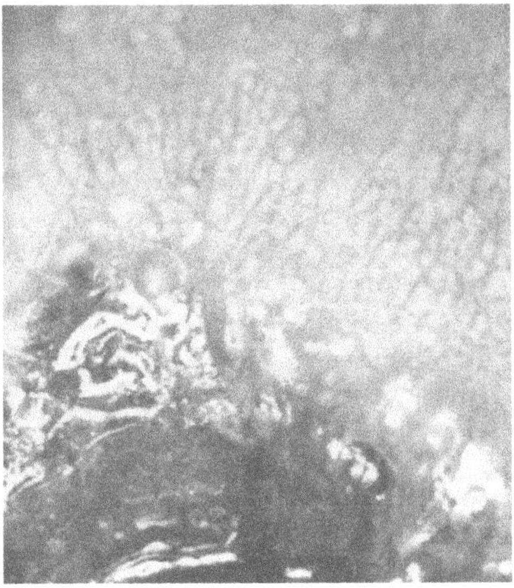

Fig. 73

Fig. 72. Resembling a punctation: right part of the picture. On the upper left side also region resembling a mosaic

Fig. 73. Resembling mosaic

Resembling Leukoplakia. The epithelium is slightly thickened. This condition could be called a "slight keratinization". The spot often becomes noticeable only after the acetic acid test. These areas are iodine-light or iodine-negative in Schiller's iodine test. They are sometimes discovered only during a second examination after application of the iodine solution (Fig. 71).

Resembling a Punctation. This is a relatively common finding; in most cases it involves very small areas with dense accumulations of vascular dots, without demonstrable thickening of the epithelium or differences in color from the surrounding tissue. It may prove difficult to differentiate between this condition and the vascular pattern of vaginitis. The outlines are usually blurred. The picture becomes better differentiated after application of acetic acid. Such an area usually stands out because of its low content of glycogen after application of iodine solution.

The iodine test often makes it possible to differentiate between pictures resembling a punctation and those of colpitis, namely in cases of spotty colpitis that are iodine-positive, with only small specks that appear iodine-negative (Fig. 72).

Resembling Mosaic. In this condition the epithelial thickening is often absent, only the vascular pattern exhibiting a mosaic-like arrangement. This finding frequently becomes apparent only after application of acetic acid. These areas remain iodine-negative or iodine-light with Schiller's Iodine test (Fig. 73).

The Atypical Transformation Zone

This finding has been described by Glatthaar (1955). It consists of transformation zones with the epidermidalization or the vascular pattern deviating from the normal. The decision to designate a zone of transformation as atypical or abnormal must be left to the examiner's discretion. The criteria, which vary greatly, cannot be defined unequivocally. The atypical transformation zone is considered a catchall for findings that cannot be easily classified or that deviate from the normal (Burghardt, 1959; Holtorff, 1960; Nold, 1960; Cramer, 1961; Bret, Coupez, Ganse, Nyklíček and Zinser, 1961). We call the following changes atypical transformation zone:

1. Marked vascularity within an open or closed transformation zone, without an arborescent ramification and without an observable direction of growth from the periphery towards the cervical os. The vessels are randomly arranged. Small differences of caliber are observed. The vessels do not have the shape typical of positive colposcopic findings (Fig. 74). A vascular pattern resembling the atypical transformation zone has been produced experimentally in the ear of the mouse by application of methyl cholanthrene (Kern and Zander, 1959).

The epithelium may be thin, bleeding readily on contact. It may be irregularly thickened and appear glassy and yellowish. This shade of color is brought out by acetic acid.

2. Another group to be considered atypical transformation zones are those with an open transformation zone that contains visible glandular openings with raised, mound-like edges of thickened epithelium. The epithelium around this mound often is slightly thickened also but not sufficiently to be considered a hyperkeratosis. The effect of acetic acid accentuates this picture. The glandular openings are often very close together, more so than they appear in the normal open transformation zone.

Atypical Red Area and True Erosion

The atypical red area (Wespi, 1938) is a reddened spot more or less sharply differentiated from its surroundings by its color and usually by showing no design on its surface or in its vasculature. There are no differences of levels. Red areas of this kind may have other causes, among them subepithelial inflammation.

True erosion follows the loss of surface epithelium; the subepithelial stroma is uncovered. Accordingly, true erosion is distinguished from the red area by its clear depression, especially at the edge (Fig. 75). The erosion is usually caused artificially, when squamous epithelium is torn off through manipulation of the portio (tenacula, curettage, rough swabbing, and so forth). Differentiation of the two lesions is difficult at times. Both findings stand out more clearly after the acetic acid test. The iodine test shows these areas to be iodine-light.

The atypical red area and the true erosion are rare findings.

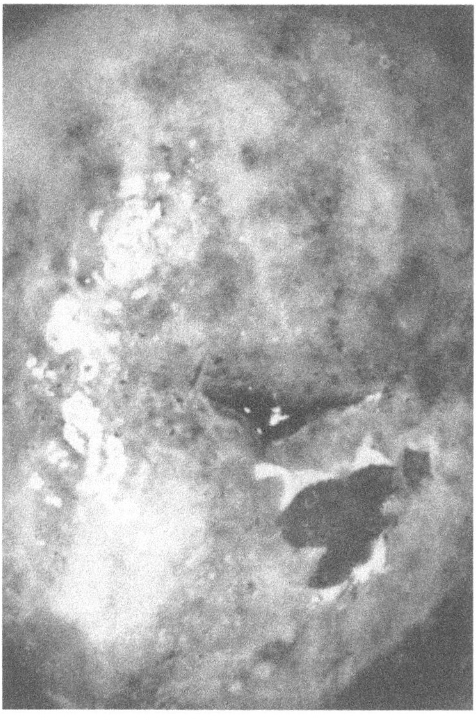

Fig. 75. True erosion, apparently artificial. At the edge of the erosion is the torn squamous epithelium. In addition, the surface of the portio has a partly closed and partly open transformation zone

Positive Colposcopic Findings

As will be discussed later, the positive colposcopic finding is always a manifestation of a malignant neoplasm of the cervix. Two distinct forms are recognized.

Pathologic Vascular Pictures from marginal areas or surfaces of epithelium involved in malignant transformation. HINSELMANN called these vascular anomalies "adaptive vascular hypertrophy", implying increased formation of vessels in response to the malignant growth (GANSE, 1952, 1954, 1957, 1959, 1960; KRÜGER, 1957; KOLLER, 1959; HOLTORFF, 1961).

How do the vessels appear? The blood vessels accompanying the neoplasm differ greatly, according to its individual growth. It is easier first to describe how they do not appear. The vessels do not ramify in reactive vascular hypertrophy, their growth is not oriented, and they do not gradually become thinner. The vascular net is more closely meshed than in the atypical transformation zone (Fig. 76). The blood vessels sometimes lie in bundles parallel to one another. Variations of caliber are quite noticeable whenever the vessels can be traced for an appreciable distance in their course near the surface. MESTWERDT described one type that should be mentioned at this point: the so-called "corkscrew capil-

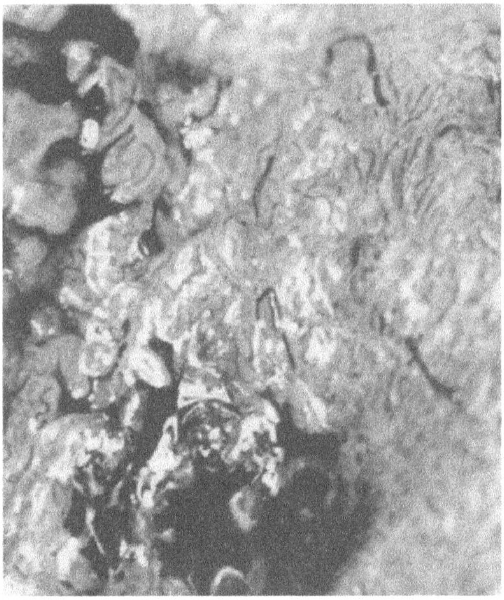

Fig. 76. Adaptive vascular hypertrophy. The vessels are neither oriented nor ramified. Development of so-called "corkscrew capillaries"

laries" that reach close to the surface, where they form two or three tight coils and then disappear again downward. The so-called "hairpin vessels" described by GANSE are similar. They are always aggregated in one area, as though a basal area suddenly exhibited hypertrophic vascular loops. The tissue in which the vessels are found may vary considerably. It may give the impression of normal squamous epithelium or it may be strikingly uneven or granular. A special subdivision of this category is the papillary punctation with distinct wart-like epithelial knobs visible in a basal area. These findings have also a common designation, "IVa areas", in HINSELMANN's histologic nomenclature.

Vascular loops like corkscrews have also been demonstrated in the experimental growth of malignant tumors in the mouse ear (KERN and ZANDER, 1959).

Because of its malignancy this lesion is easily injured and it readily bleeds.

Acetic acid stops the bleeding temporarily and causes the area to appear paler. Observation through the green filter is particularly important in such cases,

Table 24

Colposcopic designation	Explanation	Evaluation
Portio covered with normal squamous epithelium	Surface of the portio entirely covered with squamous epithelium	
Ectopy	Columnar epithelium of the endocervix on the surface of the portio	
Ectopy with transformation zone	Ectopy, slight epidermidalization on the surface of the portio, starting from the edge	negative (potentially benign)
Open transformation zone	Ectopy covered with squamous epithelium with open glandular ducts	physiologic epithelial displacements during a woman's life
Closed transformation zone	Ectopy covered with squamous epithelium. Glandular ducts closed. Development of Nabothian follicles	
Transformation zone with marked vascularity	Arborizing vessels grow into the squamous epithelium of the zone of epidermidalization	
Matrix-like findings	Characteristics of matrix areas, but only suggested	
Matrix areas:		
Leukoplakia	Whitish, thickened epithelium, Hyperkeratosis	
Mosaic	Mosaic like pattern in the thickened squamous epithelium	suspicious (questionable)
Punctation	Punctate vascular pattern on reddened or whitish base	nonphysiologic findings
Atypical transformation zone	Pictures of epidermidalization and vascularization not normal	
IV a area, (Adaptive vascular hypertrophy)	Typical vascular picture Corkscrew capillaries, varying caliber. Random vascular pattern	positive (potentially malignant)
Irregular protuberances of carcinoma	Irregular protuberances of tissue with differences of level and vascular atypias, bleeding regularly. Whitish-yellow color. Fatty or pulpy, friable	malignant lesion of the portio

because it brings out the vascular pattern. The *iodine test* always shows that these areas are iodine-light or iodine-negative.

The pictures described here afford colposcopic clarification of cases not clearly explained clinically. Carcinomas, especially if early are hidden behind these changes.

Carcinomatous Tissue. Finally, carcinomatous tissue is considered a positive colposcopic finding. The colposcopic appearance of true neoplastic tissue may assume many different forms (Fig. 77). If it is keratinizing carcinoma of the squamous epithelium, its appearance is nodular and glassy or fatty. If it is poorly differiantiated tumor, the tissue looks pulpy and friable. Photographs of adaptive vascular hypertrophy are best taken at the margin of the tumor.

Application of acetic acid also stops bleeding temporarily in these tumors, which frequently develop petechiae. Carcinomas are usually iodine-light after application of *iodine solution*.

Colposcopic findings are classified as normal, suspicious and positive. The characteristics and the evaluation of colposcopic findings are summarized in Table 24.

Efficiency of Colposcopy in Early Diagnosis of Cervical Carcinoma

The extent of application and the appreciation of colposcopy are subject to variations. In Germany, it had a monopoly in the detection of the smallest cancers and their early stages. This situation remains so, as far as experienced colposcopists are concerned; they are for the most part pupils of HINSELMANN. After the introduction of cytology both methods were often used together. Cytology was given preference in many laboratories, especially since a certain percentage of cases detected cytologically were missed by the colposcope. The development was similar in our clinic. We have had three times as many patients examined cytologically since 1957 as colposcopically, but the number of colposcopic findings in the punch card file has increased to 4,500 during the reported period. This material has been evaluated in the same way as the cytology.

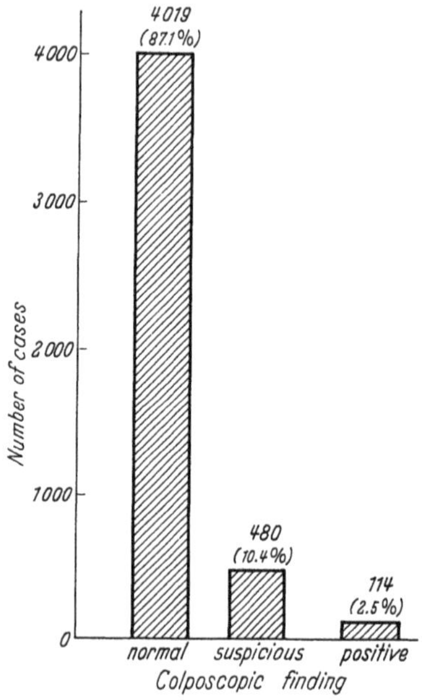

Fig. 78. Distribution of normal, suspicious and positive colposcopic findings in 4,613 examinations (KERN, RISSMANN and HUND, 1964)

A few associates are in charge of the colposcopic examination and subsequent recording. The patients from the wards and ambulatory patients are sent for colposcopy during office hours. Thus, the colposcopic material could be evaluated in a strictly uniform way, without individual errors of physicians in training. Colposcopy is, of course, in use in individual wards also, but the findings are not entered in the card file.

Colposcopic examinations were performed on 4,613 patients during the stated period. On classification of the total material into normal, suspicious and positive colposcopic categories (Fig. 78), the results are 87.1% normal, 10.4% suspicious, and 2.5% positive findings. These groups of findings are shown graphically in Fig. 79. The closed transformation zone and the portio covered with normal squamous epithelium represent the largest group among the normal colposcopic findings.

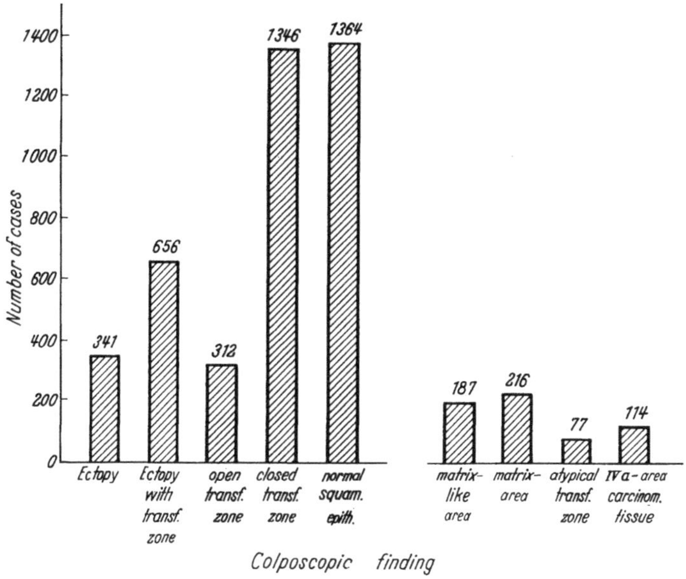

Fig. 79. Graphic representation of the colposcopic findings in the entire material (4613 cases) (Kern, Rissmann and Hund, 1964)

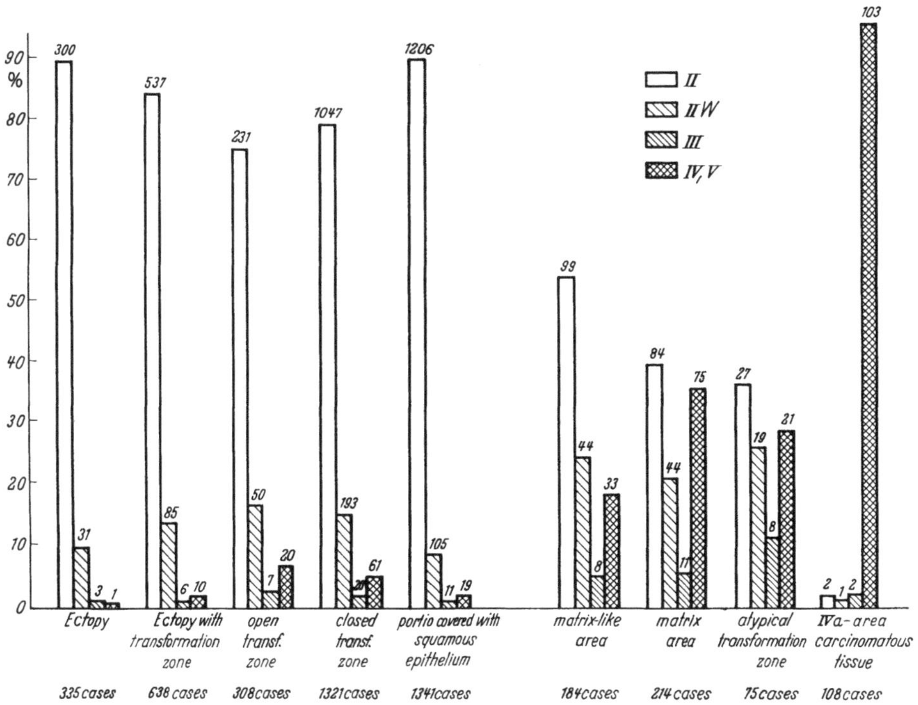

Fig. 80. Results of cytology in various colposcopic findings. (Total: 4524)

One woman out of ten had a suspicious colposcopic finding, mainly matrix areas or matrix-like areas. The correlation of normal colposcopic findings with age has been discussed on page 119. The calculation of the patients' average age with colposcopically suspicious findings shows a difference between "matrix-like" and matrix area, justifying the separation of the two kinds of findings. The resulting average age for the "matrix-like" areas (187 cases) is 36.3 years (standard deviation 11.3, with an accuracy of 95%, confidence limit 34.6—38.0), and for the matrix areas (216 cases) 39.7 years (standard deviation 10.7, accuracy 95%, confidence limit 38.2—41.2). An interval of about 1—6 years may be assumed, therefore, for the development of true matrix areas from matrix-like areas. The average age for 77 women with "atypical transformation zone" is 43.3 years (confidence limit 40.7—45.9 with an accuracy of 95%).

There were 4,524 cases available for *comparison with cytology*. That implies the availability in this group of one or more cytologic smears in addition to the colposcopic finding. The colposcopic findings have been used as a standard for comparison of the varying cytologic findings in the graphic representation (Fig. 80). It shows that cytologically suspicious or positive smears may appear for every colposcopic finding. In Table 25 the findings are more closely compared. The results of the colposcopic examinations will be discussed in the following paragraphs.

Colposcopically Normal Findings

In a group of 3,943 patients who colposcopically appeared nonsuspicious the cytologic test aroused urgent suspicion in 111 (2.8%) cases classed as "Group IV or V", and further check-up was indicated in 47 cases (1.2%) classed as "Group III".

Table 25. *Total comparable colposcopic and cytologic material* (KERN, RISSMANN and HUND, 1964)

Cyto-logic group	Colposcopic finding			Total
	Normal	Suspicious	Positive	
II/II W	96.0% 3,785 92.2%	67.0% 317 7.7%	2.8% 3 0.1%	90.7% 4105 100%
III	1.2% 47 61.8%	5.7% 27 35.5%	1.8% 2 2.7%	1.7% 76 100%
IV/V	2.8% 111 32.4%	27.3% 129 37.6%	95.4% 103 30.0%	7.6% 343 100%
Total	100% 3,943 87.1%	100% 473 10.5%	100% 108 2.4%	100% 4,524 100%

This calculation confirms our previous observations that a benign colposcopic finding does not necessarily exclude a malignant epithelial change.

MAJEWSKI and PLATEN (1962) emphasized that marked vascularity in normal colposcopic findings could contribute to the appearance of an epithelial atypia. We have examined the normal transformation zones with that concept in mind (Table 26).

The percentage incidence of cytologically positive findings is actually higher when marked vascularity has been found colposcopically than when it is not, but this difference cannot be verified statistically.

We wish to emphasize, however, that all these cases exhibit arborescent ramifications without variations of caliber, as shown by MESTWERDT (1953) as a normal finding in Fig. 50 of his Atlas.

Table 26. *Transformation zones with and without marked vascularity and their cytologic findings* (KERN, RISSMANN and HUND, 1964)

Colposcopic finding		Cytologic finding			Total
		II/IIW	III	IV/V	
Open transformation zone	without vessels	246 (92.1%)	5 (1.9%)	16 (6.0%)	267 (100%)
	with marked vascularity	29 (80.5%)	2 (5.6%)	5 (13.9%)	36 (100%)
Closed transformation zone	without vessels	869 (94.7%)	12 (1.3%)	37 (4.0%)	918 (100%)
	with marked vascularity	377 (92.4%)	8 (2.0%)	23 (5.6%)	408 (100%)

Colposcopically Suspicious Findings

Suspicious colposcopic findings (matrix-like, matrix area, atypical transformation zone) occurred in 10.56% (473 cases) of all patients examined with the colposcope. This percentage is consistent with that of many reports on its frequency, indicating that a finding of this kind may be expected in one woman out of ten. The so-called "index of malignancy" reported in the literature indicates that among all suspicious colposcopic findings one woman out of ten has an epithelial atypia.

CRAMER (1956 I, II) found in more than 10,000 cases examined colposcopically 11.2% suspicious and positive findings; 7.1% of them were verified histologically. DIETEL (1953) and DIETEL and FOCKEN (1955) found in the entire material 8—10% matrix areas, 11% of which were shown histologically to be epithelial atypias. The index of malignancy rose to 27% when special attention was paid to the "particularly marked" matrix areas.

LIMBURG (1956) reported an index of malignancy of 10.8% in more than 4,000 suspicious colposcopic findings. HOLTORFF (1957) calculated the figure of 7.2% after histologic verification among more than 4,000 suspicious and positive findings.

In our material this ratio is substantially higher, approximating the figure reported by DIETEL and FOCKEN for "particularly marked" matrix areas.

Of a total of 473 suspicious colposcopic findings 129 (27.3%) were cytologically positive and 27 (5.7%) cytologically suspicious; that means that in the material presented at least one woman in four may be expected to have an epithelial atypia.

An evaluation of the various colposcopically suspicious findings as compared with cytology is shown in Table 27, with the classic matrix areas having the highest percentage of cytologically positive results (35.1%). The matrix-like areas, on the other hand, have only 18.0%, an additional reason for the inclusion of only tentative findings of matrix in the separate group "matrix-like". The atypical transformation zone with 28.0% also includes a considerable fraction of cytologically positive findings. The differences between the percentages have been verified statistically. WAGNER (1960) and WAGNER and FETTIG (1961) reported the index of malignancy of 13.8% for the atypical transformation zone.

Table 27. *Colposcopically suspicious findings and the cytologic results* (KERN, RISSMANN and HUND, 1964)

Colposcopically suspicious findings	Cytologic finding			Total
	II/IIW	III	IV/V	
Matrix-like area	143 (77.7%)	8 (4.3%)	33 (18.0%)	184 (100%)
Matrix area	128 (59.8%)	11 (5.1%)	75 (35.1%)	214 (100%)
Atypical transformation zone	46 (61.3%)	8 (10.7%)	21 (28.0%)	75 (100%)
Total	317 (67.0%)	27 (5.7%)	129 (27.3%)	473 (100%)

The fate of matrix areas has been followed in several series over many years. It was found that the matrix areas may persist for many years without changes; they may also disappear under certain conditions (ZINSER, 1949; MESTWERDT, 1951; RECKEN, 1955; DIETEL and FOCKEN, 1955).

Colposcopically Positive Findings

Colposcopically positive findings occurred in 2.4% of the entire material that could be compared with the cytologic data. Only three cases were in cytologic groups II or IIW among the total of 108. These three cases are among the true cytologic failures in invasive carcinomas (see Table 18). A colposcopically positive finding (IVa area, carcinomatous tissue) always implies a pathologic epithelial change and requires histologic clarification.

There were 658 cases available for *comparison of the colposcopy with the histology* with regard to complete confirmation or rejection of the colposcopic finding.

Tables 28 and 29 present the colposcopic findings in 658 histologically sectioned portios, prepared according to the same strict requirements described in our considerations for cytologic examination (p. 95).

With regard to the accuracy of colposcopy, a calculation shows the colposcopic finding to be in accord with the histology in 67.8% of the cases, whereas only the expression of a suspicion may be deduced from colposcopic examination in 21.4%, and 10.8% are "false negative" findings. No "false positive" diagnoses were made with the colposcope.

Table 28. *Colposcopic finding in 658 cases completely verified histologically (serial cervical sections)* (KERN, RISSMANN and HUND, 1964)

Histologic findings	Colposcopic findings			Total
	normal	suspicious	positive	
Benign findings on the portio	342 (88.6%)	44 (11.4%)	—	386 (100%)
Early cases	62 (39.5%)	83 (52.9%)	12 (7.6%)	157 (100%)
Cervical carcinomas	9 (7.8%)	14 (12.2%)	92 (80.0%)	115 (100%)
Total	413 (62.8%)	141 (21.4%)	104 (15.8%)	658 (100%)

Table 29. *"False" or equivocal colposcopic findings, compared with 658 histologically verified cases* (KERN, RISSMANN and HUND, 1964)

Histologic findings	Colposcopic findings			Total
	"false negative"	suspicious	"false positive"	
Benign findings on the portio	—	44 (11.4%)	—	386 (100%)
Early cases	62 (39.5%)	83 (52.9%)	—	157 (100%)
Cervical carcinomas	9 (7.8%)	14 (12.2%)	—	115 (100%)
Total	71 (10.8%)	141 (21.4%)	—	658 (100%)

Table 30. *"False" colposcopic findings, compared with 658 histologically verified cases* (KERN, RISSMANN and HUND, 1964)

Histologic findings	Colposcopic findings		Total
	"false negative"	"false positive" or "suspicious"	
Benign findings on the portio	—	44 (11.4%)	386 (100%)
Early cases	62 (39.5%)	—	157 (100%)
Cervical carcinomas	9 (7.8%)	—	115 (100%)
Total	71 (10.8%)	44 (6.7%)	658 (100%)

Inclusion of the suspicious colposcopic findings (21.4%) in the positive findings changes the result as follows (Table 30).

This calculation results in a confirmation of the colposcopic finding in 82.5%, with 10.8% false negative and 6.7% "false positive" (suspicious) colposcopic findings.

We attempted to evaluate about 4,500 colposcopic findings from different points of view. Various difficulties stood in the way of such an evaluation. The material examined belonged to another group studied by another routine method (cytology) and was not representative of gynecologically healthy women; it was rather a further selection of patients from a gynecologic clinic. We feel this difficulty is especially significant in evaluation of the method.

For these reasons comparison with cytology is problematic. Search for early cases was performed primarily by cytology; colposcopy was adjunct. The colposcopic failures, therefore, may be objectively ascertained, whereas it is not possible to evaluate the advantages of this method had it been applied to the entire material. We should, nevertheless, like to attempt an interpretation.

The *colposcopically positive findings* are quite unequivocal, for they include, without exception, a histological basis for malignancy, implying that a colposcopically positive finding, without regard to the cytologic result, must be verified histologically.

The *normal colposcopic findings* also permit an unequivocal statement, since among them there were 111 (2.8%) cases with a cytologically positive finding out of a total of 3,943 patients examined colposcopically and cytologically; a normal colposcopic finding therefore does not exclude an epithelial atypia. Consistent histologic verification of the cytologically positive cases makes the relation within the colposcopically normal findings appear even more unfavorable: 10.8% "false negative" among 658 portios. This figure rises to as high as 39.5% "false negative" findings if the early cases only are considered. We have repeatedly found this percentage. Using colposcopy alone we would therefore have overlooked 62 of 157 early cases, or one out of every three cases, because they appeared normal under the colposcope. That fact is beyond doubt. Everybody interested in the early diagnosis of cervical carcinoma is disturbed by failures of "his" method. Even if our thoughts about certain failures in colposcopy are correct, there still seems to be a possibility in cytology also of overlooking one out of every three cases. Do these failures in both methods represent an area of true complementation of cytology and colposcopy? We cannot answer this question because the two methods have not been applied to the entire material (Limburg, 1958).

The great number of *suspicious colposcopic findings* is undoubtedly a real disadvantage of colposcopy (roughly 10% of the entire material or about 50% of all histologically verified early cases). What procedure should be followed if early diagnosis were performed *only* by means of the colposcope? We have assumed to date that only every tenth suspicious colposcopic finding was related to an epithelial atypia. A major procedure such as conization would not be justifiable in this case. Only removal of small bits of tissue would therefore remain, methods such as punch biopsy, Schiller's scrapings, curettage, and so forth, with all their uncertainties, for the verification of an epithelial atypia assumed to be present on the basis of the suspicious colposcopic finding. The risk of biopsies at the wrong site is great with these methods. We were able to demonstrate this fact through topographic comparison of the colposcopic finding with the histologically ascertained location of the carcinoma in situ (Kern and Bötzelen, 1961). Not every tenth but every forth suspicious colposcopic finding in our material is related to a truly pathologic epithelium. This fact signifies a substantial increase in the value of the finding. It may well be imagined that some of the cases missed cytologically could be hidden among the colposcopically suspicious findings (MESTWERDT, 1958). A malignancy ratio of 1:4 for the suspicious colposcopic findings in the material of a clinic must be given full attention. These findings should be verified by continuing cytologic check-up. If that should not be possible, SCHILLER's scrapings with a careful cervical curettage may be the method of choice.

The material available was subjected to cytologic search for early lesions of the cervix and examined colposcopically as well. Histologic studies were performed on the basis of the cytology. This method is the basis of Tables 31 and 32.

Table 31. *Errors of cytology in 999 cases and of colposcopy in 658 cases for which serial histologic cervical sections were available, that is, optimal histologic proof (benign findings of the portio, early cases, and carcinomas)* (KERN, RISSMANN and HUND, 1964)

Methods of search	Result			Total
	"false negative"	suspicious	"false positive"	
Cytology	12 (1.2%)	36 (3.6%)	15 (1.5%)	999 (100%)
Colposcopy	71 (10.8%)	141 (21.4%)	—	658 (100%)

Table 32. *Results of cytology in 178, and of colposcopy in 157 early cervical cases* (KERN, RISSMANN and HUND, 1964)

Methods of search	Result			Total
	negative	suspicious	positive	
Cytology	4 (2.3%)	12 (6.7%)	162 (91.0%)	178 (100%)
Colposcopy	62 (39.5%)	83 (52.9%)	12 (7.6%)	157 (100%)

JANISCH, KLEIN and KREMER (1959) and BRANDL and KOFLER (1959) instituted a similar comparison of cytologic and colposcopic findings in histologically confirmed early cases and grossly nonsuspicious cancers of Group I. Both groups of authors criticized especially the high rate in colposcopy of suspicious findings, that is, indefinite results.

Because it is less equivocal cytology is superior to colposcopy as a method of cancer detection in comparisons of this kind.

Comparative Localization in Colposcopic and Histologic Findings

The surgical verification of early cases as practiced at the Gynecologic Clinic of the University of Cologne and their special histologic study enable us to ascertain postoperatively the exact location and extent of the epithelial lesion in the histologic specimen.

Early changes in the cervix have been reported in 1961 in 105 cytologically detected cases (KERN, 1961, 1962; KERN and BÖTZELEN, 1961). The colposcopic finding was recorded preoperatively with an exact description of the observations made, including colored colpophotographs and sketches, and compared with the histologic picture of the cone obtained surgically.

A pair of pictures was methodically made of each individual case, placing an exact drawing of the outline of the histologic picture against a colposcopic drawing, thus affording a direct comparison of extent and location of the carcinoma in situ with the colposcopic finding. Figures 81 and 82 demonstrate how the drawings are projected upon each other in situ. Fig. 83 shows several pairs of sketches from the entire material of 105 individual cases.

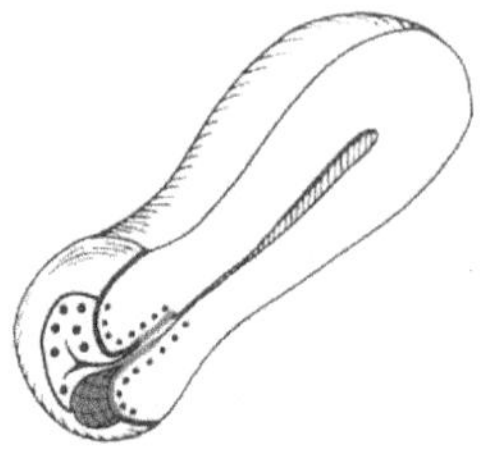

Fig. 81. This drawing explains how the colposcopic and histologic sketches were produced by analogy with vertical and horizontal projections

Table 33 recapitulates the results with regard to location of the carcinoma in situ and the colposcopic findings.

The *colposcopically positive findings* (nine cases) were always confirmed histologically as carcinomas in situ or as microcarcinomas *on the surface of the portio* (Zinser and Kern, 1958; Janisch, Klein and Kremer, 1959; Kern and Bötzelen, 1961).

A *suspicious area* was found with the colposcope in 51 cases. The abnormal epithelium was histologically within the area or in proximity to the colposcopically suspicious areas (Krüger, 1958; Vöge, 1960).

In this group, the carcinoma in situ was entirely endocervical in ten cases, but close to the colposcopically suspicious area insofar as the latter always reached the external os. The colposcopically suspicious area on the surface of the portio in these cases must be considered an *indication* only (Hinselmann, 1942; Holtorff, 1958).

Table 33

Colposcopic finding	Location of the carcinoma in situ	
	on the surface of the portio	in the cervical canal
negative	34	11
suspicious	41	10
positive	9	—
Total	84	21
	105	

Among the 41 carcinomas in situ on the surface of the portio, eleven were found histologically to be on both lips of the cervical os, whereas a suspicious finding was detected colposcopically on one lip only.

It was surprising in view of the great number of "false negative" colposcopic findings that they by no means involved only endocervical changes, but in 34 cases included carcinomas in situ clearly located on the surface of the portio that produced colposcopic findings not deviating from the norm. Not even those cases in which the boundary between squamous and columnar epithelia was on the surface of the portio were exceptions (Ganse, 1955).

The eleven endocervical lesions because of their location remained hidden from the naked eye, and hence also from the colposcope. This kind of colposcopic failure was to be expected (Lönne, 1942; Treite, 1944; Waschke, 1951; Zinser, 1951; Zinser and Diegritz, 1952; Morari and Strametz, 1953; Walz, 1955; Burghardt and Bajardi, 1956; Limburg, 1956, 1958; Navratil, Burghardt and Bajardi, 1956; Kaufmann, Runge, Ober and Stoll, 1957; Held, 1957; Navratil, Burghardt, Bajardi and Nash, 1958; Zinser, 1958 I, II; Zinser

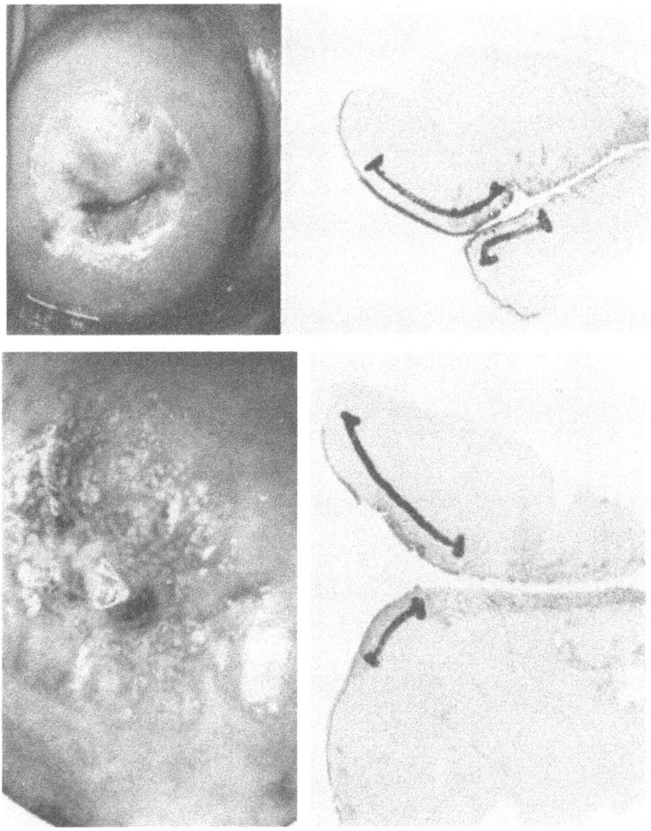

Fig. 82. Two examples of paired pictures: colposcopic finding on the left, histologic specimen on the right. The extent of the carcinoma in situ is indicated by black ink in the histologic specimen

and Kern, 1958; Wespi, 1958; Navratil, 1958; Bajardi, Burghardt, Kern and Kroemer, 1959; Janisch, Klein and Kremer, 1959; Kern and Bötzelen, 1961). It is very important, however, that 34 carcinomas in situ on the surface of the portio did not arouse suspicion. To them, eleven cases must be added in which only one lip appeared suspicious colposcopically, whereas the carcinoma in situ had spread over both lips of the cervical os.

These results seemed clear proof to us that carcinomas in situ in any location cannot always be detected with the colposcope; in other words, unequivocally benign cases cannot always be distinguished with the colposcope.

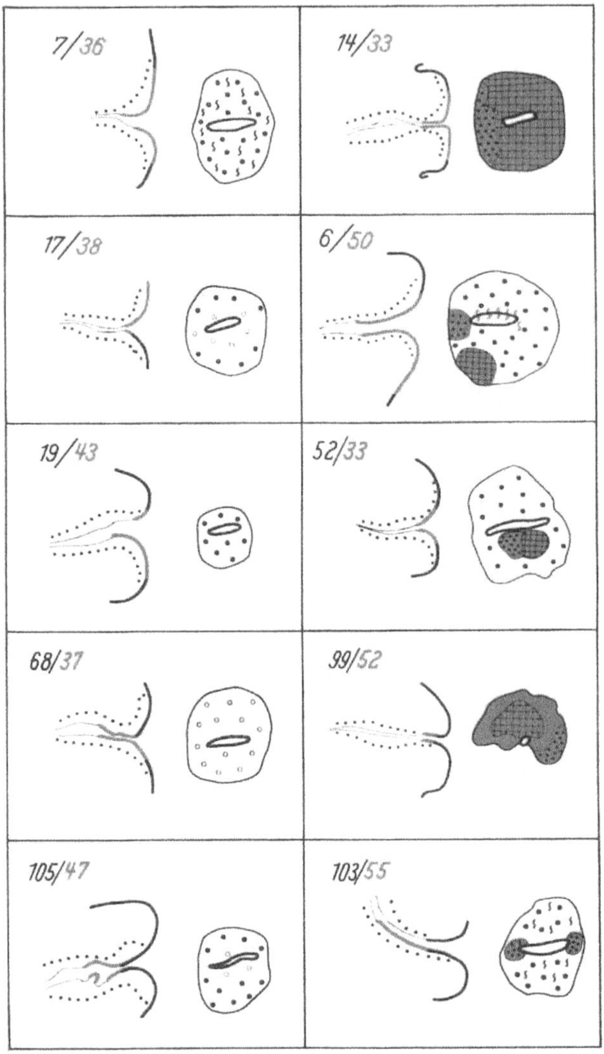

Fig. 83. Examples of drawings representative of those made of 105 carcinomas in situ, of which the colposcopic finding made preoperatively was compared with the extent of the carcinoma in situ in the serial cervical sections. (Black number: consecutive numbering. Red number: patient's age. The carcinoma in situ is indicated by a red line in the histologic drawing. The colposcopic sketch uses the symbols shown in Fig. 56) (KERN and BÖTZELEN, 1961)

We differ in this regard from other authors who believe that they are able to recognize with the colposcope unequivocally benign lesions of the surface of the portio (GLATTHAAR, 1952; DIETEL and FOCKEN, 1955; LIMBURG, 1956; CRAMER, 1958; KRÜGER, 1958). Our investigations have been given support by BURGHARDT and BAJARDI (1956), NAVRATIL and co-workers (1956, 1959), BURGHARDT (1959) and ZINSER (1962), who also found in material treated similarly that carcinomas in situ on the surface of the portio may be inacessible to colposcopic demonstration.

The histologic pictures seem to us to offer a satisfactory answer to the question why a certain number of carcinomas in situ on the surface of the portio cannot be recognized with the colposcope. In the manner of normal squamous epithelium carcinoma in situ overgrows cervical glands; it can grow around glandular ducts or occlude them. The boundary on the surface does not differ from that of normal squamous epithelium in HAMPERL's groups "simple replacing growth" and "bulky outgrowth". There is, furthermore, in most cases no special vascular pattern. The great nuclear density in carcinoma in situ might manifest itself in reflected light possibly by a difference of shade of color, but this difference is obviously not clear.

Experienced colposcopists frequently state that they have never yet seen a carcinoma that would have been undetectable colposcopically. That may be correct for invasive cancers. For the early cases that have been missed colposcopically, however, it is a fact that during the long latent period of carcinoma in situ, until the lesion becomes a true cancer (up to 15 years), it does not become detectable even upon repeated examination.

The comparison of colposcopic examinations with the histologic specimens of cytologically detected carcinomas in situ necessarily leads to the conclusion that colposcopy is not capable of singling out the unequivocally negative cases. Not only endocervical carcinomas in situ but also a certain fraction of those located on the surface of the portio cannot be recognized with the colposcope.

Schiller's Iodine Test

Historical Introduction

This remarkably simple clinical test known as "SCHILLER's Iodine Test" has, in addition to cytology and colposcopy, definite importance in early cancer detection.

WALTER SCHILLER was born in Vienna in 1887. During the twenties he worked mainly in gynecological pathology (SCHILLER, 1927 I, II, 1928 I, II, III, 1929, 1931, 1932). In the histological preparation of a large number of surgically removed uteri, he discovered several of the "smallest cervical carcinomas" that had not produced any symptoms and would be considered carcinomas in situ according to present thinking. In the course of the histological examination he noticed that the squamous carcinomas of the cervix were conspicuously lacking in large amounts of glycogen whereas normal squamous epithelium was characterized by abundance of it. He attempted to utilize this observation for an in vivo test. He tried more than 200 solutions and decided on the so-called "Iodine test". In this test, the surface of the portio is swabbed with iodine solution that stains the intermediate layers of the squamous epithelium, which contain glycogen, dark brown, whereas other kinds of tissue remain more or less unstained. According to SCHILLER's recommendation, all spots that remained light on the surface of the portio during the iodine test should be carefully scraped to permit the detection of all the abnormal epithelium. His paper on this subject appeared in 1929 in the "Zentralblatt für Gynäkologie" with the title: "Jodpinselung und Abschabung des Portioepithels". (Application of Iodine and Scraping of the Epithelium of the Portio.)

During these same years, HINSELMANN developed the colposcope. Its potentialities relegated the iodine test to the background in Germany, as an examination to be added to colposcopy.

A few years later, SCHILLER emigrated to Boston, Massachusetts, where interest in the early diagnosis of cervical carcinoma was especially high. His method took hold and came into widespread use (SCHILLER, 1933, 1934 I, II, III, 1936, 1937, 1938 I, II, 1955). Its simple technique without the use of special equipment seems, in contrast to that of colposcopy, to have greatly aided its acceptance in America. In 1937, SCHILLER wrote: "The iodine test is neither painful, nor difficult, nor expensive." Review articles from American clinics on the early diagnosis of cervical carcinoma always mention the results of the iodine test, emphasizing its reliability (YOUNGE, 1956, 1957, 1958; YOUNGE and KEVORKIAN, 1959; FRIEDELL, HERTIG and YOUNGE, 1960).

The Method of the Iodine Test

The procedure in SCHILLER's iodine test is as follows:

The vaginal walls are kept apart by two separate specula and the portio is exposed. A swab is dipped in LUGOL's solution and applied to the entire surface of the portio. Within a few seconds the glycogen-containing squamous epithelium turns a deep, dark brown. If swabbing of the surface of the portio is to be avoided,

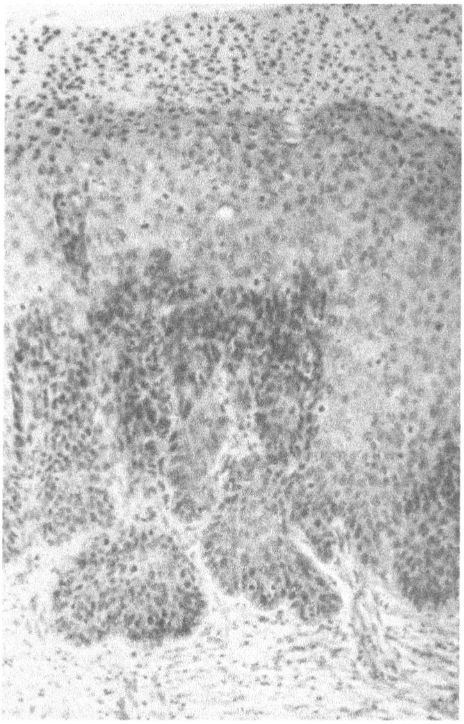

Fig. 84. Carcinoma in situ with bulky outgrowth. The aqueous iodine solution applied preoperatively was too strong. It caused a peculiar alteration of the uppermost layers (marked eosinophilia with pyknotic nuclei)

lavage of the vagina with LUGOL's solution may be performed. The solution stains the underclothing, and the spots cannot easily be removed. Residual solution in the vagina should therefore be carefully removed. Once the color has appeared it may be observed with the naked eye or through the colposcope. The coloring of the squamous epithelium persists for from 1 to 3 days. Normal inspection of the portio or a colposcopic examination may, therefore, not be repeated until this period has elapsed.

The composition of the iodine solution is quite essential. We use the following:

iodine	6.0
potassium iodide	12.0
distilled water	200.0

that is, a 3% aqueous solution. The containers must be sealed hermetically, lest the concentration increase because of evaporation.

Alcoholic solutions as well as aqueous iodine solutions of higher concentration cause necrosis of the squamous epithelium, involving the superficial and intermediate layers. If, for example, a solution of this kind with the wrong concentration is applied before conization for the purpose of ascertaining the limits of the cone, superficial artifacts are found histologically in the epithelium, rendering the diagnosis more difficult. The squamous epithelium in a case of this kind is shown in Fig. 84, after application of an aqueous 5% iodine solution.

Findings of Schiller's Iodine Test

The three distinct terms "iodine-positive", "iodine-light" and "iodine-negative" are in general use. Synonyms for iodine-positive and iodine-negative are iodine-staining and noniodine-staining, respectively (American Society for Colposcopy). An exact definition of these terms follows.

Iodine-Positive (Fig. 85). Deep brown stain of the entire surface of the portio (colposcopy: normal cervical squamous epithelium, older processes of transformation; histology: normal squamous epithelium containing glycogen).

Iodine-Light (Fig. 86 and 87). Light, red-brown stain of varying intensities. The iodine-light areas may be of greatly differing varieties. There may, for example, be regenerating squamous epithelium advancing towards the external os (colposcopy: fresh zones of transformation). This epithelium usually contains little glycogen and, therefore, becomes iodine-light. Regenerating squamous epithelium, however, may also lack glycogen, even though it does not appear iodine-negative but rather of a mixed color, because it consists of only a few layers of cells through which the red submucosa is faintly visible. A similar effect is caused by a zone of transformation with marked vascularity. The ectropion of columnar epithelium that does not contain glycogen histologically also appears iodine-light because of the red layer underneath, and because of the residual iodine solution in the epithelial crypts. The iodine-light areas are usually found around the external cervical os, mainly with blurred outlines.

Iodine-Negative (Fig. 87 and 88). Ochre to light yellow spots standing out clearly against the iodine-stained background, as well as showing a distinctly different color from the iodine-light areas, than which they are considerably paler. The size of iodine-negative areas varies greatly. They may extend as far as the external os or may be found at the periphery of the surface of the portio. They are usually sharply outlined either by smooth lines or irregularly as in a geographical map.

What is the nature of an iodine-negative area? Generally, it can be said only that it must represent tissue that contains either *no* glycogen or an amount so small that it is beyond the sensitivity of the iodine test. It is obvious that the iodine-negative spots do not permit histologic conclusions. These areas are frequently undetectable colposcopically and are noticed only after application of the iodine test.

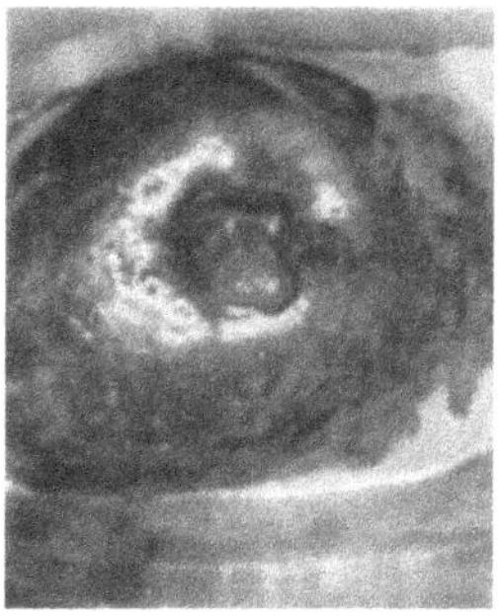

Fig. 85

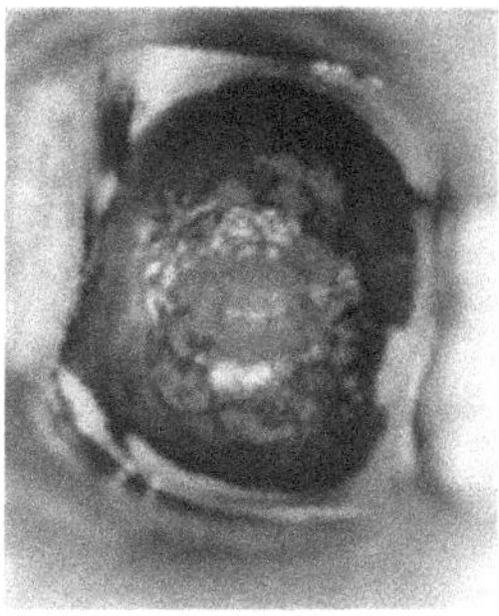

Fig. 86

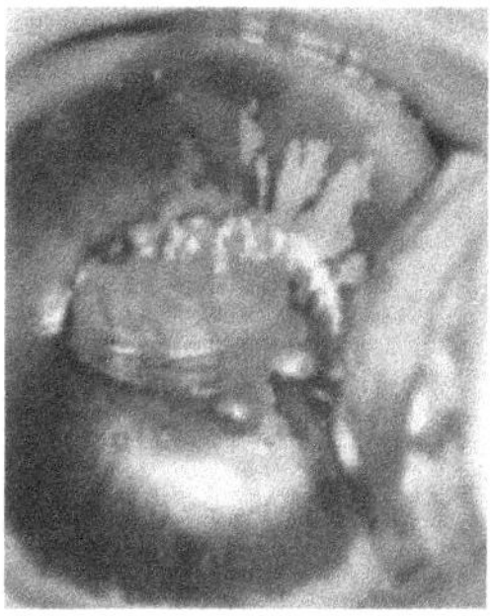

Fig. 87

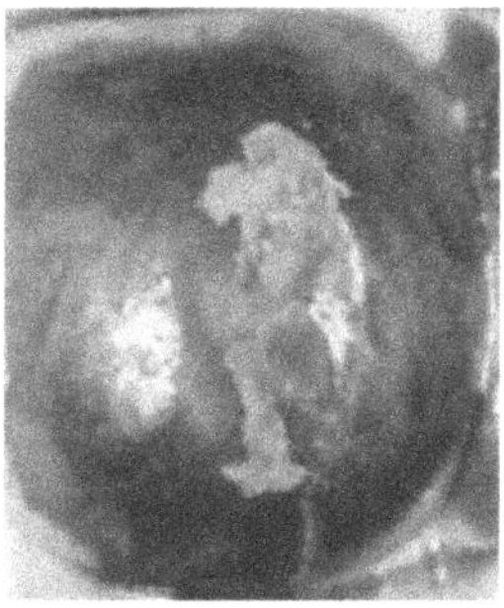

Fig. 88

Fig. 85. Iodine-stained portio, a mucous plug appears at the external os

Fig. 86. Circular iodine-light area with blurred outlines

Fig. 87. Iodine-light area adjacent to sharply outlined iodine-negative areas mainly on the anterior lip.

Fig. 88. Sharply outlined iodine-negative area on the surface of the portio (KERN, STADLER and HINDERFELD, 1962)

Our Own Investigations with Schiller's Iodine Test

We compared cytology, colposcopy, SCHILLER's iodine test, and histological results in this investigation (KERN, STADLER and HINDERFELD, 1962; KERN-BONTKE and KERN, 1962).

We attempted to approach the following problems:

1. What are the iodine findings in a large group of patients?
2. How do the iodine findings relate to simultaneously obtained colposcopic findings?
3. What is the histological basis for the iodine findings?

The division of the iodine findings into four distinct groups proved necessary in the course of evaluation of the material:

a) iodine-positive (deep brown, uniform stain of the entire surface of the portio),

b) iodine-light (iodine-light area on the surface of the portio),

c) iodine-light and iodine-negative (combination of iodine-light and iodine-negative areas on the surface of the portio; Fig. 87),

d) iodine-negative (unstained area on the surface of the portio).

Iodine Findings in the Entire Material

Fig. 89 indicates the iodine findings in the entire group of 733 cases, showing that about three-quarters of all cases have iodine-light and iodine-negative spots on the surface of the portio. The elimination of all early cases and carcinomas

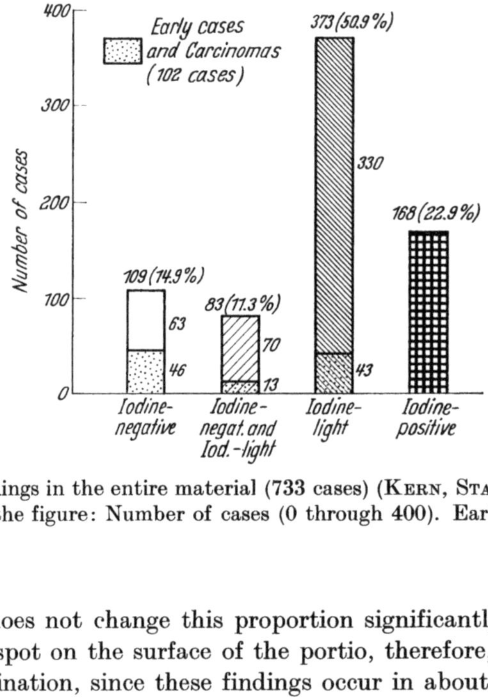

Fig. 89. Iodine findings in the entire material (733 cases) (KERN, STADLER and HINDERFELD, 1962). — Text in the figure: Number of cases (0 through 400). Early cases and carcinomas (102 cases)

from the total does not change this proportion significantly. An iodine-light or iodine-negative spot on the surface of the portio, therefore, means little without additional examination, since these findings occur in about three-quarters of all patients.

More significant is the finding of iodine-positive portios within the total group under investigation. Among these 168 patients there was not a single cytological indication of a malignant epithelial lesion. The statistically calculated probability of a carcinoma in situ or a carcinoma with an iodine-positive portio is less than 1%. If the portio is iodine-positive and if no other method of examination can be undertaken, the patients may be advised with 99% accuracy that they do not have cancer or a precancerous lesion. Even though a statement of this kind can be made with 99% accuracy only in one fourth of all patients, the fact is rather important, especially to the practicing physician. GRAVES (1933) and YOUNGE (1957) expressed the same opinion about the accuracy of an iodine-positive finding. MARTI (1939) expressed doubt, however, because he thought that an endocervical epithelial lesion could be hidden behind an iodine-positive portio. LEE, MELNICK and WALSH (1956) also consider the iodine findings unreliable in the search for carcinomas in situ. In our material, however, not a single endocervical carcinoma in situ was found among 168 cases. The iodine findings in endocervical lesions will be discussed later.

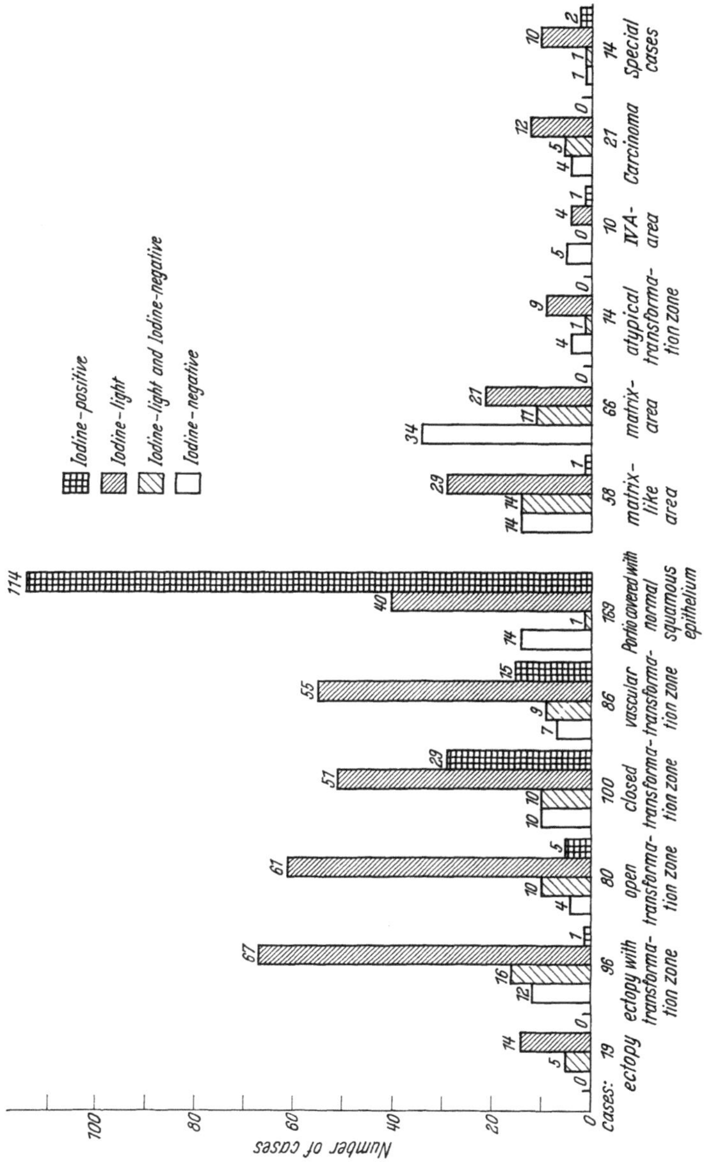

Fig. 90. Iodine findings correlated with the colposcopic findings (KERN, STADLER and HINDERFELD, 1962)

Iodine Findings and Colposcopy

Fig. 90 provides a survey of the iodine findings compared with the colposcopic findings, and Fig. 91 is an abbreviated representation on the basis of percentages. Fig. 90, using numbers of cases, first shows the numbers of the four iodine findings to differ greatly with each colposcopic finding. Portios with ectopies and early epidermidalization have a particularly high number of iodine-light areas. The more advanced the epidermidalization, up to the epidermidalized portio of old women, the more glycogen is contained in the overlying squamous epithelium and the higher is the ratio of iodine-positive portios. It is very important to point

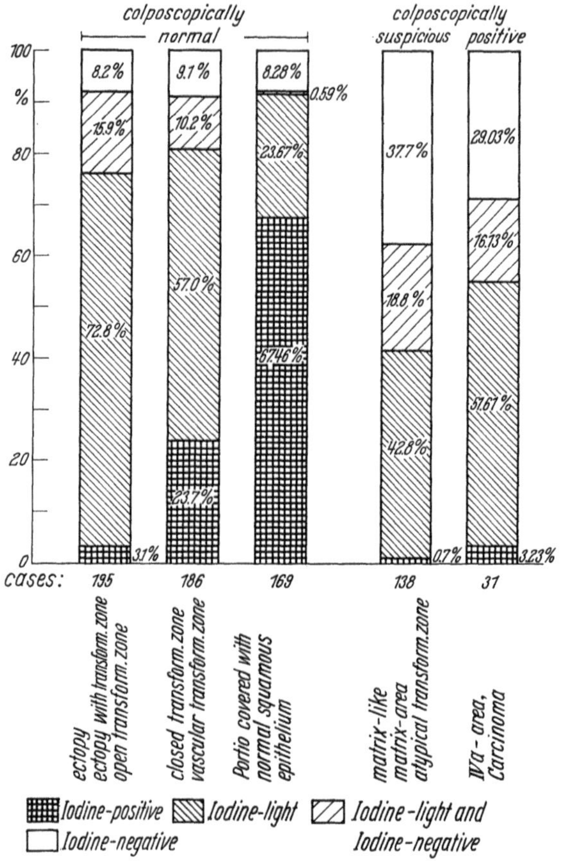

Fig. 91. Percentage distribution of the iodine findings among normal, suspicious and positive colposcopic findings (KERN, STADLER and HINDERFELD, 1962)

out, however, that 14 iodine-negative, 1 iodine-light/iodine-negative, and 40 iodine-light findings occurred on the portio among 169 cases with normal squamous epithelium. These findings are of particular significance in the detection of early cases among the colposcopic pictures known as "benign". Iodine-positive areas are almost absent from the suspicious and positive colposcopic findings, whereas the number of iodine-light or iodine-negative findings varies. The difference appears even more pronounced when expressed in percentages (Fig. 91). The proportion of iodine-negative areas in the normal colposcopic findings is somewhat less than 10% (8.2%, 9.1%, 8.28%), but in the suspicious and positive colposcopic findings it is substantially higher (37.7% and 29.03%). This difference is statistically significant, with $P = 0.001$. Within the three groups of colposcopically normal findings the differences among the four groups of the iodine test also are significant, with $P = 0.001$.

Iodine Findings in Carcinomas in Situ and in Carcinomas

The entire material contained 102 cases (13.9%) that represented malignant diseases of the squamous epithelium. These cases comprise 68 early cases (2 microcarcinomas, 58 carcinomas in situ, and 8 dysplastic epithelia) and 34 gross carcinomas. As mentioned above, not one of these cases shows an iodine-positive portio. Fig. 92 indicates the iodine findings in these cases. That 52.9% of all early cases and 29.4% of all carcinomas had definitely iodine-negative spots was noteworthy.

As the appearance of iodine-negative and iodine-light areas alone, however, does not permit adequate evaluation, because too many normal cases show findings of this kind, we tried to gain a better idea about the areas from their sizes, locations, and outlines. As shown by our investigations, small spots on the periphery of the surface of the portio obviously do not indicate much with regard to a malignant growth, whereas moderately large and large areas extending to the external os significantly more often imply a malignant epithelial disease (up to 50% in our material).

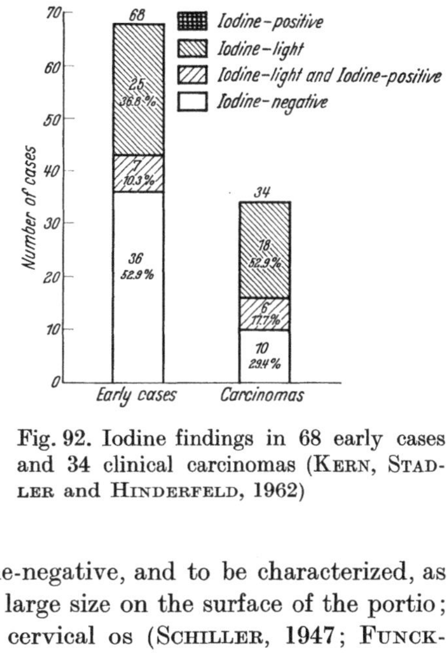

Fig. 92. Iodine findings in 68 early cases and 34 clinical carcinomas (KERN, STADLER and HINDERFELD, 1962)

The outlines of the iodine-negative areas were usually found to stand out sharply from the surroundings, whereas iodine-light areas usually have blurred outlines.

The carcinomas in situ and carcinomas within the entire material can, therefore, be said to be always iodine-light or iodine-negative, and to be characterized, as a rule, by unstained spots of moderate to large size on the surface of the portio; these spots may extend to the external cervical os (SCHILLER, 1947; FUNCK-BRENTANO, MORICARD, PALMER and DE BRUX, 1952 I, II; BERGER and WENNER-MANGEN, 1953; GEISENDORF, 1953; BERGER, 1954; FUNCK-BRENTANO, 1954; BORY and associates, 1955, 1956; PUNDEL and SCHWACHTGEN, 1956; YOUNGE 1956, 1958; MCKAY, TERJANIAN, POSCHYACHINDA, YOUNGE and HERTIG, 1959; NYBERG, TÖRNBERG and WESTIN, 1960; KOTTMEIER, VASQUEZ-FERRO, WACEK, JENNY and WENNER-MANGEN, 1961; WYSS, 1961).

What is the Histological Basis of the Iodine Findings?

As in our investigation of colposcopy, it became possible in the course of our histologic preparation of all surgical specimens in serial sections to compare the extent of the iodine finding with that of zones not containing glycogen in the histologic specimen (Kern-Bontke and Kern, 1962).

The periodic acid-leukofuchsin reaction (PAS reaction/periodic acid-Schiff reaction) according to the method of Hotchkiss and McManus was performed on the serial cervical sections for this purpose. The tissue had been fixed in Stieve's solution, which kept the glycogen well-preserved. As a check on the presence of glycogen, a parallel section was treated with diastase in each case as a control.

We attached a drawing of the histologic picture to the sketches of the colposcopy and the iodine test. In the composite the extent of epithelium not containing glycogen as well as that of markedly atypical epithelium was shown. We investigated, moreover, the manner in which the glycogen was distributed within the epithelium. An evaluation was feasible in 197 cases (117 normal cervices, 61 early cases and 19 carcinomas).

With the exception of only a few cases, an explanation of the iodine finding could always be found in the survey sections of all *normal cervices* (117 cases) by means of the PAS reaction. All iodine-light and iodine-negative areas corresponded to areas of squamous epithelium with little or no glycogen and with a normal structure of the surface of the portio. Ectopies were found in a few cases. Histologically, the surfaces of all iodine-positive portios were epidermidalized by squamous epithelium that contained glycogen. The quantities of glycogen in the epithelium vary greatly. Presence of glycogen in a few cellular layers of the squamous epithelium apparently suffices to achieve a positive reaction in the iodine test.

Summarizing the comparative investigation (colposcopy, iodine test, and histology) of 61 early cases (53 carcinomas in situ and 8 dysplastic epithelia), we find this result: in 34 cases carcinoma in situ shows the same extent of growth as the area with little or no glycogen on the surface of the portio, as indicated by the iodine test (Oki, 1927; Boschetti, 1929; Foraker and Marino, 1956; Henry and Latour, 1957; Botella-Llusiá, 1958; Manglano, 1961). Colposcopy, on the other hand, showed a suspicious area of the same size only in eight cases. The extent of the iodine-negative area was not consistent with the location of the carcinoma in situ in 27 cases. When the carcinoma in situ was on the surface of the portio, it was substantially smaller than the iodine finding and located in the midst of squamous epithelium of normal structure with little glycogen.

Of special interest is the situation found in eleven endocervical carcinomas in situ. Iodine-light or iodine-negative areas were visible on the surface of the portio in all cases and corresponded to squamous epithelium of normal structure with little or no glycogen, respectively. This finding means that normal squamous epithelium with little glycogen abuts the endocervical carcinoma in situ and spreads onto the surface of the portio.

All carcinomas (19 cases) were iodine-light or iodine-negative, as expected. Here again eight endophytic tumors showed an iodine-light or iodine-negative spot on the surface of the portio, because morphologically normal squamous epithelium with little or no glycogen was spreading there.

In a histologic section, the findings "iodine-light" or "iodine-negative" are not synonymous with "containing little glycogen" or "containing no glycogen". Areas that appear iodine-negative may contain some glycogen, and vice versa. The visual impression is apparently determined not only by the content of glycogen but also by the contrast with the surrounding normal squamous epithelium, and by the faintly red submucosa shining through from below (Table 34).

Table 34. *Content of glycogen in the histological section compared with Schiller's iodine test*

Content of glycogen with PAS reaction		Dysplastic epithelium			Carcinoma in situ			Carcinoma		
		0	(+)	+	0	(+)	+	0	(+)	+
Result of iodine test	iodine-light	1	2	—	12	3	3	7	2	—
	iodine-light/ iodine-negative	1	—	1	1	2	2	3	1	—
	iodine-negative	1	2	—	17	12	1	5	1	—
Number of cases		3	4	1	30	17	6	15	4	—
			8			53			19	

Summary

The study comparing SCHILLER's iodine test, colposcopy, and histology permits the conclusion that an iodine-light or iodine-negative finding alone does not mean much because too many normal portios exhibit this reaction. Combined with a cytological finding indicating an epithelial disease, it points to the location of the diseased epithelium in more than half the cases. The epithelial lesion is a small area within the unstained area of the iodine test in one-fourth of all cases. In the remaining cases the carcinoma in situ must be expected to be endocervical. Iodine-positive portios exclude an epithelial atypia with a statistical accuracy of 99%.

We consider the iodine test to be a valuable additional method of localizing carcinoma in situ whenever cytological findings indicate an epithelial atypia.

Biopsies and Their Significance

The initiation of therapy for cancer has been and still is dependent on histopathologic diagnosis. Since microscopic anatomy has evolved, the trust of the clinician in the judgment of the pathologist has generally been unlimited. If his diagnosis is "cancer", rather extensive therapy is usually begun. Only those who have with their own hands been responsible for the biopsy and for its histologic preparation, with all the inherent problems, can comprehend how difficult the diagnosis often is for the pathologist when he is faced with a minuscule piece of tissue, usually without knowing the clinical picture and frequently without more than the rather meager information that the specimen in question consists, for example, of tissue from the portio.

The clinician's routine forces him automatically to turn to major surgery as soon as the term "cancer" or "carcinoma" appears in the report. The diagnosis of carcinoma in situ also produces this automatic effect frequently because of its terminology. We questioned the head of a large surgical pathology laboratory that was attached to an institute of pathology. He replied that unfortunately in 90% of all cases diagnosed as carcinoma in situ the entire internal genital tract of the patient was sent to him. He added that he saw practically no conizations.

Many mistakes may be made in removal of tissue and they render the diagnosis difficult for the pathologist. On the other hand, the histological diagnosis is often unfortunately misunderstood by the clinician. As a result, wrong steps are taken.

In the following section we shall discuss the conditions under which biopsies are indicated, as well as techniques and possible errors. These discussions are the result of our collaboration with K. G. Ober.

The removal of a biopsy specimen in clinical carcinoma is basically different from that in clinically nonsuspicious so-called early cases.

Biopsy of the Cervix for Diagnostic Purposes

Sampling of fragments
Cervical curettage
Excision of specimen
Punch biopsy (usually more than one)
Schiller's scrapings
Ring biopsy
Conization

Sampling of Fragments

Sampling of fragments is the method of choice in lesions from which something can actually be "broken off" for histological verification of clinical carcinomas. Various instruments may be used for the sampling of fragments.

Punch biopsy forceps are instruments that remove an oval piece of tissue when two halves, which are shaped like sharp spoons, are closed. This instrument is best suited for exophytic tumors. It removes a piece of tissue large enough for diagnosis. It offers the technical advantage of removing the tissue safely from the vagina, if the instrument remains closed.

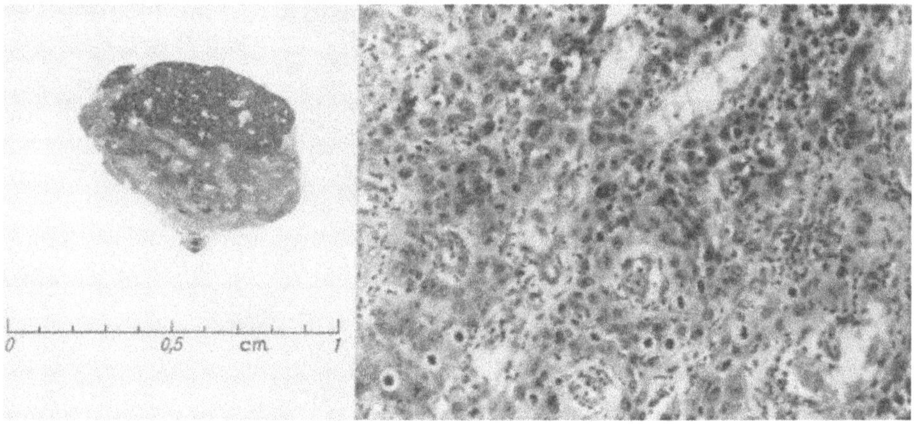

Fig. 93. Sampling of fragments. The left half of the picture shows the piece of tissue removed with the biopsy forceps as seen through a magnifying glass. Each division represents 1 millimeter. The histological picture of the case under examination is shown in the right half of the picture

Pieces of tumors may be removed equally successfully also with the *sharp spoon forceps*, which is actually one of the two halves of the biopsy forceps described above. A small sharp spoon forceps permits entering the cervical canal, where tissue from an endocervical tumor may be removed. The same may be said of a small *sharp curette*, which also permits the easy sampling of fragments from endocervical or exophytic tumors (Fig. 93).

Cervical Curettage

Cervical curettage is indicated when an endocervical carcinoma is suspected; this suspicion is sometimes based on cytological findings. A small, sharp curette is used for the curettage of the endocervix, without prior dilatation and *without* passing beyond the internal os. If the carcinoma is in an advanced stage, the intended curettage becomes a sampling of fragments as described above, but if the growth of the cancer has not spread to that extent, the curettage should be performed quickly and carefully. This procedure is at times not simple, for removal of the tissue may be difficult and profuse bleeding may carry away the small fragments of tissue. A small piece of linen placed on the posterior blade of the speculum retains the particles of tissue.

The evaluation of the tissue collected by cervical curettage may cause considerable difficulty. No decision is possible about the question whether merely

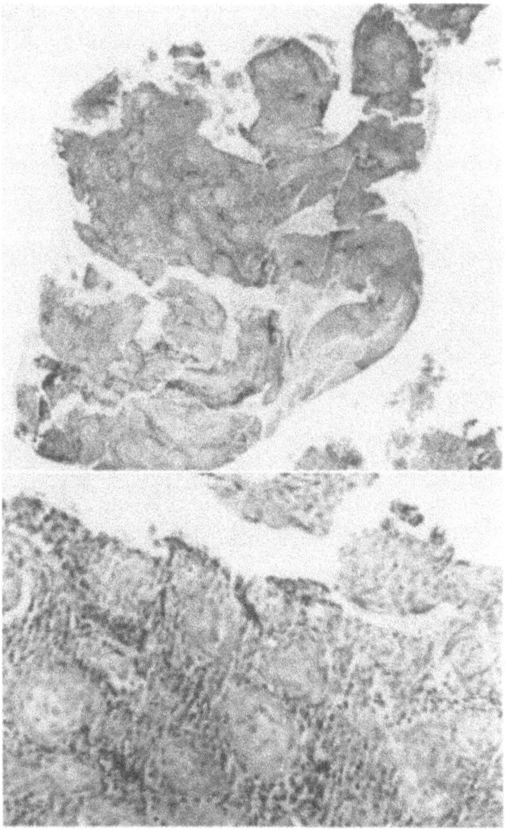

Fig. 94. Survey and histological picture of a cervical curettage from which cancer may be diagnosed without difficulty

carcinoma in situ is present, or true cancer, if only strips of atypical squamous epithelium without recognizable stroma have been collected (Fig. 94, 95). One case in our material shows how unproductive a cervical curettage can be: no tissue could be collected from the cervical canal although an endocervical, largely scirrhous carcinoma the size of a cherry was located there, clinging closely to the cervical wall because of its manner of growth (Fig. 96). In a case of this kind, the pathologic diagnosis is of value only if a definitive diagnosis of cancer can be made from the tissue. We do not consider a cervical curettage to be indicated if an early case is suspected.

Excision of Specimen

The excision of a specimen differs from the previously described methods of collection of tissue, since the piece removed from the portio with the scalpel is

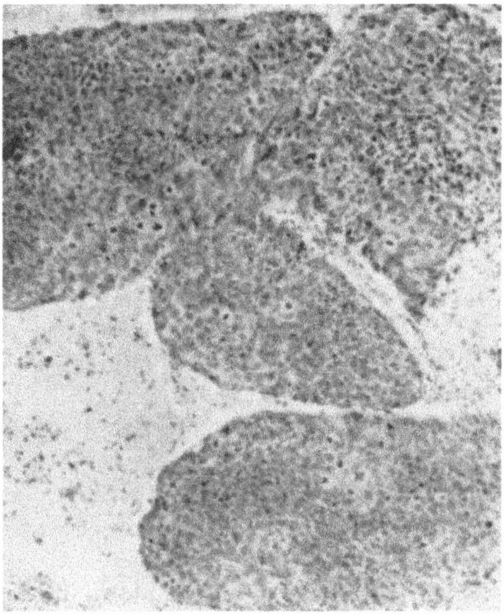

Fig. 95

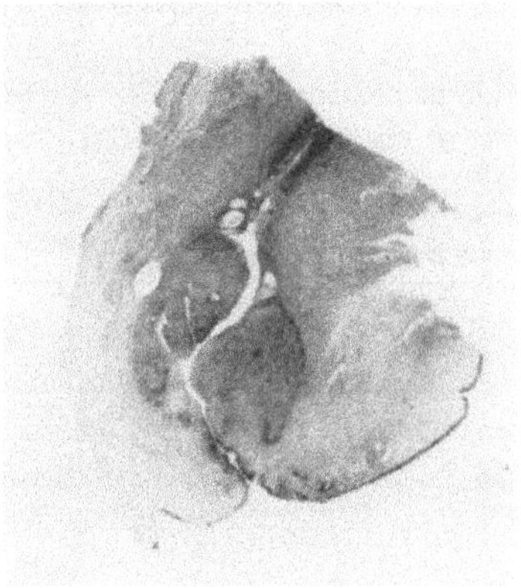

Fig. 96

Fig. 95. Cervical curettage. A definite decision with regard to carcinoma or carcinoma in situ cannot be made. The strips of markedly atypical epithelium do not bear any relation to the stroma

Fig. 96. Survey section through a cervix with a largely scirrhous cancer the size of a cherry growing into the cervical canal; here the cervical curettage remained unproductive. Approximately natural size

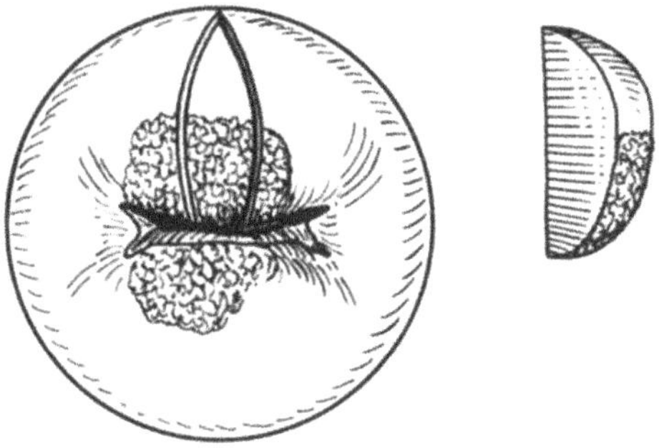

Fig. 97. Excision of specimen. Technique of removal and size of the piece of tissue removed

generally larger. An effort is often made in this procedure to extend the excision into the healthy tissue. This method is not required for clinically unequivocal cancer. It was intended mainly for the considerable number of portios that cannot be clearly evaluated grossly. Technically it has been recommended to excise a piece of tissue shaped like a segment of an orange from the 12 o'clock position, if the lesion has developed in a circular area, or from the area most suspicious grossly, from the external os to the periphery of the surface of the portio. The resulting wound is closed with two or three sutures (Fig. 97).

The excision of specimens has serious disadvantages:

If only histologically nonsuspicious tissue is excised, the result reveals nothing with regard to the conditions of other parts of the portio or of the endocervix. The uncertainty of finding the most serious lesion after excision of a specimen has been pointed out repeatedly (DE WATTEVILLE, GEISENDORF, DANON, 1952; BAJARDI and BURGHARDT, 1957; HOHLBEIN, 1958; HÜTER and MÜLLER, 1959; GRÜNBERGER, 1960; KRONE, 1960, 1962; PALMER, 1961). If a carcinoma in situ is found histologically, a second operation must be performed for total removal. The uncertainty remains, furthermore, of a true cancer possibly hidden in the remaining surrounding tissue, the incision having perhaps been made only in the marginal area of that cancer.

We consider the excision of specimens to be dispensable. The factors of uncertainty are too large in this method. It may have some justification in rare tumors of the portio (papillomas and so forth). Sampling of fragments or cervical curettage is decisive for clinical carcinomas. The early case should be detected by methods of early diagnosis. The elements of uncertainty mentioned before are not reduced significantly if the excision of a specimen is performed under the colposcope. It has been proved that use of the colposcope does not always provide an indication of where the most severe lesion is located (see p. 137). Table 35 summarizes records gathered for three different years at the gynecological clinic of the University of Cologne within the last 10 years; it shows the extent to which excisional biopsy of the cervix has been replaced by other methods. The records indicate that all biopsies performed during 1959 were special cases. The number of biopsies has decreased even further during the last 4 years.

Table 35. *Number of excisions of specimens recorded in three years at the Gynecological Clinic of the University of Cologne*

Year	Number of excisional biopsies
1952	178
1955	65
1959	17

Punch Biopsy

The punch biopsy, usually from multiple areas, is very extensively employed in America. The multiple biopsy aims at minimizing the danger of removal at the wrong place. The "four quadrant biopsy" is, therefore, often used. The punch biopsy is performed with rather delicate forceps for the removal of a piece of tissue a few millimeters in diameter (Fig. 98). The arrangement of the sharp edges of the forceps permits the removal of a piece of tissue that is generally triangular.

This manner of removal of tissue is used in America for ambulatory patients without colposcopy in iodine-negative areas. The accuracy is said to be high, partly perhaps because the tissue is collected from several areas on the surface of the portio. BICKENBACH, SOOST, CAMPOS, FIDLER, and BOYES (1961) in a symposium pointed to the possibilities of failure of the punch biopsies. BERGER (1959) considered the four-quadrant biopsy insufficient.

Punch biopsies are frequently performed under the colposcope (LIMBURG, 1956; HILLEMANNS and VESTNER, 1956); their purpose is only the histological verification of early cases.

We do not remove tissue in this manner for this reason: if the cytologic smear is positive and suggests carcinoma in situ, then the diagnosis is correct in 90% of the cases. If the cytological diagnosis is verified with the help of the punch biopsy, a therapeutic operation must follow. If the result of the punch biopsy is negative, it means nothing because the lesion may have been missed. The problems inherent in the removal of small pieces of tissue become clear if survey sections are used

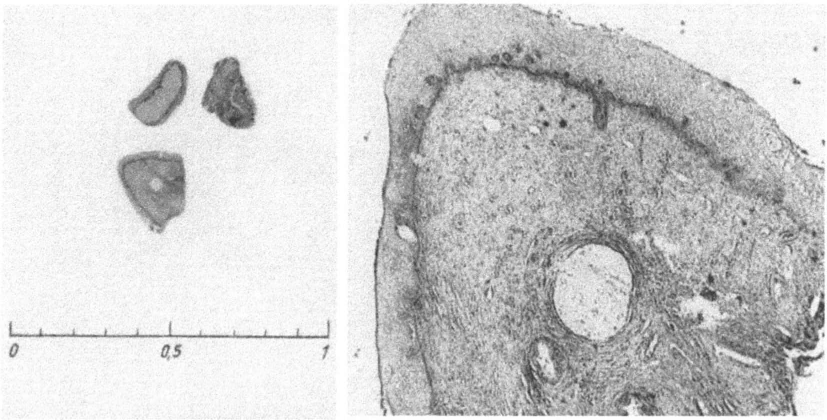

Fig. 98. Small pieces of tissue collected by punch biopsy. A survey of the material collected is shown on the left. Each division represents 1 millimeter. The histological picture is shown on the right. It is normal squamous epithelium overlying cervical stroma

for the verification of the extent of a carcinoma in situ. Small areas in particular appear relatively often. The diagnostic accuracy of punch biopsies is generally not better than that of diagnosis by cytology. We prefer the combination of diagnosis and therapy in one operation.

Schiller's Scrapings

This manner of collecting tissue actually represents a "curettage of the surface of the portio". SCHILLER described this method in connection with the iodine test and recommended the use of sharp spoon forceps to shave that part of the surface of the portio that did not turn brown with iodine. The instrument to be used must be well sharpened to avoid destructive shearing of the epithelium and obliteration of its structure. SCHILLER's scrapings, if performed solely on the basis of the iodine test, would result in very many benign findings because about 80% of the iodine-negative and iodine-light areas result from lack of glycogen in morphologically normal epithelium. Combined with a careful cervical curettage performed on the basis of an indicated cytological finding, however, this procedure can be recommended. The scrapings of tissue offer considerable chance of detecting diseased epithelium (BEHRENS, 1957/58; BERGER, 1959; JENNY and WACEK, 1961). The uncertainty inherent in small samplings of tissue naturally characterizes this method also. The lesion may be more severe than indicated by the scrapings, since it is not generally possible to ascertain the relation of the epithelial fragments to the stroma (Fig. 99).

The danger of not finding the diseased epithelium is less than in the excision of a specimen or in punch biopsy. The use of this method is advisable if no decision can be reached about major surgery on the basis of a cytologically positive smear

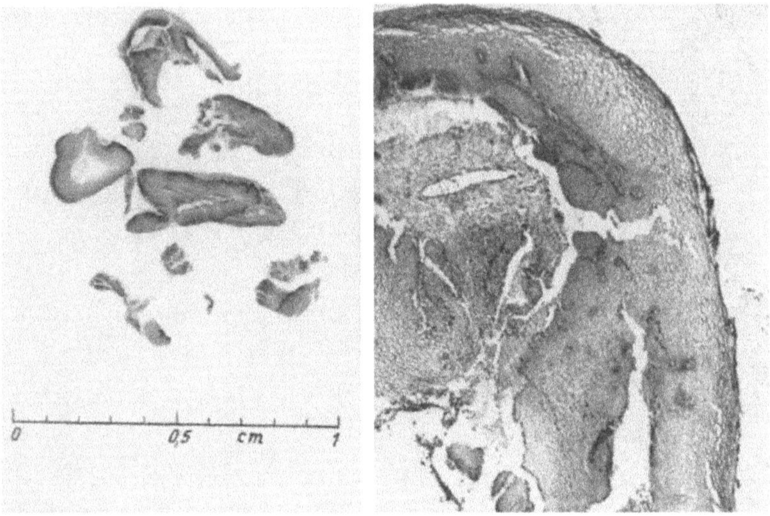

Fig. 99. Tissue collected by SCHILLER's scrapings. On the left, a survey of the collected material. Each division represents 1 millimeter. On the right, the histological picture. It is normal squamous epithelium overlying cervical stroma

and if histological data appear desirable for additional verification. If the desired result has been obtained, further therapeutic intervention is necessary. The accuracy of the results of SCHILLER's scrapings combined with cervical curettage is undoubtedly good. HELD has presented several reports on this subject.

We do not, however, use this method because we rely on the safety of cytology and, therefore, proceed immediately with conization, in consideration of two advantages of this procedure:

1. The patient is spared a second operation.

2. The structure of the tissue in the cone remains uninjured. Many artifacts are produced by SCHILLER's technique in the epithelium of the surface of the portio and in the endocervix, making exact classification according to HAMPERL's groups difficult.

Ring Biopsy

The ring biopsy is one of the *diagnostic* kinds of collection of tissue. Its use is based upon recognition that most early cases are located around the external cervical os at the junction between squamous and columnar epithelia. Its technique varies. A flat cone-shaped piece of tissue may be removed around the os, or an electrocautery may be used for the incision. The ring biopsy is either a conization in miniature or a flat ring a few millimeters in thickness that is excised from the area of the epithelial boundaries. The dimensions are shown in comparison with conization in Fig. 100.

This method also is useful for the histological verification of evidence obtained by methods used in detection of early cancer. The ring biopsy leads also to the detection of a more advanced change in the direction of carcinoma. Most early

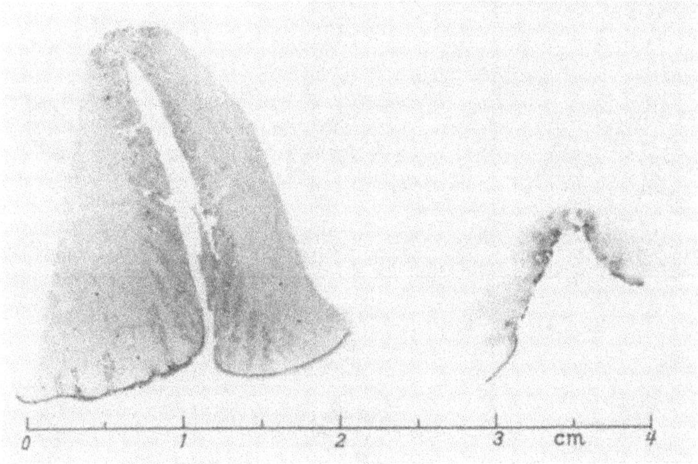

Fig. 100. Comparison of the sizes of conization and ring biopsy. Each division represents 0.5 centimeter

cases undoubtedly are confirmed by means of ring biopsy. Carcinomas in situ that are located high within the endocervix may be missed, unless the obligatory cervical scraping follows. Ring biopsy as a diagnostic sampling of tissue is recommended by numerous authors: Ayre (1948), Carter, Cuyler, Thomas, Creadick, and Alter (1952), Grünberger (1956), Clauss (1956), Krüger (1957, 1958), Winter (1958), Berger (1959), Hüter and Müller (1959), Palmer (1961).

For ring biopsy as well as for the other previously described methods of collecting tissue it is necessary to follow through with a second therapeutic procedure because the spread of the carcinoma in situ in most cases extends beyond the fragment of tissue excised. Only a thorough histologic preparation of the ring biopsy can indicate complete or incomplete removal of the lesion. For this reason we use this method only in exceptional cases.

Conization

This operation is the annular removal of tissue of the portio in the shape of a cone around the external os. The requirements with regard to the size of this piece of tissue vary considerably from clinic to clinic. The sizes actually range from that of a ring biopsy to that of the cone depicted in Fig. 100. This variation, of course, implies considerable differences in indication, use, and success of conization in different clinics. Authors who emphasized diagnostic conization as the method of choice are: KRIMMENAU (1958), PEALE (1959), BEECHAM and EMICH (1959), OBER and BÖTZELEN (1959), LEONHARDT (1959), HOHLBEIN and KRIMMENAU (1959), NEVINNY-STICKEL (1960), LEEB and ULM (1960), KRONE (1960, 1962), HESTER and READ (1960), GRAY, BARNES and Lee (1960), FLUHMANN and LYONS (1960), FETTIG and HILLEMANNS (1960), BICKENBACH, KRONE, and

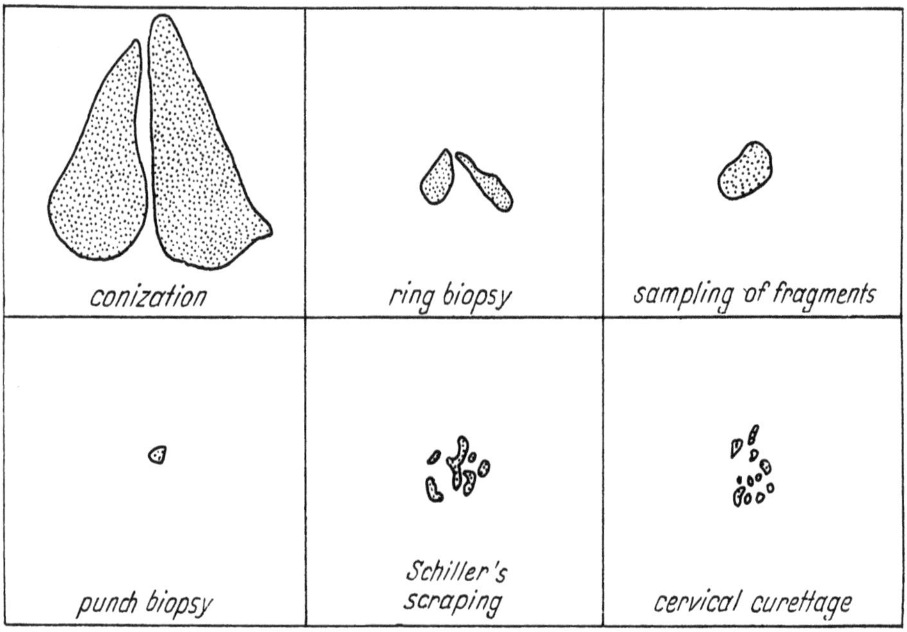

Fig. 101. Comparison of sizes of the specimens of tissue collected by conization, ring biopsy, sampling of fragments, punch biopsy, SCHILLER's scrapings and cervical curettage. The sketches were made by tracing the outlines of the histological preparations, natural size

JANS (1960), BOYES and FIDLER (1960), BICKENBACH, SOOST, CAMPOS, FIDLER, and BOYES (1961), WADDELL, WELCH, and DECKER (1961), KRÜCKEMEYER (1961), EMIG and HUNTER (1961), KOSS and DURFEE (1961), SCOTT and BALLARD (1962), BURGHARDT (1963).

We consider *conization a surgical procedure that is indicated particularly in early cases and that affords optimal histologic diagnosis as well as optimal therapy.* Consequently, the lesion in the great majority of cases may be removed completely by conization.

In consideration of the special importance ascribed to conization in every sense, its problems will be discussed in detail in the following chapter on the treatment of the early stages.

The samples of tissue collected by the various methods are arranged for comparison of their true sizes in Fig. 101. The possibilities of evaluation and the reliability of these biopsies may be easily visualized from the picture.

Treatment of the Early Stages

Historical Introduction

The ideas about the treatment of the early stages are closely related to their detection and diagnosis. Since the end of the twenties, these ideas varied between radical surgical or radiation therapy and simple local excision. They were more or less radical depending on the author's views of carcinoma in situ as true cancer or a precancerous stage.

Since the beginning of his method of early diagnosis, HINSELMANN represented the school of opinion that for carcinoma in situ a high cervical amputation or even the excision of a lip of the os and of suspicious areas under the colposcope was adequate therapy. SCHILLER, on the other hand, considered a radical removal of the internal genitalia by WERTHEIM's method or radiation therapy to be indicated. In view of the age of young patients, he was willing in 1938 to aim at less radical therapy, but found local surgery of the cervix insufficient. A few years later, STOECKEL (1942) expressed the opinion of many gynecologists: "But whoever has the opportunity at present to look at seemingly entirely normal cases of the earliest variety without any abnormal clinical finding instinctively shrinks from the idea of subjecting these women to radical surgery, especially if they are still young. The question arises: Is this therapy, this enormous operation, this total genital mutilation really necessary in cases of this kind?" TREITE, his pupil, then reported a simplified therapy consisting in simple extirpation of the uterus. STOECKEL's clinic refrained from using subsequent radiation because of the resulting castration. MESTWERDT (1951) considered conservative therapy for microcarcinoma only in exceptional cases and advised extreme caution. REICHEN (1952) spoke for conservative surgery in carcinoma in situ in younger women, as did SCHUBERT and SCHMERMUND (1954) as well as SCHEFFEY and LANG (1954). JORDAN, BADER and DAY (1956/57) advised individual minimal definitive therapy with an optimum of safety. Conization was considered adequate in clearly intraepithelial growth by LATOUR, BROWN and TURNBULL (1957) and NOVAK (1957), but any kind of microinvasion was to be treated radically. The leading German-speaking gynecologists in 1957 held a detailed symposium in Heidelberg on the problems of therapy. SCHMIDT-ELMENDORFF proposed electrocauterization of the markedly atypical epithelium, but did not meet with approval because of the objection that this procedure would destroy all means of histologic verification. DE WATTEVILLE recommended radical local removal of the superficial carcinoma without discussing technical details. NAVRATIL was in favor of a graded therapy that varied from amputation of the portio to total extirpation of the uterus, unless there were signs of invasion. ANTOINE thought that radical local removal by conization or amputation of the portio, if performed in a way

Table 36. *Therapy of early stages of cervical carcinoma*

Author	Type of management
KOTTMEIER (1959)	Mainly conization, possibly hysterectomy
KRIEGER and MCCORMACK (1959)	Depending on age, conization or hysterectomy
KIRCHHOFF and WITT (1959)	Avoidance of all mutilating therapy
TOWNSEND and BEISCHER (1960)	Mainly hysterectomy, some cases radical operation, a few conservative
MUSSEY (1960)	Conization, amputation of the portio, cauterization, radium therapy
MCLAREN (1960)	Depending on age, amputation of the portio or hysterectomy
MARTINS and DREICON (1960)	Conization in young women, but radical operation for even the smallest invasive microcarcinoma
HOHLBEIN and GANSE (1960)	Conization for young women, hysterectomy over 45
LATOUR (1961)	Conization in young women, otherwise hysterectomy with vaginal cuff but conservation of the ovaries
FUNCK-BRENTANO (1961)	Depending on age, removal of the portio or hysterectomy, possibly with lymphadenectomy
SOKOLOVSKY, DERAGNE and MALISHEVA (1961)	Diathermy excision
MOORE, MORTON, APPLEGATE and HINDLE (1961)	Conization for young women
ROGOVENKO (1961)	Cone-shaped diathermy excision
KRONE (1960)	Electroconization, some cases radiation therapy, a few hysterectomy
HUGUIER (1961)	High amputation of the portio, conization insufficient
EMIG and HUNTER (1961)	Hysterectomy with 2.5 cm long vaginal cuff
WADDELL, WELCH and DECKER (1961)	Depending on age, conization or hysterectomy
CAMPOS, SCHÜLLER and TAYLOR (1961)	Conization
OBER, KAUFMANN and HAMPERL (1961)	Depending on age, conization or hysterectomy
GÜNTHER and STOLL (1962)	Sturmdorf-cone
ZINSER (1962)	Depending on age, conization or hysterectomy
BOYD, ROYLE, FIDLER and BOYES (1963)	As conservative as possible, with careful cytologic follow-up
LISSE (1963)	SCHAUTA's radical operation or radiation with carcinoma dose
MICHALKIEWICZ, PRZYBORA, SIMM and WOLNA (1963)	As conservative as possible, with careful cytologic follow-up
WAY (1963)	Depending on age, conization or hysterectomy

that removed the entire lesion, would render superfluous any further therapy. KOTTMEIER reported on 225 conizations with clinical carcinoma found in the cone in 17%, whereas the other cases remained free of recurrence without further treatment. HELD suggested a very conservative procedure (conization) in young women but removal of the uterus in older women (KAUFMANN, RUNGE, OBER and STOLL, 1957).

Seven years have elapsed since that symposium. In those clinics that are interested in the problem of early diagnosis and that give it their attention, the local total removal of the markedly atypical epithelium is recognized with increasing frequency as the therapy of choice. Their aim is modification of the therapy according to the age of the patient. Table 36 lists various groups of researchers and the therapy practiced by them in early cases during the last 5 years.

Conization or Hysterectomy as Treatment of the Early Stages of Cervical Carcinoma

If the use of one of the methods of early diagnosis yields a definite indication of an early case, removal is indicated. The decision about adding histological verification depends on the accuracy of the method of search used.

Conization of the cervix aims at removal in toto of the diseased epithelium. This operation is indicated in all sexually mature women whose internal genitalia are normal. It is difficult to state an upper age limit, since it depends on the total picture presented by the individual woman. If a woman of 45 still menstruates regularly and appears relatively well-preserved, we perform a conization. If we are faced with a prematurely aged woman in her early forties with several children, the decision to perform hysterectomy is likely to be made. Basically, conization preserves the menstrual cycle and the possibility of conception.

In pregnant women with early cases, pregnancy and delivery have until very recently been allowed to continue before conization was performed. Even today this procedure can undoubtedly be defended in view of the long duration of the latency of carcinoma in situ. Recent published reports from BEECHAM and ANDROS (1960), FERGUSON and BROWN (1960), AYRE and SCOTT (1961) demonstrated, however, the feasibility of a conization without endangering the pregnancy unless too extensive an operation is performed. We followed that suggestion with the same success, performing conizations on several pregnant women without disturbing the pregnancy. Operations on the portio do not seem to stimulate labor in the pregnant uterus, as may be observed after SHIRODKAR's operation also. In pregnancy, the cone is usually kept quite flat because of the ectropion.

Hysterectomy with the adnexa left in place is indicated for the older woman in the menopause or later, if her internal genitalia are normal. This operation is performed vaginally if possible. Hysterectomy is performed in younger women if in addition to the epithelial atypia, other pathologic conditions of the genitalia are present, such as myomas or adnexal tumors, among others, and if this complication renders preservation of the genitalia impossible.

The extirpation of the uterus need not be discussed here technically, since it involves the usual vaginal or abdominal operations. It should be pointed out only that we are careful during the operation, particularly in the vaginal procedure, not to destroy the surface of the portio and the endocervix in grasping the cervix with tenacula and applying traction. The damage thus produced may be so severe that the histological verification of the epithelial atypia in the surgical specimen may become difficult or even impossible. For this reason, the portio is grasped laterally with bullet forceps at 3 and 9 o'clock before a circular incision is made in the vaginal mucosa without touching the surface of the portio. The subsequent operation proceeds in the customary manner. The histological preparation of the surgical specimen is the same as in conization (see p. 171).

Surgical Technique in Conization

Through conization we endeavor, as mentioned before, to remove the entire lesion, thus employing the operation as *definitive therapy*. To achieve this aim it is necessary to be familiar with the normal epithelial conditions of the cervix and their morphological changes during a woman's lifetime, because without

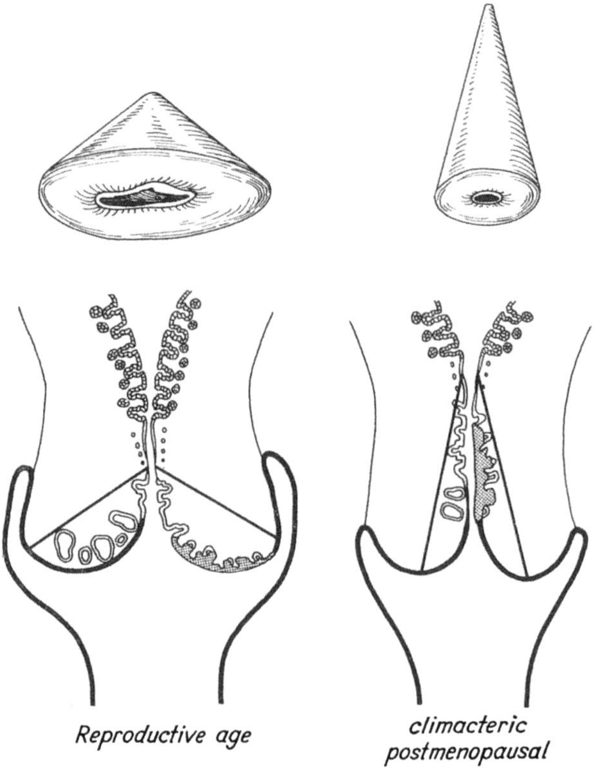

Fig. 102. Direction of incision and shapes of the cones of tissue removed by cervical conization, depending on the patient's age (modified after OBER and BÖTZELEN, 1959)

that information it is impossible to know about the possible location of an early change and to modify the shape of the cone accordingly. The cone must have its base in the normal squamous epithelium of the surface of the portio, its apex extending to the uppermost cervical glands. Investigations by OBER have shown that the length of the endocervical mucosa is nearly constant, notwithstanding the morphologic changes of the cervix and the migration of the boundary between squamous and columnar epithelia. Carcinoma in situ always spreads from that boundary towards the cervical glands. Carcinoma in situ in sexually mature women is therefore logically found more often on the surface of the portio, and in women in the menopause or later more often in the endocervix. The cone to be excised in women in the reproductive age group must, therefore, have a broad base with a flat shape and a wide angle, and in older women a small base with a narrow shape with a sharp angle (Fig. 102).

The condition of the surface of the portio determines the shape of the cone that is to be excised. The location of the most peripheral cervical gland is ascertained preoperatively on the surface of the portio, even though it may be visible only as a retention cyst.

The grossly visible reddened spot, the so-called erythroplakia, gives a good indication. If gross inspection only is made of the surface of the portio, the line of incision must include the reddened area. Processes of transformation will usually be visible on the surface of the portio. Colposcopic inspection may facilitate the localization of the "last cervical glands". They must be within the lines of incision. The depth of the fornices provides another lead. If the fornices are deep, the "last cervical glands" are usually located near the periphery of the surface of the portio. If the fornices are shallow, cervical glands are almost never visible on the surface of the portio.

Another safeguard is the iodine test performed with a considerably diluted iodine solution. All iodine-light or iodine-negative areas should be within the line of incision. This indicator may meet with difficulties in certain exceptional cases, when, for example, iodine-negative areas extend deep into the fornices, or even onto the vaginal mucosa. OBER and BONTKE (1959) reported a case of this kind (No. 1 of the 150 cases) in which the carcinoma in situ extended to the lower third of the vagina. ZINSER also observed several cases of this kind (ZINSER, MEISSNER and BÖTZELEN, 1963). The surgeon cannot tell from the iodine test whether the iodine-negative areas originate in morphologically normal squamous epithelium that is poor in glycogen or in markedly atypical epithelium. If the iodine-light or iodine-negative area does not extend too far into the fornix, the vaginal mucosa may be excised as well. If the area is large, the actual extent of the lesion must be ascertained by collection of small specimens of tissue (punch biopsy or, preferably, SCHILLER's scrapings) before further surgery is started. The extent of iodine-negative areas and their histologic basis are ascertained preoperatively in cases of this kind in the course of routine early diagnosis.

In the surgical technique of conization the portio is exposed with separated specula. Surgical preparation of the vagina or swabbing of the portio should be avoided in order to prevent damage to the superficial epithelium. The visual orientation with regard to the location of the last cervical gland and the iodine test follow (Fig. 104). Then the portio is grasped at 3 and 9 o'clock without touching its surface and is pulled forward. This procedure renders unnecessary the application of lateral retractors. The circular line of incision for the base of the cone is then made with a narrow scalpel to a depth of a few millimeters. A Hegar dilator may be used to explore the shape of the cervical canal. Starting at 12 o'clock, a hole is then made with a narrow scalpel at the height indicated by the incision, thereby attempting to remove a conical piece of tissue with a sawlike movement of the scalpel peripherally through the indicated line of incision, while the point remains in the cervical canal. If the purpose of the conization is the removal of a larger cone, the excision usually does not succeed at the first attempt. In that case, the indicated line of incision is deepened to about 5 millimeters and bullet forceps are applied to the surface of the cone at 3 and 9 o'clock without touching the superficial epithelium. If as much as possible of the cervical wall is to be preserved in very young patients, the specimen should preferably be taken at a depth of about 0.5 to 1.0 centimeter in the cervical stroma beneath the epithelium that is to be removed; thus, not a regular cone but a round, flat piece of tissue with a centrally superimposed small cone results. Upon removal of the cone from the site of excision, a thin piece of silk is drawn through the upper edge at 12 o'clock and loosely tied for orientation (Fig. 109). The cone is immediately immersed in STIEVE's fixative. The glass containing the fixative must be large enough for the cone to move freely.

The resulting wound usually bleeds heavily. The internal os is, nevertheless, first dilated with Hegar dilators and the corpus curetted. In this procedure, the wound is closed anteriorly and posteriorly with two Sturmdorf sutures of chromic catgut, without mobilization of the vaginal mucosa.

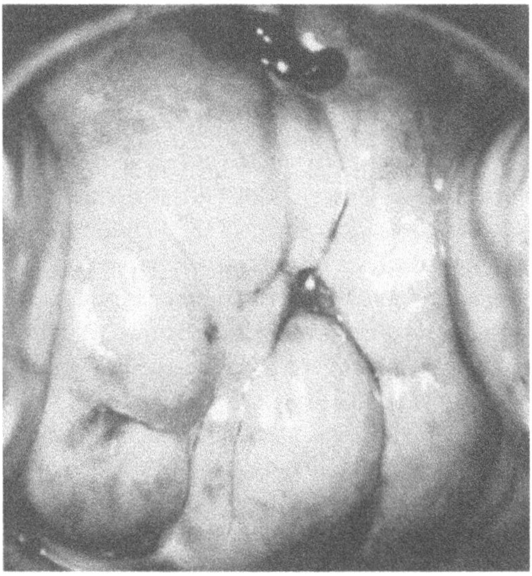

Fig. 103. Portio after conization and covering of the wound area with Sturmdorf sutures. Years later the grooves where the sutures had been placed may still be seen

In very deep conizations, two additional lateral sutures of chromic catgut are advisable at times.

The technique of excision of the cone as described with subsequent closing with Sturmdorf sutures has some disadvantages. OBER and BÖTZELEN (1959) described this technique with its advantages and disadvantages in detail. These are the disadvantages:

1. There is a danger of postoperative bleeding that occurs between the seventh and twelfth day after surgery in 8 to 10% of all cases. This bleeding is usually rather massive and requires exposure of the vagina and inspection of the area of the wound. The loss of blood may require replacement (VÁSQUEZ-FERRO, 1959; HESTER and READ, 1960).

2. Two weeks of hospitalization are necessary because of the relatively frequent postoperative bleeding. This period of hospitalization does not cause difficulties in Germany, but may be a serious problem where the patients must pay the bills themselves.

3. The cosmetic result of the newly formed portio is often not good. The catgut sutures frequently cut into the tissue, and the poor appearance of the surface of the wound is an unpleasant surprise on the day the patient is discharged. The spontaneous healing of the portio is, however, astonishing, and it is adequately reformed. Years after the wound has completely healed, the grooves caused by the Sturmdorf sutures may still be clearly noticed in most cases. The portio may immediately be recognized as "surgically altered" (Fig. 103).

SCOTT, WELCH and BLAKE (1960) reported on a bloodless method of conization or annular biopsy. A description of SCOTT's technique follows:

The portio is exposed and grasped at 3 and 9 o'clock, its surface is inspected as described above, and SCHILLER's iodine test is performed (Fig. 104). (Or the iodine test may be delayed until after the injection described below.) The cervix is then infiltrated with a dilute solution of epinephrine, which is prepared by adding 10 drops of epinephrine to 100 ml. of physiological saline. About 200 ml. of this solution are needed. The solution is drawn into a 20 ml. syringe and a needle of medium size (No. 1) with bayonet joint. A longer needle may also be used, but its insertion into the firm cervical tissue is more difficult. The periphery of the portio outside the area to be excised is then punctured in the direction of the cone, and 10 to 20 ml. are injected through each site of puncture by moving the needle back and forth. The infiltration of the firm cervical tissue requires considerable force. It is facilitated substantially by puncturing the channel before the procedure. Without a bayonet joint the connection between needle and syringe comes apart easily, because the pressure applied is too great. The edge of the portio around the cervix is punctured in this manner at regular distances six to eight times, and 50 to 150 ml are infiltrated. The portio swells substantially and turns glassy white where it is not covered with iodine (Fig. 105). Unless this color effect has been attained the attempt to reduce subsequent hemorrhage is unsatisfactory (BURGHARDT, 1963).

The patient's blood pressure must be watched during the infiltration, since in almost all cases it undergoes a short period of fluctuation to systolic pressures of 160 to 200 mm Hg. Patients with high pressure or myocardial damage and those in danger of apoplexy must therefore be excluded from this procedure.

If the iodine test has not been performed before the infiltration the portio is very carefully swabbed with LUGOL's solution to make visible the extent of the iodine-negative areas. The uptake of the iodine stain is not impaired by the infiltration. The distention of both lips of the os by the infiltration sometimes causes the size of the area that is poor in glycogen to change.

The excision of the cone is performed as described (Figs. 106, 109). The difference between this procedure and the bloodier method is striking: the incised surfaces remain almost free of bleeding and are yellowish-white. Thus, the area of the operation is ideally exposed for inspection. The excision of the cone is followed by dilatation of the internal os and curettage of the corpus, while the site of the wound remains bloodless (Fig. 107). Upon completion of the curettage the wound site is subjected to electrocoagulation, starting from the apex of the cone. During this procedure the portio undergoes a visible reshaping as a result of the uniform coagulation of the cervical tissue by heat (Fig. 108). If the hole in the tissue of the portio measures 3 cm in diameter, after the cauterization is

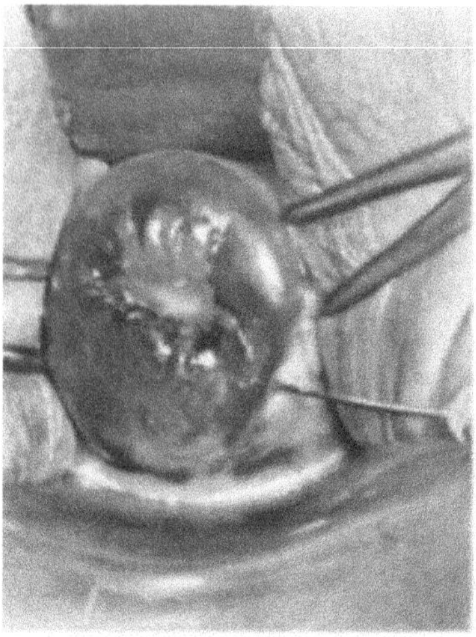

Fig. 104

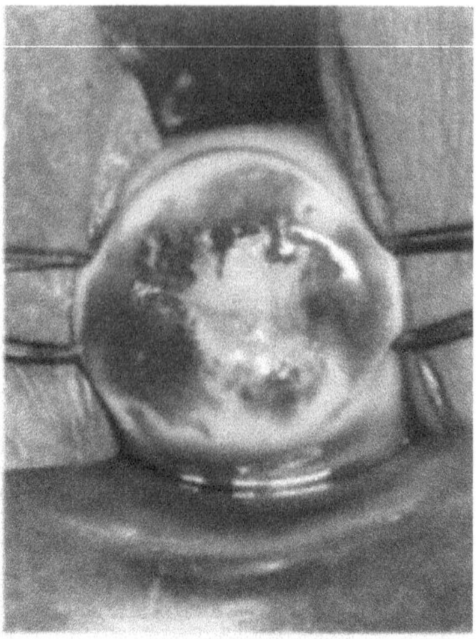

Fig. 105

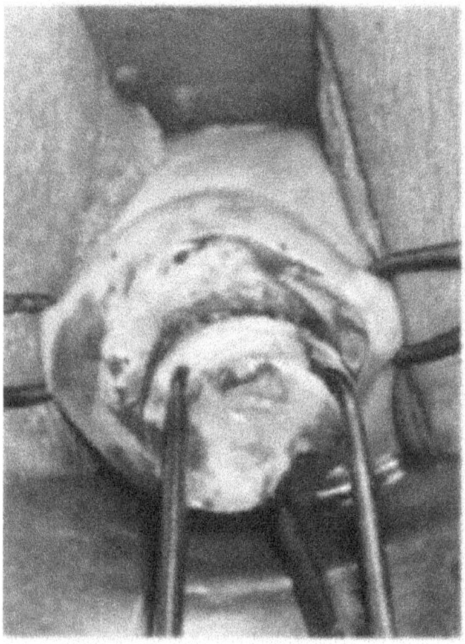

Fig. 106

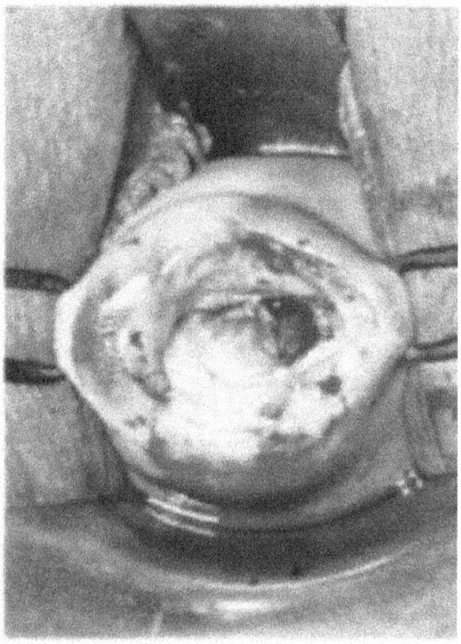

Fig. 107

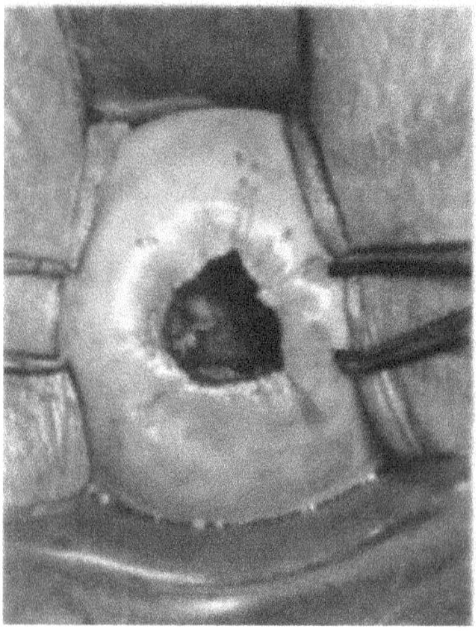

Fig. 108

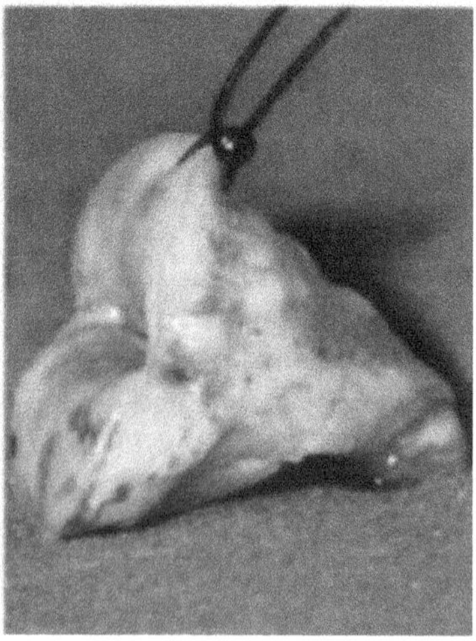

Fig. 109

(For Legends see p. 169)

completed it is only 1 to 2 cm. The small crater remaining in the tissue is filled with Leukocyllase powder and the vagina lightly packed with a tampon.

Hemorrhages occurring later after surgery seem to be considerably less common in this method, but they are not entirely excluded. The cosmetic result is so good that it is difficult to demonstrate the result of operation on the healed portio (Fig. 110). SCOTT recommended a periodic dilatation of the internal os after the operation to prevent stenosis. We have to date not seen any stenosis, without having used this procedure.

OBER in a few cases refrained from electrocauterization of the wound without noting any disadvantage. Moderate bleeding a few hours after conization occurred in only one case. The cosmetic result in the healing of the wound is the same.

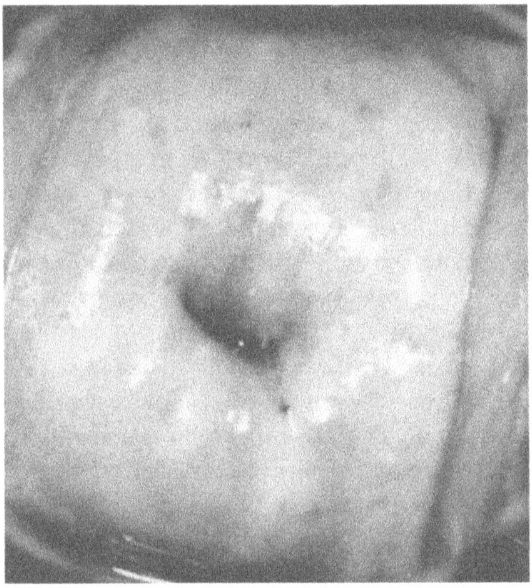

Fig. 110. Cervix after conization by SCOTT's technique. The cosmetic result is very good

The form of the external os during electrocoagulation, however, can be very well controlled even as the procedure is being completed; this factor seems to be an advantage.

Fig. 104. The portio is grasped at 3 and 9 o'clock after SCHILLER's iodine test. At 4 o'clock, puncture for infiltration with solution of epinephrine

Fig. 105. Distended, glassy-white portio after infiltration has been completed. The swelling caused by the infiltration of both lips of the os changes the size of the circular iodine-negative area around the external os

Fig. 106. Cone almost entirely removed. Wound areas are almost free of blood. The cone is removed between two bullet forceps in the cervical stroma, while the surface of the portio is left intact

Fig. 107. Wound area after excision of the cone. The wound area can be easily inspected and is largely free of blood

Fig. 108. Reshaping of the external os after careful cauterization of the wound area

Fig. 109. Cone of tissue with a thread inserted at 12 o'clock for identification

Bickenbach, Krone and Jans (1960), among others, use the electric knife rather than the scalpel for conization, thus achieving relative ischemia even without infiltration of epinephrine. The therapeutic and cosmetic results are also very good. We do not use this method because the cone may be so severely coagulated on all sides to a depth of about 1 to 2 mm that a histologic evaluation of the area of the wound is made difficult, as well as the means of ascertaining whether the carcinoma in situ has been removed. The cone, furthermore, cannot be shaped so well with the electric knife as with the scalpel.

Other Therapeutic Operations on the Portio Leading to the Removal of an Epithelial Atypia

In addition to conization two other kinds of operations on the cervix also provide adequate treatment of an epithelial atypia under certain conditions: amputation of the portio and Bonney's plastic surgery.

Amputation of the Portio. Hinselmann suggested this surgical method for the removal of superficial carcinomas. His was an extraordinarily modern point of view, when elsewhere at least hysterectomy was being recommended. In the amputation of the portio the cervix is cut off straight, and the wound covered by means of Sturmdorf's plastic operation. This operation is still in use with the Manchester-Fothergill procedure. The amputation of the cervix in older women should be performed at a very high level, in accordance with our consideration of conization; yet, it cannot be performed to technical satisfaction because of the involution of the uterus. The amputation of the cervix in younger women may be performed more flatly since the atypia is usually located on the surface of the portio.

Bonney's plastic surgery. Bonney devised this operation as treatment for discharge in cases with severe, often inflammatory, exudation from the surface of the portio. A flat disc of the portio is removed from the entire surface, which is then covered by Sturmdorf's operation. The result is not good cosmetically. Hinselmann devised a very similar method: the removal of the so-called "Portio-scheibe". This operation is still being performed by his pupils. His colposcopic studies convinced Hinselmann that in the majority of cases carcinoma in situ is located on the surface of the portio. He devised this method as a diagnostic procedure, however, because he disapproved of the removal of a small specimen of tissue, and rightly so. It may be seen readily that the cervical canal remains nearly untouched in this operation. A cervical curettage performed at the same time is subjected to the same possible errors as are all other small samplings of tissue. For this reason, Bonney's plastic procedure should not be considered therapy for early cases.

The only remaining therapeutic operation that can compete with conization is high amputation of the cervix. Both methods effect local but total removal of an early lesion. The local treatment aims at the preservation of the menses and, to a large extent, of fertility, in sexually mature women. In both methods the cycle is unimpaired, as is the ability to conceive, even though the so-called "cervical factor" is missing (Fettig and Kühn, 1963). On the other hand,

removal of cervical mucosa that is frequently altered by inflammation has a favorable effect on conception. The results of the two methods differ, however, in regard to the mechanism of cervical competence that is of great importance in a developing pregnancy. Fig. 111 demonstrates this difference schematically.

The muscular parts of the cervical wall are preserved in conization, leaving the external portions of the cervix for the regeneration of the remainder of the organ. The reformed cervical canal is lined by squamous epithelium. The regenerated cervix remains relatively competent.

In the amputation of the portio the peripheral parts of the cervix also are removed, although they need not be in the early cases because no cervical glands are involved. After this procedure the endometrial cavity is protected by only a short stump that tends to open readily upon increasing pressure from above.

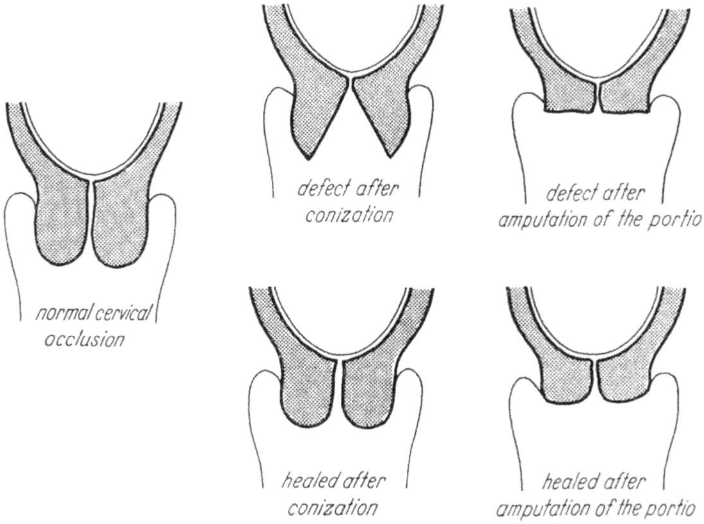

Fig. 111. Schematic illustration of the capacity of the cervix to remain competent during pregnancy after various operations on the portio

Removal of the peripheral cervical wall is not necessary for the treatment of the abnormal epithelium, whereas it is very detrimental to the preservation of moderately adequate cervical competence.

The foregoing considerations must result in the recognition that during the reproductive years conization is the most appropriate therapy for a woman with a carcinoma in situ of the cervix.

Histological Preparation of the Removed Tissue

Histological study of the removed tissue (cone or uterus) should reveal the kind of lesion and its location, and ascertain whether the lesion has been removed completely.

Difficulties may be encountered in the histological examination of tissue to confirm findings of other methods of detection, especially cytology. The reliability of the method of detection is disparaged unjustly after all steps in verification have been taken, when the pathology laboratories that receive the tissue are not familiar with the questions posed and optimal techniques for histological examination of the cervix. Unfortunately, it happens not infrequently that the pathologist in an overburdened laboratory performs his own "biopsy" from the specimen of portio submitted, prepares a frozen section, and informs the clinician that there is no indication of cancer in the tissue submitted. The remaining material is usually discarded. Histological diagnosis reached in this manner cannot serve as evidence in the early diagnosis of cervical carcinoma.

The histological preparation of the cervix has often been taken over by a gynecologist trained in pathology, who was interested in the case.

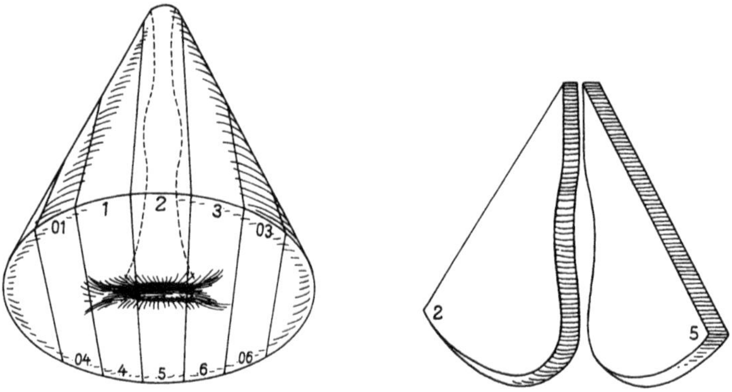

Fig. 112. Lines of gross sectioning of the fixed cone or cervix for histologic studies; numbering of the tissue slices before embedding in paraffin

Our laboratory has developed a histological technique that has led to optimal results thanks to the skill of our technical assistant, M. von Matuschka.

The excised cone or extirpated uterus while still warm is immersed in Stieve's fixative. There must be enough of the liquid to allow the tissue to float and to be surrounded by it on all sides. Its composition is as follows:

hot saturated aqueous solution of chloride of mercury	760 ml
40% formalin	200 ml
glacial acetic acid	40 ml

The advantage of this fixation is a uniformly rapid penetration of the firm cervical tissue.

After 12 to 24 hours, the tissue is hard enough to be cut grossly, without distortion. It must then be transferred into formalin; otherwise it becomes too hard. If the specimen is a uterus, the internal os is marked by a shallow incision and the cervix severed from the fundus uteri a few millimeters above the mark. The cone has been marked previously by the surgeon with a thread at 12 o'clock. The thread is removed. To mark the histological section in conizations, a small incision is made in the cervical tissue at 12 o'clock about 1 cm from the surface of the portio (Figs. 82 and 113). The cervix is then cut with a sharp, broad knife into slices about 0.5 to 0.7 cm thick. The cervix or cone is held tightly against a wooden board with thumb and index finger of the left hand, and the central slice is cut first, including the cervical canal if possible. The procedure is illustrated in Fig. 112.

Three to five slices are obtained in this manner, or in very large portios sometimes as many as seven. In most cases, however, three slices are sufficient. They are numbered uniformly, as shown in Fig. 112. Slice 2/5 usually breaks in two if the cervical canal is wide. The lateral portions of the cervical canal are often contained in slices 1/4 and 3/6 on the (medial) side of the slice facing the center. The middle slice 2/5 is not marked for sectioning because both of its sides are equally important. On slices 1/4, 3/6, and those more lateral, the medial side is marked for sectioning.

The following procedure of embedding in paraffin is the method of M. von Matuschka, who reported (1962) this procedure for the preparation of large histologic

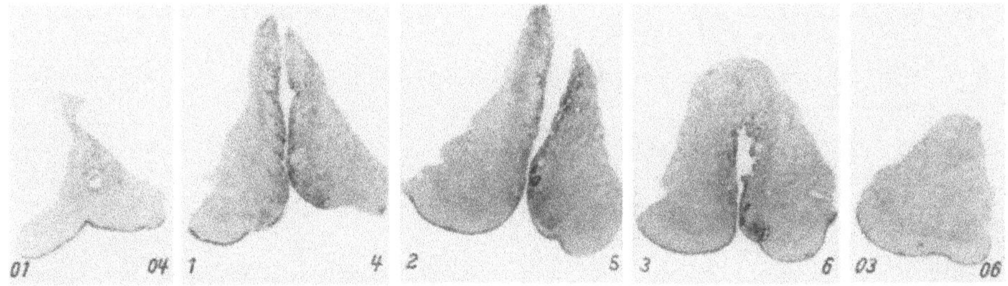

Fig. 113. Preparation of multiple serial sections of cervix. Numbering facilitates three-dimensional reconstruction. Approximately natural size. The small notch in the cervical wall made for orientation is visible in the three middle sections

sections. After fixation and cutting of the tissue blocks, without washing they are immersed in the following solutions:

1. 70% alcohol, 2 to 3 hours at 70°, or better, overnight at room temperature.
2. 96% alcohol, 1 hour at 70°.
3. Absolute alcohol, 3 hours at 70° with three changes.
4. Acetone/alcohol, 1:1, 1 hour at 70°.
5. Acetone, 1 hour at 70°.
6. Paraffin (melting point 58°), over night at 70°.
7. Preparation of paraffin blocks.

The individual times vary somewhat according to the size and thickness of the tissue.

The paraffin blocks may be sectioned at 6 to 8 μ with an ordinary paraffin microtome. Five sections are prepared first from each block; the extent of the carcinoma in situ is then examined and more sections are cut as needed. Generally, however, an adequate survey of the kind of lesion is obtained from the three to five sections at uniformly distributed planes through the surface of the portio. The sections are stained with iron hematoxylin-eosin; the PAS stain with and without diastase is routinely performed in every case to ascertain whether there is glycogen in the squamous epithelium. A series of sections from one cone prepared according to this method is shown in Fig. 113.

What are the advantages of this method of histological preparation of large histological sections?

1. The exact location and extent of the abnormal epithelium can be easily ascertained. The arrangement of the sections can be reconstructed satisfactorily.

2. The direction of the section is always vertical through the squamous epithelium, excluding tangential sections, which may possibly be deceptive.

3. This method provides the ideal opportunity to ascertain whether the lesion has been removed completely. Furthermore, the location of possibly suspicious remnants may be ascertained. SCHULMAN and CAVANAGH (1961), on the other hand, were not able to arrive at definite conclusions from the prepared cone.

4. The procedure confirms or disproves with the utmost objectivity whatever has been indicated by other methods of search.

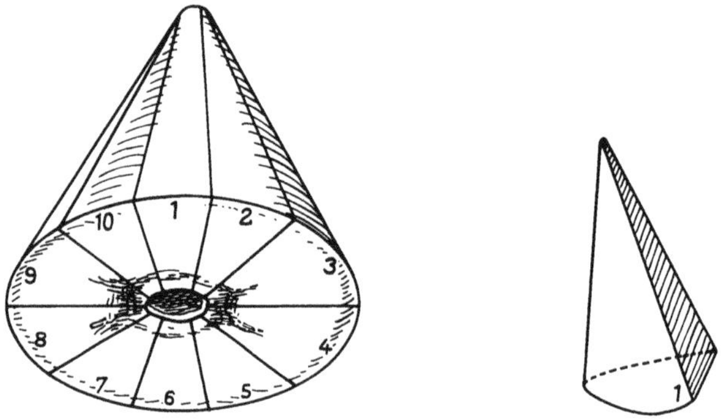

Fig. 114. Division of a cervix into sectors for embedding in paraffin

There is one limitation to our material prepared in this manner: in most cases the survey sections have been prepared as mentioned. The remaining material is in the paraffin blocks, from which the sections have been made, and they still contain tissue about 0.2 to 0.5 cm in thickness. This material has not yet been studied. Two errors may result:

First, a few so-called "false positive" cytological cases might still have a histological basis, were the whole material thoroughly studied. Second, the histological diagnosis in the classification of HAMPERL's groups was made from the most severe change found in all sections. It is therefore possible that some cases classified in a group would advance to a higher group if the remaining material were serially sectioned and studied (BURGHARDT, 1962). We believe, however, that such an error is small because early invasion of the stroma, for example, is always spread out and therefore appears in the survey sections also.

This kind of large histologic section is used similarly by BURGHARDT and BAJARDI in Graz, and by MORICARD in Paris. MACMILLAN (1960) also pointed out that only multiple serial cervical sections can confirm or disprove a cytological suspicion.

Another widely used histological technique for portios should be mentioned here, namely, the division of the portio into sectors, as illustrated in Fig. 114.

The portio is divided into eight to twelve sectors to obtain eight to twelve wedgelike segments. The narrow side of the wedge faces the cervical canal. It is usually very thin and tends to be slightly distorted and uneven during fixation and embedding. As a consequence, when the paraffin blocks are planed for final sectioning, a section of the cervical canal is lost from each block; that is, eight to twelve sections may be lost. For this reason we do not favor this method (Krone, 1960; Boyes and Fidler, 1960; Mestwerdt and Wespi, 1961).

Results of Treatment, Recurrence, Follow-Up

As mentioned previously, the **treatment** of carcinoma in situ at the gynecological clinic of the University of Cologne consisted either in conization or hysterectomy, depending on the patient's age. In Fig. 115 a summary of 161 cases

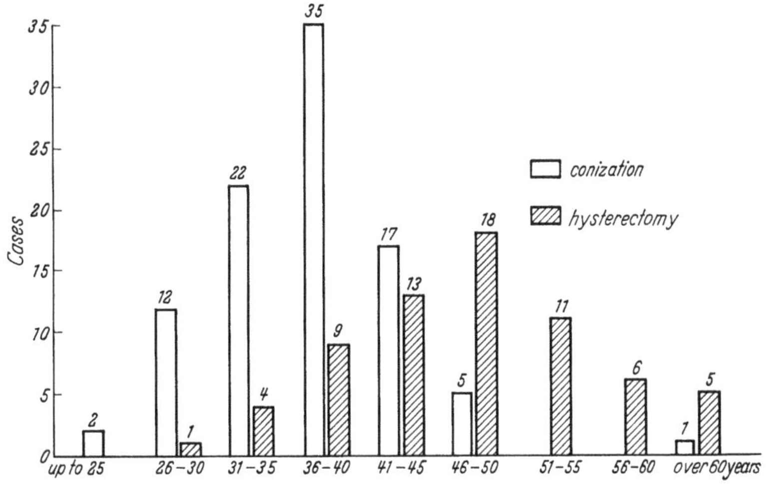

Fig. 115. Surgical operations for treatment of carcinoma in situ according to the patient's age (Theiss, 1963)

demonstrates the relation between conization and hysterectomy. Whenever a hysterectomy was performed prior to the fortieth year of age, other incidental genital diseases played a role in the indication for hysterectomy.

The histological preparation of the cervix of all patients who had been treated by hysterectomy proved that the lesion was totally removed. All these patients are to date in good health with no indication of recurrence.

In 89% of all cases treated by conization, the histological preparation indicated that the lesion was removed completely (Ober and Bötzelen, 1959). This percentage appears to be very high in comparison with other reports. We ascribe this high percentage to the shape of the cone excised, individually adapted in each case to ensure definitive therapy. The lesion had not been removed completely by Scott and Reagan (1956) in about 60%, and by Grünberger and Margreiter in 40% of the cases. Fettig and Hillemanns (1962) reported that more than 34.5% had not been removed completely by conization.

Our patients in whom conization had not totally removed the carcinoma in situ remained under close cytological observation. In most patients, the cytological result was, to our surprise, negative. Our explanation is that the remnant was small and therefore destroyed during healing of the wound, or that the spread of the carcinoma in situ coincided precisely with the edge of the incision. The cytological follow-ups revealed two cases with remnants of the epithelial lesion still present. Hysterectomy was subsequently performed in both cases. WAGNER (1961) reported that in 17% of his cases a "cytological recurrence" appeared after ring biopsy, conization, or amputation of the portio. A second excision in the shape of a cone was occasionally performed in young women, whereas hysterectomy was performed in the other cases of this kind.

None of the patients treated by conization shows any indication of a recurrence.

In summary, it can be said that in our entire group of patients the early treated cases to date show neither local recurrence nor indication of distant metastases.

Reports on **recurrences** after treatment of carcinoma in situ are difficult to compare because the term "recurrence" has been subjected to various interpretations. Remnants of markedly atypical epithelium cannot actually be termed recurrences. Those cases should be considered recurrences in which a carcinoma in situ develops again, even though the entire primary lesion was definitely removed. The question of definition of a recurrence is closely related to the care exercised and the method used in histologic studies. KOTTMEIER (1961), for example, reports 13 infiltrating carcinomas after 144 amputations of the portio had been performed for carcinoma in situ. KOSS, MELAMED and DANIEL (1961) found seven carcinomas in situ from 1 to 17 years after the treatment of cervical carcinoma had been completed. A carcinoma in situ 2.5 cm^2 in size was found on the posterior vaginal wall by CARTER, SALVAGGIO and JARKOWSKI (1961) 6 months after hysterectomy had been performed for carcinoma in situ. GRAHAM and MEIGS as early as 1952 reported three cases of recurrences 6, 7 and 10 years after hysterectomy for carcinoma in situ.

Recurrences may undoubtedly develop wherever squamous epithelium abuts columnar epithelium; that is, in the same circumstances that obtained prior to the appearance of the primary carcinoma in situ. To prevent the reapproximation of squamous and columnar epithelia and the resulting "unrest" at the border, we endeavor to remove the entire area of the cervical glands during conization. There is, of course, no such proximity after a hysterectomy; other etiological factors must therefore be present in the secondary malignant transformation of the squamous epithelium when recurrences occur in the vaginal vault. Generally, however, the danger of cervical carcinoma is eliminated in any patient in whom the boundary between squamous and columnar epithelia has been removed.

PEMBERTON and SMITH expressed this idea as early as 1929, when they considered the removal of any condition furthering the development of a neoplasm, by means of the prophylactic plastic surgery of EMMET, cauterization, or amputation of the portio. Similar efforts were also reported by other authors (GREENTREE, 1951; SCHMIDT-ELMENDORFF, 1954; GRÜNBERGER, 1959; JUNGHANS and WAITZ, 1960; and BREITNER, 1962).

An interesting consideration was reported by JUNGHANS and SACHS (1962), who contrasted a group of patients treated prophylactically with a group of untreated patients. The prophylactic treatment consisted in removal of the cervical glandular area with its usually inflammatory changes. No cervical carcinomas appeared in the first group, but there was a high morbidity rate equal to that of neoplasms in other locations. This idea is pertinent to the basic principles of early diagnosis of cancer, as well as to the meaning of all medical care in general.

The success of treatment after conization consists not only in the removal of the epithelial atypia, but also in the preservation of the menstrual cycle and of fertility.

The cycle remained undisturbed in all of our patients, and we have to date not observed stenosis of the internal os after conization. Complaints of dysmenorrhea or dyspareunia are very rare. Intermenstrual bleeding occurs occasionally.

The evaluation of fertility is influenced by the patient's age. The largest percentage of patients is within the fourth decade of life, when fertility is generally declining. BURGHARDT (1961) studied the problem of fertility after conization and after flat as well as high amputation of the portio. He summarized his observations as follows:

> After operation, 42 (18.1%) out of 232 women of childbearing age conceived. Half of the pregnancies occurred during the first year after operation. A total of 57 pregnancies occurred (26 births at full term, 10 premature births, 13 miscarriages, 1 tubal pregnancy, and 7 pregnancies still in progress at the time of the observation). The tendency to abort seemed greater after high amputation of the portio than after flat amputations or conization.

YOUNGE and KEVORKIAN (1959) emphasized the capacity for childbearing after conization. The possibility of giving birth is often of decisive significance to the individual patient.

Follow-up on Patients. Women treated by conization or hysterectomy for an early lesion need careful follow-up as much as patients with clinical cancer do. A card file is kept on our patients, who are checked every three months during the first year, semiannually in the second and third years, and once a year thereafter. The examination at follow-up includes inspection of the vaginal vault or the portio with the speculum, colposcopy, cytology, and SCHILLER's iodine test with subsequent manual pelvic examination.

Suggestions to the Clinician Regarding the Search for Incipient Gynecological Cancer

YOUNGE (1957) entitled one of his papers on the early stages of cervical carcinoma: "Cancer of the uterine cervix. A preventable disease". Cervical carcinoma could indeed be a preventable disease if comprehensive early detection were practicable. Unfortunately, however, a chasm still divides theory from practice, a chasm created by ignorance as well as by difficulties with organization and personnel. All concerned with early detection agree that as many women as possible over 30 should be examined prophylactically. For those, however, who have seen a 19 year old with a far advanced cervical carcinoma, comprehensive prophylaxis would have to include considerably younger women (COPENHAVER, 1960; HELD, 1960). Observations made by FERGUSON (1961), who found positive cytologic smears in young girls, also indicate the advisability of a lower age limit.

What are the ideas advanced in the cause of cancer prevention?

Many examples prove that specialists in gynecology as well as general practitioners employ good methods of early detection in their offices. ZIMMER (1957 I, II; 1959 I, II) proved by several comparative studies the efficiency of one physician's practice in the fields of cytology and colposcopy. FARK and SPRANGER (1959) and MARTIN and HARRICHHAUSEN (1961) urged that every doctor's office become a center for cancer prevention.

It is true that there is a prevalent impression that the detection of the early stage of cancer is, in practice, a "hobby", whereas most practicing physicians for various reasons do not or cannot work in this area. The opinion is widely held that the general practitioner cannot be expected to take on this additional burden, and it is for this reason that the organization of information centers for cancer has been promoted. BICKENBACH (1954) has discussed their problems in detail. PHILIPP (1955) spoke in their support, declaring that information centers for cancer will be necessary until the examination of healthy women is encompassed by the respective health plan. He considered the information centers for cancer to be in no sense competitive with the office practice of the physician. NEVERMANN (1955) pointed to the undercurrent of distrust of practicing physicians for information centers and thought that such centers would be unnecessary if the practitioner were paid for his advice on cancer; this plan has, unfortunately, not yet been put into effect.

According to DITTRICH, SCHMERMUND and SIEGEL (1956) the best results were obtained by collaboration between practitioner and cancer center, consisting in screening by the practitioner and special examination at the cancer center (DEIS, 1952; SCHROEDER, 1953; WASCHKE, 1952, 1954; BURGHARDT, 1957). v. MIKULICZ-RADECKI (1957) expressed the opinion that the early detection of cancer was not the realm of the practitioner, and that his contribution would be sufficiently important were he to recognize clinical carcinoma that permitted diagnosis on first sight in 80% of cases. CRAMER, FRITSCH and GEPPERT (1957) requested that more cancer information centers be organized, because those already in operation had demonstrated their efficiency but were too few in number. The number of cancer information centers in Nordrhein-Westfalen had risen to 179 by 1959 (WEBER, 1959). Nevertheless, only a fraction of the female population undergoes examination.

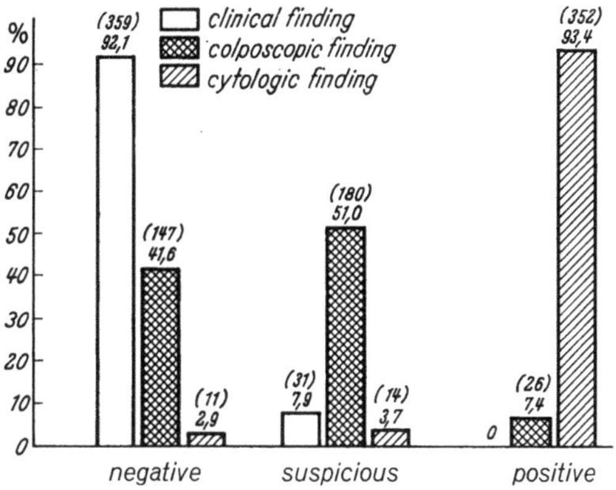

Fig. 116. Clinical, colposcopic, and cytologic findings in early lesions of the cervix uteri (THEISS, 1963)

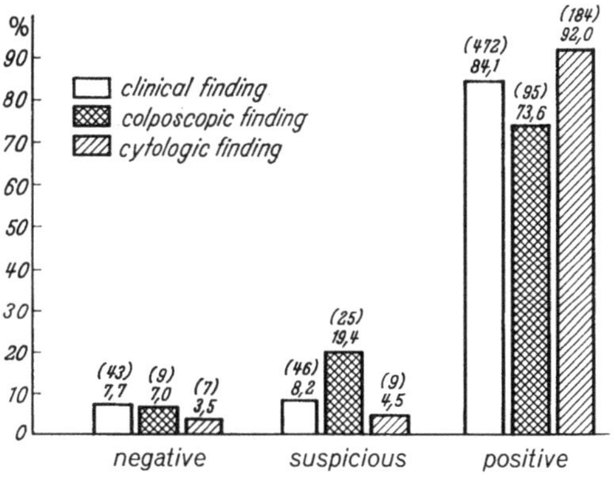

Fig. 117. Clinical, colposcopic, and cytologic finding in clinical carcinomas of the cervix (THEISS, 1963)

Progress has been achieved in the dispute about "how and by whom" early detection should be pursued by the organization of laboratories, similar to institutes of pathology, for the study of cytological material sent to them. Some of them are affiliated with institutes of pathology; others are independent. Thus, the argument that cytology, in comparison with colposcopy, is too expensive for the practicing physician is in part invalidated (WESPI, 1959; KRAKE, 1960). Sampling of the cytological material is not more time-consuming than the colposcopic examination, although the time needed for transportation must be added. Excellent suggestions for the practical collection of smears and their transportation have been made by KAUFMANN and FIEGE (1950), FREMONT-SMITH and GRAHAM (1952), BACH and STOLL (1953), SMOLKA (1958), BOSCHANN (1960), SOOST (1960 I, II), GRAHAM (1960) and ANTOINE (1960).

In conclusion, we shall try to make suggestions for a meaningful attack by the practicing physician on the early detection of cancer and the sequence of the steps to be taken if indicated by the findings.

Once more, the decisive differences between clinical, colposcopic, and cytologic findings in carcinoma in situ and cervical carcinoma are shown in Figs. 116 and 117. Cervical carcinoma permits a diagnosis on first direct examination in 80% of the cases. Carcinoma in situ cannot be detected thus. The detection of this precancerous condition of the cervix is the aim of any prophylactic examination.

What Can the Practicing Physician Do?

1. Every woman in the childbearing age when consulting her physician should be advised of the necessity of a prophylactic gynecological examination.

2. When the portio is exposed with the speculum but a colposcopic or cytologic examination is not feasible, the iodine test should definitely be performed. If the entire surface of the portio turns brown-black, the certainty that there is no malignancy on the portio is 99%. If there are iodine-negative or iodine-light areas, the patient should be referred to the appropriate place for additional examination (a specialist or a cancer information center) (MAMZACK, 1955; WEILL and DELAGE, 1959). The number of women who can be eliminated as entirely healthy is, unfortunately, not very large — only one fourth of all patients.

3. If inspection of the surface of the portio with the colposcope is feasible, suspicious findings must be checked very carefully. Positive findings require histological clarification. It is very important to recognize that endocervical lesions remain hidden from the colposcope and that even those carcinomas in situ that are on the surface of the portio cannot be distinguished with certainty from normal epithelium colposcopically. Thus, clearly benign changes cannot be differentiated with the colposcope. The colposcope is very helpful in the evaluation of SCHILLER's iodine test.

4. If cytologic smears can be sent out for examination, very useful information may thus be gained, but the smears must be taken very carefully in contact with the epithelium, fixed, and protected from damage during transportation.

If the cytologic examination points to Groups I or II, the patient should be advised to return after one or two years. If the diagnosis is Group III, the smears must be repeated until an unequivocal cytological report is obtained, positive or negative. If the diagnosis Group III is combined with the indication of dysplastic epithelium, a cytologic check must be performed every 3 months. If the result is Group IV or V, there is more than 90% certainty of a malignant neoplasm on the portio, and histologic verification is required.

5. If histologic verification becomes necessary on the basis of a positive colposcopic or cytologic finding, it should be entrusted to a special clinic. Any small biopsy is unreliable. Conization must be considered the method of choice. The histologic preparation for the verification of the diagnosis should be performed in laboratories specially experienced in this area of gynecological histo-

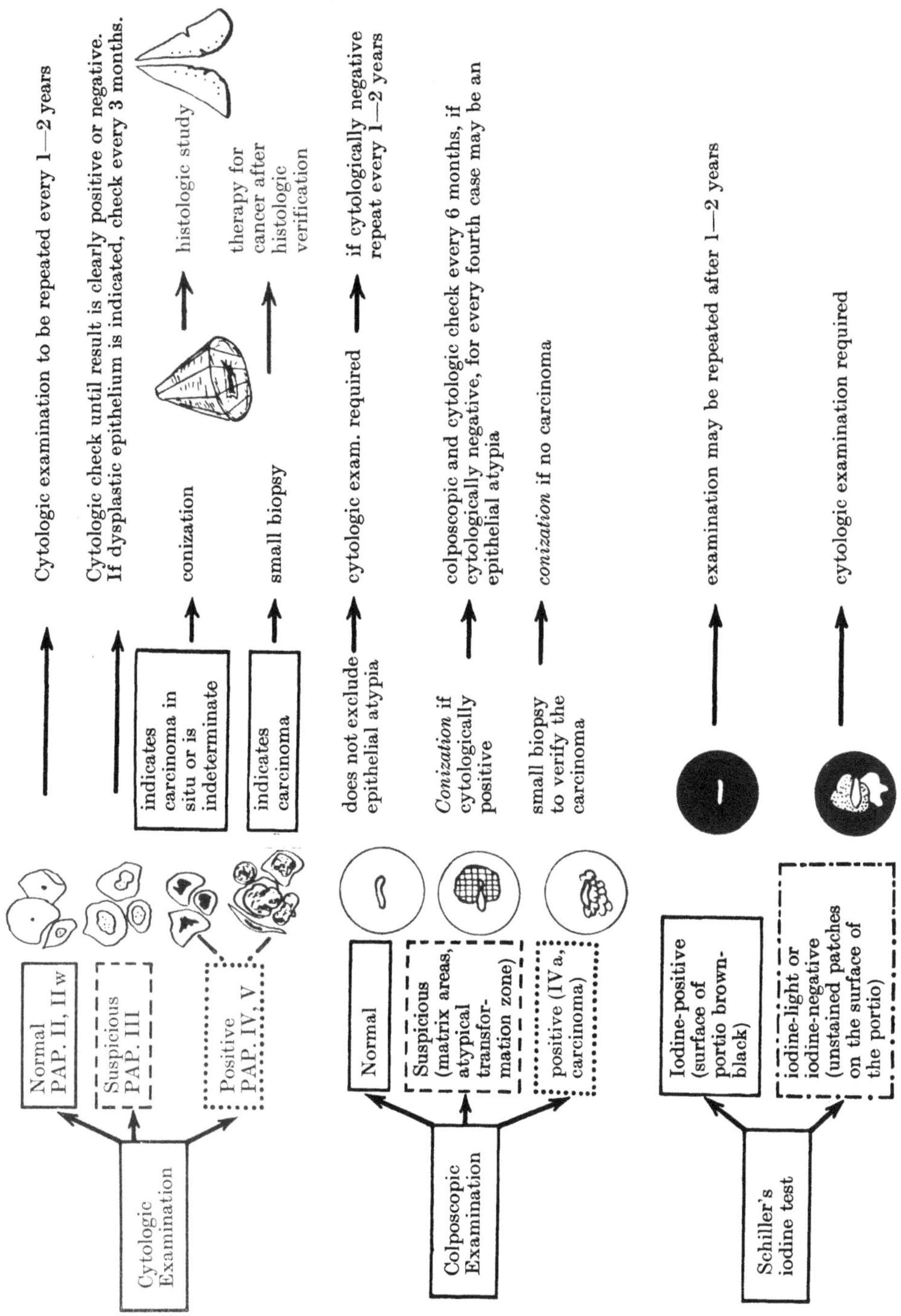

Fig. 118. Summary of examinations for early detection, their results, and their practical significance

pathology. The preparation of multiple serial histologic sections of the cervix uteri should be obligatory to confirm or refute a finding indicative of malignancy. Fig. 118 shows the steps to be taken in the search for incipient cancer.

References

ACHENBACH, R. R., R. E. JOHNSTONE, and A. T. HERTIG: The validity of vaginal smear diagnosis in carcinoma in situ of the cervix. Amer. J. Obstet. Gynec. **61**, 385—392 (1951).

ANDERSON, A. F.: The occurrence of dyscaryotic cells in carcinoma in situ. Acta cytol. (Chic.) **1** (1), 44 (1957).

— The management of the cytology test. J. Obstet. Gynaec. Brit. Emp. **66**, 239—246 (1959).

ANDERSON, W. A. D., and S. A. GUNN: Cytologic detection of cancer — consideration of its future: A comparative examination of the Papanicolaou and Acridin-Orange technics. Acta cytol. (Philad.) **6**, 468—470 (1962).

ANTOINE, T.: Zytodiagnostisches gynäkologisches Zentrum. Krebsarzt **14**, 477—478 (1959).

— Was kann der Praktiker von der Zytologie erwarten? Krebsarzt **15**, 233—234 (1960).

— K. BRANDL, V. GRÜNBERGER, E. KOFLER, H. KREMER, and W. WALZ: Inspection technics for carcinoma in situ. (Symposium.) Colpomicroscopy of carcinoma in situ. Acta cytol. (Philad.) **5**, 412—415 (1961).

— A. GRABNER u. V. GRÜNBERGER: Die Kolpomikroskopie. Mikroskopie 8, 73—83 (1953).

—, u. V. GRÜNBERGER: Atlas der Kolpomikroskopie. Stuttgart: Georg Thieme 1956.

AYRE, J. E.: A simple office test for uterine cancer diagnosis. Canad. med. Ass. J. **51**, 17—22 (1944).

— Vaginal cell examination as a routine in diagnosis. A study of vaginal and cervical cytology as related to abnormal growths. Sth. med. J. (Bgham, Ala.) **39**, 847—852 (1946).

— Vaginal and cervical cytology in uterine cancer diagnosis. Amer. J. Obstet. Gynec. **51**, 743—748 (1946).

— Selective cytology smear for diagnosis of cancer. Amer. J. Obstet. Gynec. **53**, 609—617 (1947).

— Diagnosis of preclinical cancer of the cervix. Cervical cone knife: Its use in patients with a positive vaginal smear. J. Amer. med. Ass. **138**, 11—13 (1948).

— The vaginal smear. "Precancer" cell studies using a modified technique. Amer. J. Obstet. Gynec. **58**, 1205—1219 (1949).

— Cancer cytology of the uterus. Introducing a concept of cervical cell pathology. New York: Grune & Stratton 1951.

— Early cancer detection: prediction of preclinical and preinvasive stages by cytology. Acta Un. int. Cancr. **15**, 289—295 (1959).

— Role of the halo cell in cervical cancerigenesis. A virus manifestation in premalignancy? Obstet. and Gynec. **15**, 481—491 (1960).

—, and W. B. AYRE: Progression from "precancer" stage to early carcinoma of cervix within one year. Combined cytologic and histologic study with report of a case. Amer. J. clin. Path. **19**, 770—778 (1949).

—, and E. DAKIN: Cervical cytology tests in cancer diagnosis: Glycerine technique for mailing. Canad. med. Ass. J. **54**, 489—491 (1946).

—, and J. W. SCOTT: Carcinoma in situ in pregnancy. J. Amer. med. Ass. **176**, 102—105 (1961).

BACH, G. H., u. P. STOLL: Gynäkologische Zytologie in der Sprechstunde. Münch. med. Wschr. **95**, 1149—1151 (1953).

BAHRENBERG (1895): Zit. nach G. N. PAPANICOLAOU. Acta Un. int. Cancr. (Brux.) **14**, 249—254 (1958).

BAJARDI, F.: Beitrag zur Frage der prospektiven Bedeutung des nicht invasiven atypischen Plattenepithels des Collum uteri. Z. Geburtsh. Gynäk. **152**, 340—348 (1959).

— Material obtained by cervical scraping only. Symposium. Acta cytol. (Chic.) **4**, 242—245 (1960).

BAJARDI, F.: Über Wachstumsbeschränkungen des Collumcarcinoms in seinem invasiven und auch präinvasiven Stadium. Zugleich ein Beitrag zur formalen Genese pathologischen Gebärmutterhalsepithels. Arch. Gynäk. **197**, 407—454 (1962).

— J. A. BRET, F. COUPEZ, W. R. LANG, and W. WALZ: Colposcopy of leucoplakia. Symposium. Acta cytol. (Philad.) **5**, 115—124 (1961).

— J. A. DE BRUX, J. DUPRÉ-FROMENT, E. SIEGLER, C. SIRTORI, and C. W. TAYLOR: Histomorphology of carcinoma in situ. Symposium. Acta cytol. (Philad.) **5**, 271—284 (1961).

—, u. E. BURGHARDT: Ergebnisse von histologischen Serienschnittuntersuchungen beim Carcinoma colli 0. Arch. Gynäk. **189**, 392—403 (1957).

— — H. KERN et H. KROEMER: Nouveaux résultats de la cytologie et de la colposcopie systématiques dans le diagnostic précoce du cancer du col de l'utérus. Gynéc. prat. **10**, 315—329 (1959).

— M. GAUDEFROY, R. KRIMMENAU, and C. W. TAYLOR: Symposion on probable or malignant cervical lesions-carcinoma in situ. I. Histology of carcinoma in situ. What is not carcinoma in situ? Symposium. Acta cytol. (Philad.) **5**, 331—339 (1961).

—, and C. SIRTORI: The atypical non-invasive zones around invasive cervical carcinoma. Symposium. Acta cytol. (Philad.) **5**, 355—358 (1961).

BANGEN, H., A. FOCKEN u. G. FRANZ: Neue Gesichtspunkte zum Problem der Frühdiagnostik des Collumcarcinoms. Arch. Gynäk. **196**, 67—95 (1961).

BANGLE, R., M. BERGER, and M. LEVIN: Variations in the morphogenesis of squamous carcinoma. Cancer (Philad.) **16**, 1151—1159 (1963).

BEALE, L. S. (1860): Zit. nach G. N. PAPANICOLAOU. Acta Un. int. Cancr. (Burx.) **14**, 249—254 (1958).

BECHTOLD, E., and N. B. REICHER: The relationship of trichomonas infestations to false diagnoses of squamous carcinoma of the cervix. Cancer (Philad.) **5**, 442—457 (1952).

BEDOYA, J. M., L. R. RICO y G. RIOS: Problemas de la tricomoniasis genital. II. Causas de las resistencias al tratamiento y de las recidivas. Acta gynaec. obstet. hisp.-lusit. **5**, 324—329 (1956).

BEECHAM, C. T., and G. J. ANDROS: Cervical conization in pregnancy. Obstet. and Gynec. **16**, 521—526 (1960).

—, and J. P. EMICH Jr.: Carcinoma in situ. Obstet. and Gynec. **13**, 653—656 (1959).

BEHRENS, H.: Was leistet die Probeabschabung von der Portio uteri bei der Diagnose des Frühcarcinoms? Arch. Gynäk. **190**, 126—145 (1957/58).

—, u. K. TIETZE: Über das Regeneratepithel an der Portio vaginalis uteri und seine Abgrenzung gegenüber dem sogenannten „Oberflächencarcinom". Arch. Geschwulstforsch. **15**, 8—18 (1959).

BEJANCON et DE JONG (1913): Zit. nach G. N. PAPANICOLAOU. Acta Un. int. Cancr. (Brux.) **14**, 249—254 (1958).

BERGER, J.: Wahl und Leistungsfähigkeit der Methoden in der Früherfassung des Collumkarzinoms. Schweiz. med. Wschr. **84**, 860—867 (1954).

— Importance de l'examen histologique des biopsies au niveau du col utérin et des coupes en série. (Localisation topographique.) Gynéc. et Obstét. **58**, 134—137 (1959).

—, et H. WENNER-MANGEN: La colposcopie. Son importance dans l'examen du col. Son intérêt dans le dépistage du cancer au début. Gynéc. et Obstét. **52**, 303—324 (1953).

BERIĆ, B., u. H. SMOLKA: Über den Einfluß der in der Kolposkopie angewandten Reagenzien auf das Zellbild des Portioabstriches. Geburtsh. u. Frauenheilk. **18**, 852—864 (1958).

BERTALANFFY, F. D.: Fluorescence microscope method for detection of pulmonary malignancies. Canad. med. Ass. J. **83**, 211—212 (1960) (I).

— Cytodiagnosis of cancer using acridine orange with fluorescence microscopy. Cancer Bull. (Amer. Cancer Soc.) **10**, 118—123 (1960) (II).

— Cytological cancer diagnosis in gynecology by fluorescence microscopy. Mod. Med. Can. **15**, 55—65 (1960) (III).

— Fluorescence microscopy for cytodiagnosis of cancer. Postgrad. Med. **28**, 627—633 (1960) (IV).

— A new method for cytologic diagnosis of cancer. Spectrum (Pfizer Laboratories) 8, 170—174 (1960) (V).

BERTALANFFY, L. v.: Eine fluorescenzmikroskopische Schnellmethode zur Diagnose des gynäkologischen Carcinoms. Klin. Wschr. **37**, 469—471 (1959).
—, and I. BICKIS: Identification of cytoplasmic basophilia (ribonucleic acid) by fluorescence microscopy. J. Histochem. Cytochem. **4**, 481—493 (1956).
— F. MASIN, and M. MASIN: Use of acridine orange fluorescence technique in exfoliative cytology. Science **124**, 1024—1025 (1956).
— M. MASIN, F. MASIN, and L. KAPLAN: Detection of gynecological cancer. Use of fluorescence microscopy to show nucleic acids in malignant growth. Calif. Med. **87**, 248—251 (1957).
— — — — A new and rapid method for diagnosis of vaginal and cervical cancer by fluorescence microscopy. Cancer (Philad.) **11**, 873—887 (1958).
BICKENBACH, W.: Landarzt und Früherfassung gynäkologischer Karcinome. Landarzt **30**, 7—12 (1954).
— H. A. KRONE u. W. JANS: Bericht über 430 Elektrokonisationen der Portio. Geburtsh. u. Frauenheilk. **20**, 97—107 (1960).
—, and H. J. SOOST: Material obtained by three techniques: (a) Vaginal smears, (b) cervical smears and (c) endocervical smears. Symposium. Acta cytol. (Chic.) **4**, 252—256 (1960).
— — J. R. DE C. CAMPOS, H. K. FIDLER, and D. A. BOYES: What percentage of cervices show early invasion in serial histological sections in uteri which were removed under the biopsy diagnosis of "carcinoma in situ"? Symposium. Acta cytol. (Philad.) **5**, 340—344 (1961).
BLAIKLEY, J. B., H. L. KOTTMEIER, H. MARTIUS, and J. V. MEIGS: Classification and clinical staging of carcinoma of the uterus. A proposal for modification of the existing international definitions. Amer. J. Obstet. Gynec. **75**, 1286—1291 (1958).
BLANCHARD, O.: Carcinoma "in situ" del cuello uterino? J. int. Coll. Surg. **34**, 387—391 (1960).
BLUMENTHAL, E. D., and E. L. HECHT: Cellular changes associated with inflammation. Ann. N.Y. Acad. Sci. **63**, 1270—1279 (1956).
BOCK, E.: Zur mikroskopischen Diagnose von Geschwülsten der Pleura aus Punktionsflüssigkeit. Klin. Wschr. **4**, 651—652 (1925).
BODDINGTON, M. M., R. H. COWDELL, and A. I. SPRIGGS: Development of carcinoma of the cervix uteri. Observations resulting from cytological examination of 10000 cervical smears. Brit. J. Cancer **14**, 151—164 (1960).
BOEGELICK (1878): Zit. nach G. N. PAPANICOLAOU. Acta Un. int. Cancr. (Brux.) **14**, 249—254 (1958).
BONTKE, E., G. KERN u. N. SCHÜMMELFEDER: Die Akridinorange-Fluorochromierung in der gynäkologischen Zytodiagnostik. Geburtsh. u. Frauenheilk. **20**, 24—34 (1960).
BORY, R., et J. CURTZ: Les lésions dystrophiques du col et le glycogène cervical. Rev. franç. Gynéc. **51**, 121—127 (1956).
—, et H. WENNER-MANGEN: Test de Schiller et frottis vaginaux. Rev. franç. Gynéc. **50**, 161—164 (1955).
BOSCHANN, H. W.: The modus operandi of a cytology center. Acta Un. int. Cancr. (Brux.) **14**, 386—392 (1958).
— Praktische Zytologie. Berlin: W. de Gruyter & Co. 1960.
BOSCHETTI, M.: Il glicogene e le biopsie uterine. Atti Soc. ital. Obstet. **27**, 517—521 (1929).
BOTELLA LLUSIÁ, J.: Histoquimica de las atipias epiteliales del cuello uterino y del carcinoma grado 0. Obstet. Ginec. lat.-amer. **16**, 43—47 (1958).
BOYD, J. R., D. ROYLE, H. K. FIDLER, and D. A. BOYES: Conservative management of in situ carcinoma of the cervix. Amer. J. Obstet. Gynec. **85**, 322—327 (1963).
BOYES, D. A., and H. K. FIDLER: A technique to increase the value of a cone biopsy from the cervix. Cancer (Philad.) **13**, 634—635 (1960).
— — Cervical cancer control program in British Columbia. Amer. J. Obstet. Gynec. **85**, 328—331 (1963).
— — and D. R. LOCK: Significance of in situ carcinoma of the uterine cervix. Brit. med. J. **27**, 203—205 (1962).
BRANDL, K., u. E. KOFLER: Die Krebsfrüherkennungsmethoden bei 230 Fällen mit Kollumkarzinom. Geburtsh. u. Frauenheilk. **19**, 415—420 (1959).

BREITNER, J.: Zur Prophylaxe der Genitalkarzinome der Frau. Münch. med. Wschr. **104**, 118—122 (1962).
BRET, J., et F. COUPEZ: Colposcopie. Paris: Masson & Cie. 1960.
— — R. GANSE, O. NYKLIČEK, and H. K. ZINSER: Colposcopy of Ectopy, Ectropion and Epidermization. Acta cytol. (Philad.) **5**, 83—90 (1961).
BRODERS, A. C.: Carcinoma in situ contrasted with benign penetrating epithelium. J. Amer. med. Ass. **99**, 1670—1674 (1932).
BRUNSCHWIG, A.: A method for mass screening for cytological detection of carcinoma of the cervix uteri. Cancer (Philad.) **7**, 1182—1184 (1954).
BRUX, J. DE: Diskussionsbemerkung zu: The occurence of dyscaryotic cells in carcinoma in situ. Acta cytol. (Chic.) **1** (1), 45 (1957).
—, et J. DUPRÉ-FROMENT: Le carcinome intra-épithélial du col utérin doit-il être démembré? Étude histologique et cytologique. Gynéc. et Obstét. **59**, 457—477 (1960).
— — J. R. DE C. CAMPOS, and B. C. HOPMAN: Exfoliative cytology and experimental cytology of carcinoma in situ. Symposium. Can carcinoma in situ be differentiated from invasive carcinoma by means of exfoliative cytology? Acta cytol. (Philad.) **5**, 439—445 (1961).
— — R. M. GRAHAM, E. v. HAAM, and E. E. SIEGLER: Exfoliative cytology and experimental cytology of carcinoma in situ. Symposium. Cytomorphology of carcinoma in situ. Acta cytol. (Philad.) **5**, 422—436 (1961).
— A. RAUZY, and J. DUPRÉ-FROMENT: Occurrence of spindle-shaped-squamoid cells in carcinoma in situ. Acta cytol. (Chic.) **2**, 248—258 (1958).
BUCHHOLZ, H. F.: Beitrag zur breiteren Anwendung der Vaginalzytologie durch eine Trockenfixierung. Zbl. Gynäk. **81**, 498—501 (1959).
BÜNGELER, W.: Der Begriff der Praecancerose. Strahlentherapie **96**, 296—305 (1955).
—, u. W. DONTENWILL: Über den Begriff der Präcancerose unter besonderer Berücksichtigung der Mastopathie und des atypischen Portioepithels. Med. Klin. **39**, 1589—1601 (1954).
BURGHARDT, E.: Die vorbeugende Untersuchung beim Portiokarzinom als Aufgabe in der Allgemeinpraxis. Wien. klin. Wschr. **69**, 253—255 (1957).
— Das Verhalten des Stratum basale des Portioepithels in der Peripherie präinvasiver und invasiver Portiokarzinome. Krebsarzt **13**, 287—292 (1958).
— Über die atypische Umwandlungszone. Geburtsh. u. Frauenheilk. **19**, 676—683 (1959).
— Graviditäten nach Ringbiopsien, Konisationen und Portioamputationen. Geburtsh. u. Frauenheilk. **21**, 225—236 (1961).
— Die bioptische Abklärung der suspekten Portio. Wien. med. Wschr. **112**, 738—742 (1962).
— Die diagnostische Konisation der Portio vaginalis uteri. Operationstechnik, histologische Diagnostik und klinische Ergebnisse. Geburtsh. u. Frauenheilk. **23**, 1—30 (1963).
— Zur Operationstechnik der diagnostischen Konisation. Geburtsh. u. Frauenheilk. **23**, 548—551 (1963).
—, u. F. BAJARDI: Ergebnisse der Früherfassung des Collumcarcinoms mittels Cytologie und Kolposkopie an der Universitäts-Frauenklinik Graz 1954. Arch. Gynäk. **187**, 621—637 (1956).
CAMPOS, J. R. DE C., E. SCHÜLLER, and C. W. TAYLOR: What constitutes a definite diagnosis of carcinoma in situ with special reference to the amount of histological sections required ("serial sections") and type of material? Symposium. Acta cytol. (Philad.) **5**, 284—289 (1961).
CARTER, B., K. CUYLER, L. A. KAUFMANN, W. L. THOMAS, R. N. CREADICK, R. T. PARKER, C. H. PEETE, and W. B. CHERNY: Clinical problems in stage 0 (intraepithelial) cancer of the cervix. Amer. J. Obstet. Gynec. **71**, 634—652 (1956).
— — W. L. THOMAS, R. CREADICK, and R. ALTER: The methods of management of carcinoma in situ of the cervix. Amer. J. Obstet. Gynec. **64**, 833—849 (1952).
CARTER, E. R., A. T. SALVAGGIO, and T. L. JARKOWSKI: Squamous cell carcinoma of the vagina following vaginal hysterectomy for intraepithelial carcinoma of the cervix. Amer. J. Obstet. Gynec. **82**, 401—404 (1961).
CHAPPAZ, G., CHATELLIER, BAZELAIRE et GRUET: Comment évolue le "problème" de la trichomonase génitale? Gynéc. et Obstét. **54**, 87—113 (1955).
CHRISTOPHERSON, W. M., and J. E. PARKER: A study of the relative frequency of carcinoma of the cervix in the Negro. Cancer (Philad.) **13**, 711—713 (1960).

CITTI, U.: La "diskariosis" nella citologia cervicale. Ann. Ostet. Ginec. **83**, 147—161 (1961).

CLAUSS, J.: Zur histologischen Sicherung zytologischer Befunde, insbesondere durch Ringexzision. Geburtsh. u. Frauenheilk. **16**, 1104—1111 (1956).

— Möglichkeiten und Grenzen der Zytologie in Klinik und Praxis. Geburtsh. u. Frauenheilk. **18**, 90 (1958).

COPENHAVER, E. H.: The pathology, diagnosis and management of preinvasive carcinoma of the cervix. Lahey Clin. Bull. **11**, 214—223 (1960).

COUTIFARIS, B., u. L. COUTIFARIS: Die „Dyskariose" im Zusammenhang mit „Dysplasie" und präinvasivem Kollumkarzinom. Zbl. Gynäk. **81**, 744—748 (1959).

CRAMER, H.: Zytologische Befunde im zervikalen Smear bei Endometritis und Cervicitis tuberculosa. Geburtsh. u. Frauenheilk. **11**, 809—816 (1951).

— Die Stellung der Kolposkopie innerhalb der Methoden zur Diagnose des Kollumkarzinoms. Dtsch. med. Wschr. **81**, 1553—1557, 1544, 1549 (1956).

— Ergebnisse mit der Krebsfrühdiagnostik am Collum uteri in den Jahren 1950—1955. Strahlentherapie **100**, 72—79 (1956).

— Vergleich zwischen Zytologie und Colposkopie in der Entdeckung von Frühkarzinom. Acta Un. int. Cancr. (Brux.) **14**, 337—339 (1958).

— Kritisches zum Begriff der sogenannten atypischen Umwandlungszone. Geburtsh. u. Frauenheilk. **21**, 706—712 (1961).

— Die Kolposkopie in der Praxis. Einführung in die gynäkologische Krebsfrühdiagnostik, 2. Aufl. Stuttgart: Georg Thieme 1962.

— K. FRITSCH u. M. P. GEPPERT: Die Bedeutung der Krebsberatungsstellen für die Früherfassung des gynäkologischen Karzinoms. Medizinische **1957**, 1161—1167.

—, u. E. LIND: Die endocervicale Lokalisation des Karzinoms und sog. Oberflächenkarzinoms am Gebärmutterhals unter diagnostischen Gesichtspunkten. Geburtsh. u. Frauenheilk. **22**, 161—171 (1962).

—, u. D. STAMM: Ein einfaches und zweckerfüllendes Färbeverfahren für die zytologische Krebsdiagnose aus dem Vaginal- und Zervixsekret. Geburtsh. u. Frauenheilk. **10**, 676—684 (1950).

CULLEN, T. S.: Cancer of the uterus. New York: D. Appleton & Co. 1900.

— Early squamous-cell carcinoma of the cervix. Surg. Gynec. Obstet. **33**, 137—144 (1921).

CUYLER, W. K.: Diskussionsbemerkung zu: The occurrence of dyscaryotic cells in carcinoma in situ. Acta cytol. (Chic.) **1** (1), 45 (1957).

— L. A. KAUFMANN, B. CARTER, R. A. ROSS, W. L. THOMAS, and L. PALUMBO: Genital cytology in obstetric and gynecologic patients. A four-year study. Amer. J. Obstet. Gynec. **62**, 262—275 (1951).

DART, L. H., and T. R. TURNER: Fluorescence microscopy in exfoliative cytology. Report of acridine orange examination of 5491 cases, with comparison by the Papanicolaou technic. Lab. Invest. 8, 1513—1522 (1959).

DECKER, W. H.: Minimal invasive carcinoma of the cervix with lymph node metastases. Report of a case. Amer. J. Obstet. Gynec. **72**, 1116—1119 (1956).

DEIMEL, H.: Ergebnisse zytologischer und kolposkopischer Untersuchungen im Rahmen der Karzinomprophylaxe. Zbl. Gynäk. **82**, 1735—1739 (1960).

DEIS, H.: Die Früherfassung des Uteruskarzinoms nach PAPANICOLAOU in Klinik und Praxis. Zbl. Gynäk. **74**, 418—429 (1952).

DICKINSON (1869): Zit. nach G. N. PAPANICOLAOU. Acta Un. int. Cancr. (Brux.) **14**, 249—254 (1958).

DIETEL, H.: Was wird aus dem nichtbehandelten atypischen Portioepithel? Arch. Gynäk. **183**, 557—558 (1953).

—, u. A. FOCKEN: Das Schicksal des atypischen Epithels an der Portio. Geburtsh. u. Frauenheilk. **15**, 593—606 (1955).

DITTRICH, W., H.-J. SCHMERMUND u. P. SIEGEL: Ergebnisse und Probleme der vorbeugenden Krebsberatung in der Gynäkologie. Dtsch. med. Wschr. **81**, 1856—1859 (1956).

DONNÉ (1838): Zit. nach G. N. PAPANICOLAOU. Acta Un. int. Cancr. (Brux.) **14**, 249—254 (1958).

DUBRAUSZKY, V., u. J. JAEGER: Akridinorange-Fluorochromierung in der vaginalen Zyklusdiagnostik. Med. Welt **1962**, 1359—1361.

DUDGEON, L. S., and C. V. PATRICK: New method for rapid microscopical diagnosis of tumours with account of 200 cases so examined. Brit. J. Surg. **15**, 250—261 (1927).
—, and C. H. WRIGLEY: On the demonstration of particles of malignant growth in the sputum by means of the wet-film method. J. Laryng. **50**, 752—762 (1935).
DUNN, J. E., Jr.: The epidemiologic aspects of cervical carcinoma as revealed by cytologic study. J. int. Coll. Surg. **34**, 720—725 (1960).
—, and P. BUELL: Association of cervical cancer with circumcision of sexual partner. J. nat. Cancer Inst. **22**, 749—764 (1959).
DUSTIN, P., Jr., et R. PARMENTIER: Données expérimentales sur la nature des mitoses anormales observées dans certains épithéliomas du col utérin. Gynéc. et Obstét. **52**, 258—265 (1953).
EBNER, H.: The use of other techniques in cytology. Acta Un. int. Cancr. (Brux.) **14**, 403—405 (1958).
EHRLICH, P. (1880): Zit. nach G. N. PAPANICOLAOU. Acta Un. int. Cancr. (Brux.) **14**, 249—254 (1958).
EHRLICH, P.: Beiträge zur Ätiologie und Histologie pleuritischer Exsudate. Charité-Ann. (Berl.) **7**, 199—230 (1882).
EISEN, K.: Kolposkopie in der täglichen Praxis. Zbl. Gynäk. **77**, 1425—1427 (1955).
ELEVITCH, F. R., and J. G. BRUNSON: Rapid identification of malignant cells in vaginal smears by cytoplasmic fluorescence. Surg. Gynec. Obstet. **112**, 3—10 (1961).
EMIG, O. R., and W. C. HUNTER: Definitive diagnosis of premalignant and early malignant lesions of the cervix. West. J. Surg. **69**, 280—285 (1961).
ERICKSON, C. C., B. E. EVERETT Jr., L. M. GRAVES, R. F. KAISER, R. A. MALMGREN, I. RUBE, P. C. SCHREIER, S. J. CUTLER, and D. H. SPRUNT: Population screening for uterine cancer by vaginal cytology. Preliminary summary of results of first examination of 108,000 women and second testing of 33,000 women. J. Amer. med. Ass. **162**, 167—173 (1956).
ESCHBACH, W., u. W. BRUCKER: Betrachtungen zur Genese und Klinik des Carcinoma colli uteri. I. Dtsch. Gesundh.-Wes. **14**, 2186—2191 (1959).
— — Betrachtungen zur Genese und Klinik des Carcinoma colli uteri. II. Dtsch. Gesundh.-Wes. **15**, 1243—1247 (1960).
FANGER, H., and T. H. MURPHY: Carcinoma in situ of the uterine cervix. Surg. Gynec. Obstet. **111**, 177—182 (1960).
FARK, M., u. J. SPRANGER: Möglichkeiten der Krebsverhütung. Erfahrungen mit dem Krebsverhütungsprogramm der USA. Krebsarzt **14**, 129—133 (1959).
FENNELL, R. H., Jr.: Carcinoma in situ of the cervix with early invasive changes. Cancer (Philad.) **8**, 302—309 (1955).
— Carcinoma in situ of the uterine cervix. A report of 118 cases. Cancer (Philad.) **9**, 374—384 (1956).
—, and R. M. GRAHAM: A serial-section study of the cervix in cases with positive vaginal smears and negative biopsies. A report of ten cases. Cancer (Philad.) **8**, 310—314 (1955).
FERGUSON, J. H.: Positive cancer smears in teenage girls. J. Amer. med. Ass. **178**, 365—368 (1961).
—, and G. C. BROWN: Cervical conization during pregnancy. Surg. Gynec. Obstet. **111**, 603—606 (1960).
—, and H. LOZMAN: Fate of women with positive cervical cytology. Sth. med. J. (Bgham, Ala.) **51**, 296—301 (1958).
—, and M. H. MATZ: Material obtained by two techniques: (a) Vaginal smears and (b) cervical smears. Symposium. Acta cytol. (Chic.) **4**, 246—251 (1960).
FERREIRA, DO AMARAL C., I. MENEZES y G. SCHNEIDER: Colpocitologia e tricomoniase. An. bras. Ginec. **49**, 289—294 (1960).
FETTIG, O., u. H. G. HILLEMANNS: Zur Technik und Klinik der Portiokonisation im Rahmen der Früherfassung des Collumcarcinoms. Med. Klin. **55**, 2131 (1960).
— — Die Zervixkonisation. Ein Beitrag zur Indikation, Technik und Klinik im Rahmen der Früherfassung des Kollumkarzinoms. Dtsch. med. Wschr. **87**, 1197—1201, 1204 (1962).
—, u. C. KÜHN: Konzeptionshäufigkeit, Schwangerschafts- und Geburtsverlauf nach Zervixkonisation. Geburtsh. u. Frauenheilk. **23**, 517—527 (1963).

FEYRTER, F.: Über das Oberflächenkarzinom im Bereich des Collum uteri. Histologischer Begriff. Biologischer Begriff. Pflasterepithelkrebs und Basalzellenkrebs. Erythroplasie, Bowen und Oberflächenkarzinom. Zur Frage der Latenz und der Rückbildung des Oberflächenkarzinoms. Dtsch. med. Wschr. **1955**, 1628—1632, 1649—1650, 1686—1691.
FIDLER, H. K.: Are spindle-shaped squamoid cells derived from the surface of the lesion? Acta cytol. (Chic.) **2**, 278—281 (1958).
—, and D. A. BOYES: Patterns of early invasion from intraepithelial carcinoma of the cervix. Cancer (Philad.) **12**, 673—680 (1959).
FINN, W. F.: The postoperative recognition and further management of unsuspected cervical carcinoma. Amer. J. Obstet. Gynec. **63**, 717—727 (1952).
FLEGEL, H.: Zur Anwendung der Fluorescenzmikroskopie in der Medizin. Wiss. Z. Friedrich-Schiller-Univ. Jena, math.-nat. Reihe **3**, 475—477 (1953/54).
FLUHMANN, C. F.: The developmental anatomy of the cervix uteri. Obstet. and Gynec. **15**, 62—69 (1960).
— Carcinoma in situ and the transitional zone of the cervix uteri. Obstet. and Gynec. **16**, 424—437 (1960).
—, and H. M. LYONS: Carcinoma in situ of the uterine cervix. Diagnosis by biopsy. Calif. Med. **92**, 194—197 (1960).
FOORD, A. G., G. E. YOUNGBERG, and V. WETMORE: Chemistry and cytology at serous fluids. Clin. Med. **14**, 417—428 (1929).
FOOTE, F. W., Jr., and F. W. STEWART: The anatomical distribution of intraepithelial epidermoid carcinomas of the cervix. Cancer (Philad.) **1**, 431—440 (1948).
FORAKER, A. G.: Intraepithelial carcinoma of the uterine cervix: a histochemical and cytomorphological approach. Ann. N.Y. Acad. Sci. **63**, 1107—1116 (1956).
— Délimitation cyto-morphologique et cyto-chimique du carcinome intra-épithélial du col utérin. Rev. franç. Gynéc. **54**, 421—426 (1959).
—, and G. MARINO: Glycogen in invasive squamous carcinoma of the uterine cervix. Amer. J. Obstet. Gynec. **72**, 400—403 (1956).
—, and J. W. REAGAN: Nuclear mass and allied phenomena in normal exocervical mucosa, squamous metaplasia, atypical hyperplasia, intraepithelial carcinoma and invasive squamous cell carcinoma of the uterine cervix. Cancer (Philad.) **12**, 894—901 (1959).
FRANKEL, P. E.: Leukoplakie, Leukoplakiegrund und Felderung — Gedanken zur Pathogenese. Dtsch. med. J. **11**, 134—136 (1960).
FRANQUÉ, O. v.: Leukoplakie und präcanceröse Veränderung des Plattenepithels. Zbl. Gynäk. **51**, 898—901 (1927).
— Anatomie, Histogenese und anatomische Diagnostik der Uteruscarcinome. In: VEIT-STÖCKEL, Handbuch der Gynäkologie. München: J. F. Bergmann 1930.
FREMONT-SMITH, M., and R. M. GRAHAM: Screening for cervical cancer in internist's office by routine vaginal smears. J. Amer. med. Ass. **150**, 587—590 (1952).
FRICK, H. C., N. A. JANOWSKI, S. B. GUSBERG, and H. C. TAYLOR: Early invasive cancer of the cervix. Amer. J. Obstet. Gynec. **85**, 926—939 (1963).
FRIEDELL, G. H., and J. B. GRAHAM: Regional lymph node involvement in small carcinoma of the cervix. Surg. Gynec. Obstet. **108**, 513—517 (1959).
— A. T. HERTIG, and P. A. YOUNGE: The problem of early stromal invasion in carcinoma in situ of the uterine cervix. Arch. Path. **66**, 494—503 (1958).
— — — Carcinoma in situ of the uterine cervix. A study of 235 cases from the Free Hospital for Women. Springfield (Ill.): C. C. Thomas 1960.
FROST, J. K.: Trichomonas vaginalis and cervical epithelial changes. Ann. N.Y. Acad. Sci. **97**, 792—799 (1962).
FUNCK-BRENTANO, P.: Prophylaxie du cancer du col. Son diagnostic à son stade noninvasif. Rev. franç. Gynéc. **49**, 1—15 (1954).
— Le problème actuel de l'épithélioma intra-épithélial du col utérin. Gynéc. et Obstét. **59**, 5—17 (1960).
— Des indications de l'hystérectomie totale et de l'hystérectomie élargie dans les cancers intra-épithéliaux. Rev. franç. Gynéc. **56**, 831—836 (1961).
— R. MORICARD, R. PALMER et J. DE BRUX: Diagnostic et traitement de l'épithélioma pavimenteux intra-épithélial du col utérin. Sem. Hôp. Paris **1952**, 2791—2800.

FUNCK-BRENTANO, P., R. MORICARD, R. PALMER et J. DE BRUX: L'épithélioma pavimenteux intra-épithélial du col utérin. Bull. Féd. Soc. Gynéc. Obstét. franç. **4**, 80—144 (1952).

GÁBOR, P., et M. SZEGVÁRI: L'examen des cellules du cancer par la coloration "méthylevert-pyronin" dans les frottis vaginaux. Gynéc. et Obstét. **57**, 197—199 (1958).

GANSE, R.: Atypische Gefäßentwicklung beim Portiokarzinom. Zbl. Gynäk. **74**, 749—752 (1952).

— Kolpofotogramme zur Einführung in die Kolposkopie, Bd. I und II. Berlin: Akademie Verlag 1953.

— Über die Gefäßdarstellung kolposkopischer Befunde mit der Quecksilberdampflampe und dem Kolpophot. Zbl. Gynäk. **76**, 81—86 (1954).

— Vertiefung der Kolposkopie. Zbl. Gynäk. **76**, 1541—1554 (1954).

— Über das schnelle Entstehen von gesteigert atypischem Epithel auf dem Boden einer Ektopie. Oncologia (Basel) **8**, 323—333 (1955).

— Die atypische Gefäßneubildung bei Karzinom. Zbl. Gynäk. **79**, 519—524 (1957).

— Die Erleichterung der Frühdiagnose des Portiokarzinoms durch die erweiterte Kolposkopie. Z. ärztl. Fortbild. **52**, 64—67 (1958).

— Das normale und pathologische Gefäßbild der Portio vaginalis uteri. Berlin: Akademie Verlag 1958.

— Hinweise zur Verbesserung der kolposkopischen Diagnostik. Arch. Geschwulstforsch. **15**, 24—38 (1959).

— Die Bedeutung der Gefäße beim Portiokarzinom. Krebsarzt **14**, 87—93 (1959).

— Gefäßneubildung beim präinvasiven und fertigen Karzinom. Geburtsh. u. Frauenheilk. **20**, 694—697 (1960).

GEISENDORF, W.: Die Frühdiagnose des Kollumkarzinoms. Wien. med. Wschr. **1953**, 643—649.

GIACCAI, L.: Il problema diagnostico e terapeutico del carcinoma in situ del collo uterino. Radiol. med. (Torino) **42**, 366—377 (1956).

GLATTHAAR, E.: Über Versuche zur zytologischen Differenzierung des atypischen Portioepithels mit Hilfe von Gewebezüchtung und Phasenkontrastmikroskopie. Schweiz. med. Wschr. **78**, 720—724 (1948).

— Studien über die Morphogenese des Plattenepithel-Karzinoms der Portio vaginalis uteri. Basel: S. Karger 1950.

— Die Vor- und Frühstadien des Portiokarzinoms. Morphogenese, Klinik (speziell Früherfassung) und Therapie. Oncologia (Basel) **5**, 196—219 (1952).

— Épithélium atypique et cancer du col. Leurs rapports à la lumière de l'étude colposcopique répétée. Rev. franç. Gynéc. **49**, 320—331 (1954).

— Kolposkopie. In: SEITZ-AMREICH, Biologie und Pathologie des Weibes, Bd. 3, S. 911—980. München u. Berlin: Urban & Schwarzenberg 1955.

GLOYNE, S. R.: Cytology of sputum. Tubercle (Edinb.) **18**, 292—297 (1936).

GORGA, P., M. APPARECIDA-PAAL u. A. GASTIN: Die Stellung der Kolposkopie in der Propädeutik des Cervixcarcinoms. An. Clin. ginec. Fac. Med. S. Paulo **5**, 225—230 (1953).

GRAHAM, J. B., and J. V. MEIGS: Recurrence of tumor after total hysterectomy for carcinoma in situ. Amer. J. Obstet. Gynec. **64**, 1159—1162 (1952).

GRAHAM, R. M.: The definition of a dyscaryotic cell. Acta cytol. (Chic.) **1** (1), 23 (1957).

— Occurrence of dyscaryotic cells in dysplasia of the uterine cervix. Acta cytol. (Chic.) **1** (1), 42 (1957).

— Occurrence of spindle-shaped squamoid cells in invasive carcinoma. Acta cytol. (Chic.) **2**, 259—263 (1958).

— Cancer detection, including exfoliative cytology. Acta Un. int. Cancr. **16**, 377—381 (1960).

— The small histiocyte: Its morphology and significance. Acta cytol. (Philad.) **5**, 77—82 (1961).

—, and J. MCGRAW: An investigation of "false positive" vaginal smears. Surg. Gynec. Obstet. **90**, 221—230 (1950).

GRAVES, W. P.: The detection of the clinically latent cancer of the cervix. With a report on SCHILLER's Lugol test. Surg. Gynec. Obstet. **56**, 317—322 (1933).

GRAY, L. A., M. L. BARNES, and J. J. LEE: Carcinoma in situ and dysplasia of the cervix. Ann. Surg. **151**, 951—960 (1960).

GREENTREE, L. B.: Cancer of the cervix. A realistic program of cancer control for the general practitioner. Amer. J. Obstet. Gynec. **61**, 178—182 (1951).

GROSS, K., J. POSPÍŠIL, J. VIKLICKÝ, and M. ZAVADIL: Problems in the histological diagnosis of precancer of the cervix. Čs. Gynek. **24**, 523—526 (1959).
GRÜNBERGER, V.: Zur Technik der Biopsie bei Erosionen. Z. Geburtsh. Gynäk. **147**, 71—75 (1956).
— Die Elektrokoagulation der Erosio portionis als Krebsprophylaxe. Wien. klin. Wschr. **71**, 243—245 (1959).
— Nachweis der Heilung eines präinvasiven Kollumkarzinoms durch Elektrokoagulation. Zbl. Gynäk. **82**, 716—718 (1960).
—, u. K. BRANDL: Mit dem Kolpomikroskop erkannte Kollumkarzinome. Zbl. Gynäk. **76**, 254—256 (1954).
—, u. H. KREMER: Eine Schnellfärbemethode zytologischer Abstriche. Zbl. Gynäk. **82**, 1472—1475 (1960).
—, u. H. MARGREITER: Nachuntersuchungen nach Portioamputationen und Konisationen. Zbl. Gynäk. **81**, 193—203 (1959).
GÜNTHER, O., u. P. STOLL: Die Prognose des im Sturmdorf-Kegel festgestellten Frühkarzinoms. Geburtsh. u. Frauenheilk. **22**, 346—349 (1962).
GUSBERG, S. B., and D. B. MOORE: The clinical pattern of intraepithelial carcinoma of the cervix and its pathological background. Obstet. and Gynec. **2**, 1—14 (1953).
HAAM, E. v.: Dyscaryotic cells in experimentally produced carcinoma of the uterine cervix. Acta cytol. (Chic.) **2** (1), 19 (1958).
HAENSZEL, W., and M. HILLHOUSE: Uterine-cancer morbidity in New York City and its relation to the pattern of regional variation within the United States. J. nat. Cancer Inst. **22**, 1157—1181 (1959).
HALFPAP, E., u. H. HOSEMANN: Rationelle klinische Krebsstatistik. Krebsforsch. u. Krebsbekämpf. **41**, 280—283 (1959).
HALL, J. E., and I. H. ROSEN: Significance of the class III cervical smear. Amer. J. Obstet. Gynec. **79**, 709—717 (1960).
HAMPELN, P. (1876 u. 1887): Zit. nach G. N. PAPANICOLAOU. Acta Un. int. Cancr. (Brux.) **14**, 249—254 (1958).
HAMPERL, H.: Definition and classification of the so-called carcinoma in situ. Ciba Foundation Study Group Nr. 3, pp. 2—19. London: J. and A. Churchill Ltd. 1959.
— Ausbreitung und Wachstum der Tumoren. Langenbecks Arch. klin. Chir. **295**, 22—40 (1960).
— Über die Progression des sog. Carcinoma in situ der Cervix uteri zum invasiven Carcinom. Arch. De Vecchi Anat. pat. **31**, 141—147 (1960).
— Épithélioma pavimenteux intra-épithélial et micro-épithélioma. Essai d'une classification du "cancer in situ" du col utérin. Rev. franç. Gynéc. **56**, 633—644 (1961).
—, u. C. KAUFMANN: Das sogenannte Oberflächencarcinom der Portio. Z. Krebsforsch. **61**, 255—258 (1956).
— — u. K. G. OBER: Histologische Untersuchungen an der Cervix schwangerer Frauen. Die Erosion und das Carcinoma in situ. Arch. Gynäk. **184**, 181—280 (1954).
— — — Das Problem der Malignität unter besonderer Berücksichtigung des Carcinoma in situ an der Cervix uteri. Klin. Wschr. **32**, 825—831 (1954).
— — — u. P. SCHNEPPENHEIM: Die „Erosion" der Portio. (Die Entstehung der Pseudoerosion, das Ektropion und die Plattenepithelüberhäutung der Cervixdrüsen auf der Portiooberfläche.) Virchows Arch. path. Anat. **331**, 51—71 (1958).
HELD, E.: Das Oberflächencarcinom. (Nicht invasives atypisches Plattenepithel.) Arch. Gynäk. **183**, 322—364 (1953).
— Considérations sur l'épithélioma pavimenteux intra-épithélial du col utérin. Gynéc. et Obstét. **52**, 233—250 (1953).
— Das Oberflächenkarzinom (nicht-invasives atypisches Plattenepithel) der Cervix uteri. Schweiz. med. Wschr. **84**, 277—278 (1954).
— Rückbildung von atypischem und abnormem Plattenepithel der Portio im histologischen Präparat. Gynaecologia (Basel) **144**, 27—31 (1957).
— Intracervicale Lokalisation des nicht invasiven, atypischen Pflasterepithels (Oberflächenkarzinom, Carcinoma in situ) und des beginnenden Pflasterzellcarcinoms. Arch. Gynäk. **188**, 376—390 (1957).

HELD, E.: Frühdiagnose des Collumkarzinoms. Schweiz. med. Wschr. **89**, 69—72 (1959).
— Probleme der Krebsfrüherfassung in der Gynäkologie. Schweiz. med. Wschr. **90**, 965—967 (1960).
— W. E. SCHREINER u. I. OEHLER: Bedeutung der Kolposkopie und Cytologie zur Erfassung des Genitalkarzinoms. Schweiz. med. Wschr. **84**, 856—860 (1954).
HENRY, J. S., and P. A. LATOUR: Glycogen in the squamous epithelium of the cervix uteri. Amer. J. Obstet. Gynec. **74**, 610—615 (1957).
HERTIG, A. T.: What is carcinoma in situ? Proc. 3rd Nat. Canc. Conf. **1957**, p. 667—670.
—, and P. A. YOUNGE: What is cancer in situ of the cervix? Is it the preinvasive form of true carcinoma? Amer. J. Obstet. Gynec. **64**, 807—815 (1952).
HESTER, L. L., Jr., and R. A. READ: An evaluation of cervical conization. Amer. J. Obstet. Gynec. **80**, 715—721 (1960).
HILLEMANNS, H. G.: Zur formalen Genese des Carcinoma colli uteri. Arch. Gynäk. **191**, 235—270 (1958).
—, u. K. RHA: Quantitative Untersuchungen über den Beginn bösartigen Wachstums an der Portio uteri. Z. Krebsforsch. **64**, 245—252 (1961).
— — Die Cytoplasma-Kernrelation bei der Krebsentstehung am Collum uteri. Z. Krebsforsch. **64**, 262—266 (1961).
—, u. H. VESTNER: Über eine ambulatorisch durchführbare Gewebsentnahmemethode zur histologischen Beurteilung von Portioveränderungen. Geburtsh. u. Frauenheilk. **16**, 931—941 (1956).
HINSELMANN, H.: Verbesserung der Inspektionsmöglichkeiten von Vulva, Vagina und Portio. Münch. med. Wschr. **72**, 1733 (1925).
— Die Ätiologie, Symptomatologie und Diagnostik des Uteruscarcinoms. In: VEIT-STOECKEL, Handbuch der Gynäkologie München: J. F. Bergmann 1930.
— Die Diagnose des Uteruscarcinoms. Klin. Wschr. **1930 II**, 1507—1510.
— Ausgewählte Gesichtspunkte zur Beurteilung des Zusammenhanges der „Matrixbezirke" und des Carcinoms der sichtbaren Abschnitte des weiblichen Genitaltraktes. Z. Geburtsh. Gynäk. **104**, 228—243 (1933).
— Einführung in die Kolposkopie. Hamburg: Paul Hartung 1933.
— Die klinische Differenzierung der Matrixbezirke. Zbl. Gynäk. **57**, 1682—1687 (1933).
— Der Begriff der Prämatrix. Zbl. Gynäk. **57**, 2402—2406 (1933).
— Reflexionen über die Verhütung des Portiokrebses. Mschr. Krebsbekämpf. **2**, 354—364 (1934).
— Approximative Frequenz des atypischen Portioepithels. Zbl. Gynäk. **60**, 1750—1751 (1936).
— In welchem Stadium möchten wir das Portiokarzinom klinisch diagnostizieren? Münch. med. Wschr. **85**, 1071—1073 (1938).
— Kleinfeldriger Grund, ein neuer selbständiger Matrixbezirk. Zbl. Gynäk. **62**, 899—903 (1938).
— Die Bedeutung der Kolposkopie für die Bekämpfung des Portiocarcinoms. Wien. klin. Wschr. **53**, 88—90 (1940).
— Zur Theorie der kolposkopischen Frühdiagnose und der Verhütung des Carcinoms am Muttermund. Schweiz. med. Wschr. **21**, 320—323 (1940).
— Der Nachweis der aktiven Ausgestaltung der Gefäße beim jungen Portiokarzinom als neues differentialdiagnostisches Hilfsmittel. Eine Folge der Kombination des Kolposkops mit der Natrium- und der Quecksilberspektrallampe. Zbl. Gynäk. **64**, 1810—1814 (1940).
— Können wir das Carcinom am Muttermund vermeiden und wie? Mschr. Krebsbekämpf. **9**, 201—214 (1941).
— Über die Bedeutung des „Erosionscarcinoms" für die Genese des Plattenepithelcarcinoms am Muttermund. Klin. Wschr. **21**, 152—155 (1942).
— Die netzförmige Umwandlungszone der Portio. Zbl. Gynäk. **66**, 873—877 (1942).
— mit Beiträgen von T. KOLLER u. T. ANTOINE: Über die Geschichte der Kolposkopie. Z. ärztl. Fortbild. **46**, 702—731 (1952).
— Die Grundlagen einer wirksamen Prophylaxe des Kollumkarzinoms mittels der Kolposkopie. Krebsarzt **8**, 1—7 (1953).
— Contribución al diagnóstico precoz del carcinoma del cuello del utero. An. Clin. ginec. y Cir. abdom. Policlin. Mejia **3**, 35—37 (1954).

HINSELMANN, H.: Zur Frühdiagnose des Plattenepithelkarzinoms am Collum uteri. Dtsch. med. Wschr. **79**, 1637—1638 (1954).

— Frühdiagnose und diagnostische Prophylaxe des Kollumkarzinoms. Zbl. Gynäk. **76**, 1527—1536 (1954).

— Kolposkopische Studien in zwangloser Folge, H. 1—6. Leipzig: Georg Thieme 1954—1959.

— Die Kolposkopie in ihrem vierten Jahrzehnt. Z. ärztl. Fortbild. **49**, 474—478 (1955).

— Zur Prophylaxe des Kollumkarzinoms. Prophylaxe **1**, 423—426 (1955).

— Mon procédé actuel pour diagnostiquer dans tous les cas l'épithélium atypique du col de l'utérus. Gynéc. prat. **7**, 343—348 (1956).

— Aktuelle Probleme der praktischen und wissenschaftlichen Kolposkopie. Jena: Gustav Fischer 1956.

— Das Kolposkop in der Hand des praktischen Arztes ist ein unentbehrlicher Faktor einer wirksamen Prophylaxe des Portiokarzinoms. Münch. med. Wschr. **99**, 1013—1014 (1957).

— Eine allen klinischen Gesichtspunkten Rechnung tragende Inspektionsmethode. An. bras. Ginec. **44**, 339—342 (1957).

— Die Prophylaxe des Portiokarzinoms. Der gerade Weg dazu! Z. ärztl. Fortbild. **52**, 566—568 (1958).

— Moderne Methoden der Kolposkopie zur Diagnose des Portiocarcinoms. An. bras. Ginec. **48**, 189—202 (1959).

—, u. KÖHLER: $3^1/_3$ Jahre „Krebssprechstunde" mit dem Kolposkop. Münch. med. Wschr. **84**, 1082—1086 (1937).

—, u. A. SCHMITT: Die Kolposkopie. Wuppertal-Elberfeld: W. Girardet 1954.

HÖRMANN, G., u. U. FREESE: Portiokarzinom und atypisches Epithel. Geburtsh. u. Frauenheilk. **17**, 121—137 (1957).

HOHLBEIN, R.: Lokalisation der kolposkopischen Hauptbefunde bei gesteigert atypischem Epithel und Mikrokarzinom. Zbl. Gynäk. **80**, 738—743 (1958).

—, u. R. GANSE: Die Therapie des gesteigert atypischen Epithels am Collum uteri und ihre Ergebnisse. Z. Geburtsh. Gynäk. **155**, 182—196 (1960).

—, u. R. KRIMMENAU: Die Zweckmäßigkeit diagnostischer Eingriffe bei atypischem Epithel am Collum uteri. Münch. med. Wschr. **101**, 1824—1829 (1959).

HOLLAND, J. C., and M. R. ACKERMANN: Fluorescent microscopy in the diagnosis of cervical carcinoma, its application in office practice. Obstet. and Gynec. **17**, 38—40 (1961).

HOLTORFF, J.: Über die Leistungsfähigkeit der Kolposkopie bei der Früherkennung des Kollumkarzinoms. Z. ärztl. Fortbild. **51**, 670—676 (1957).

— Über das Schicksal des einfach atypischen Epithels (HINSELMANN) an der Portio. Zbl. Gynäk. **80**, 1480—1492 (1958).

— Kolposkopische Kriterien der „atypischen" Umwandlungszone. Geburtsh. u. Frauenheilk. **20**, 931—941 (1960).

— Kolposkopische und histologische Befunde an der Portio vaginalis uteri beim Trichomonadenbefall der Scheide. Arch. Gynäk. **195**, 59—71 (1961).

— Beitrag zur kolposkopischen Gefäßdiagnostik an der Portio. Gynaecologia (Basel) **151**, 417—427 (1961).

HOPMAN, B. C.: Exfoliative cytology and experimental cytology of carcinoma in situ. Symposium. Fluorescence microscopy on exfoliated cells of carcinoma in situ. Acta cytol. (Philad.) **5**, 437—438 (1961).

HORN, W. S., and C. T. ASHWORTH: Evaluation of methods for obtaining cervical smears for cytology and the introduction of an improved scraper for obtaining surface cells. Amer. J. Obstet. Gynec. **74**, 1007—1010 (1957).

HUBER, A.: Uteruskarzinom und Zirkumzision. Untersuchungen in Äthiopien. Wien. med. Wschr. **110**, 571—574 (1960).

HÜTER, K. A., u. H. G. MÜLLER: Zur histologischen Sicherung verdächtiger kolposkopischer und zytologischer Befunde durch die Ringbiopsie. Medizinische **1959**, 466—467.

HUGUIER, J.: Des indications de l'amputation du col. Rev. franç. Gynéc. **56**, 827—830 (1961).

HUNTER, D. T., Jr., and N. BROWN: Morphology of benign cells as observed through the acridine orange fluorescence technic. Acta cytol. (Philad.) **5**, 250—252 (1961).

IGEL, H.: Die Diagnose des Uteruskarzinoms durch Vaginalabstrich. Zbl. Gynäk. **69**, 1369—1371 (1947).

IGEL, H., u. W. MÜLLER: Ergebnisse der vaginalen Krebsdiagnostik bei der gynäkologischen Krebssuche an der Universitäts-Frauenklinik der Charité. Zbl. Gynäk. **78**, 1257—1269 (1956).

ISAAC, J. P., et T. A. WURCH: Une nouvelle technique de coloration différentielle des frottis vaginaux. Rev. franç. Gynéc. **47**, 275—286 (1952).

— — Technique rapide de coloration cytologique différentielle pour la recherche des cellules néoplastiques exfoliées dans les liquides biologiques. Strasbourg méd. **112**, 322—326 (1952).

ISBELL, N. P., and E. GROVER: The vaginal smear in office practice, the swab technique. An evaluation of 10,000 smears. Amer. J. Obstet. Gynec. **81**, 784—791 (1961).

JAEGER, J.: Krebsfährtensuche durch Zytodiagnostik mittels Vaginaltampons. Bericht über 500 Untersuchungen. Medizinische **1957**, 479—482.

—, u. S. ERDENEN: Ergebnisse der Zytodiagnostik zur Früherkennung der Uteruskarzinome aus der Klinik und von auswärtigen Einsendungen (Sechsjahresbericht). Zbl. Gynäk. **83**, 976—987 (1961).

JANISCH, H., R. KLEIN u. H. KREMER: Die Früherfassung des Gebärmutterhalskrebses — ihre Organisation und Problematik. Geburtsh. u. Frauenheilk. **19**, 63—69 (1959).

—, u. H. KREMER: Die zytodiagnostischen Ergebnisse im Rahmen der Karzinomsuche an der I. Universitäts-Frauenklinik in Wien (Juli 1956 bis Dezember 1958). Krebsarzt **14**, 349—354 (1959).

—, u. R. ULM: Zur Problematik der Karzinomfrühdiagnostik während der Gravidität. Krebsarzt **18**, 242—251 (1963).

JENNINGS, E. R., E. DALE, H. M. NELSON, O. A. BRINES, and G. WILSON: Uterine cytology; the "false-positive" report. J. Amer. med. Ass. **170**, 1896—1898 (1959).

JENNY, J., u. A. WACEK: Zur Frage der Treffsicherheit des cytologischen Abstriches verglichen mit der Schillerschen Probeabschabung. Gynaecologia (Basel) **151**, 84—88 (1961).

JONES, H. W., G. A. GALVIN, and R. W. TE LINDE: Re-examination of biopsies taken prior to the development of invasive carcinoma of the cervix. Proc. 3rd Nat. Canc. Conf. **1956/57**, p. 678—681.

JORDAN, M. J., G. M. BADER, and E. DAY: Carcinoma in situ: Diagnostic observation or immediate definitive treatment. Proc. 3rd Nat. Canc. Conf. **1956/57**, p. 674—677.

JOSEFSON (1901): Zit. nach G. N. PAPANICOLAOU. Acta Un. int. Cancr. (Brux.) **14**, 249—254 (1958).

JUNGHANS, E., u. V. SACHS: Über die Prophylaxe des Kollumkarzinoms. Ärztl. Forsch. **16**, 300—308 (1962).

—, u. R. WAITZ: Die Prophylaxe des Kollumkarzinoms unter besonderer Berücksichtigung der Verschorfung von Portioerosionen. Münch. med. Wschr. **102**, 1284—1289 (1960).

KAISER, R. F., M. M. BOUSER, S. C. INGRAHAM II, and A. W. HILBERG: Uterine cytology. Publ. Hlth Rep. (Wash.) **75**, 423—427 (1960).

KAST, A.: Probleme der Präputial- und Zervixkarzinome bei Tieren. Geburtsh. u. Frauenheilk, **19**, 1080—1086 (1959).

KAUFMANN, C.: Fortschritte auf dem Gebiet der Krebserkennung. Dtsch. med. J. **14**, 443—447 (1963).

—, u. K. G. OBER: Eine Einteilung der Carcinomata in situ und der präklinischen Karzinome. Geburtsh. u. Frauenheilk. **20**, 703—706 (1960).

— H. RUNGE, K. G. OBER u. P. STOLL: Früherkennung des Collumcarcinoms. Leistungen und Grenzen der Kolposkopie, Cytologie und Histologie. Berlin-Göttingen-Heidelberg: Springer 1957.

KAUFMANN, W., and H. R. FIEGE: Cytologic diagnosis of malignant disease in a general office practice. Surg. Gynec. Obstet. **90**, 451—454 (1950).

KEAN, B. H., and E. DAY: Trichomonas vaginalis infection. An evaluation of three diagnostic techniques with data on incidence. Amer. J. Obstet. Gynec. **68**, 1510—1518 (1954).

KELLY, G. L., and G. N. PAPANICOLAOU: The mechanism of the periodical opening and closing of the vaginal orifice in the guinea-pig. Amer. J. Anat. **40**, 387—411 (1927).

KERN, G.: Zelltypen im cytologischen Vaginalausstrich und ihre Zuordnung zu histologischen Bildern. Z. Krebsforsch. **63**, 149—155 (1959).

— Früherkennung des Kollum-Karzinoms. Ärztl. Mitt. (Köln) **45**, 1171—1175 (1960).

KERN, G.: Zellausbeute von zytologischen Abstrichen aus dem hinteren Scheidengewölbe, der Portiooberfläche und dem Zervikalkanal bei der Krebsfährtensuche. Geburtsh. u. Frauenheilk. **21**, 150—155 (1961).
— The early detection of cancer by vaginal smears. Cell-yield of cytological smears obtained from the posterior vaginal fornix, the portio vaginalis, and the cervical canal. Übersetzung in: Germ. med. Mth. **6**, 316—318 (1961).
— Colposcopic findings in carcinoma in situ. Amer. J. Obstet. Gynec. **82**, 1409—1414 (1961).
— Schlußwort zur Erwiderung von A. MAJEWSKI und A. PLATEN der Arbeit: Kolposkopischer Befund und Lokalisation des Carcinoma in situ. Arch. Gynäk. **196**, 634—636 (1962).
— Klassifizierung pathologischer Zelltypen und ihre Bedeutung in der gynäkologischen Krebsfährtensuche. Geburtsh. u. Frauenheilk. **22**, 1058—1060 (1962).
— Diagnostik und Therapie der Frühstadien des Collumcarcinoms. Dtsch. med. Wschr. **87**, 2068—2072, 2099—2100 (1962).
— Cytologische Vorhersage von Epithelatypien an der Cervix uteri. Arch. Gynäk. **197**, 314—350 (1962).
—, u. H. P. BÖTZELEN: Registrierung von zytologischen und kolposkopischen Befunden mit der Handlochkarte. Geburtsh. u. Frauenheilk. **19**, 871—881 (1959).
— — Kolposkopischer Befund und Lokalisation des Carcinoma in situ. Bericht über 105 Fälle von Frühveränderungen der Cervix uteri. Arch. Gynäk. **194**, 564—585 (1961).
— E. RISSMANN u. G. HUND: Gynäkologische Krebsfrühdiagnostik mit Hilfe der Cytologie. Arch. Gynäk. **199**, 502—525 (1964).
— — — Die Leistungsfähigkeit der Kolposkopie bei der Frühdiagnostik des Collumcarcinoms. Arch. Gynäk. **199**, 526—539 (1964).
— N. SCHÜMMELFEDER u. E. KERN-BONTKE: Die Acridinorange-Fluorochromierung in der Cytodiagnostik von Carcinomata in situ und Collumcarcinomen. Arch. Gynäk. **196**, 394—404 (1961).
— G. STADLER u. E. HINDERFELD: Die Schillersche Jodprobe. Bericht über 733 photographisch belegte Fälle. Arch. Gynäk. **197**, 36—56 (1962).
—, u. J. ZANDER: Gefäßveränderungen im Verlauf der Carcinogenese. Lebendbeobachtungen am Ohr der Maus nach Pinselung mit Methylcholanthren. Z. Krebsforsch. **63**, 168—183 (1959).
KERN-BONTKE, E., u. G. KERN: Die Schillersche Jodprobe im Vergleich zur Glycogenverteilung in histologischen Übersichtsschnitten der Cervix uteri. (197 photographisch belegte Fälle.) Arch. Gynäk. **197**, 57—71 (1962).
KIMMELSTIEL, P., J. F. BOS, and C. NOLEN: Community survey for uterine cancer. Obstet. and Gynec. **11**, 688—695 (1958).
KIRCHHOFF, H., u. H. J. WITT: Gesteigert atypisches Epithel und Plattenepithelkarzinom der Portio. Dtsch. med. Wschr. **84**, 979—981 (1959).
KLEIN, R., E. KOFLER u. H. KREMER: Die Stellung der Zytologie in der Diagnostik des weiblichen Genitalkarzinoms. Wien. klin. Wschr. **1957**, 653—655.
KÖNIGER, H.: Die zytologische Untersuchungsmethode, ihre Entwicklung und ihre klinische Verwertung an den Ergüssen seröser Höhlen. Jena: Gustav Fischer 1907.
KOFLER, E., u. H. KREMER: Zur Frage der Früherkennung und Behandlung des sog. präinvasiven Carcinom des Collum uteri. Arch. Gynäk. **194**, 223—234 (1960).
KOLLER, O.: The vascular patterns of cervical cancer. Acta Un. int. Cancr. **15**, 375—378 (1959).
KORTE, W.: Untersuchungen bei Trichomonas vaginalis. Arch. Gynäk. **189**, 407—410 (1957).
— Möglichkeiten und Grenzen der Kolposkopie und Kolpophotographie. Photogr. u. Wiss. **6**, 13—16 (1957).
KOŠ, J., V. MIKOLÁŠ u. V. LANĚ: Das Bild des terminalen Blutgefäßnetzes auf der karzinomatösen Cervix uteri. Zbl. Gynäk. **82**, 1487—1499 (1960).
KOSS, L. G.: Exfoliative cytology of the uterine cervix and vagina. Exfoliative Cytology, publ. by the Amer. Cancer Inc. Soc. **1961**, p. 56—67.
—, and G. R. DURFEE: Cytological changes preceding the appearance of in situ carcinoma of the uterine cervix. Cancer (Philad.) **8**, 295—301 (1955).
— — The significance of superficial cell dyskaryosis. 5. Ann. meeting of the Intersociety Cytol. Counc. Trans., Bon Air Hotel, Augusta, Georgia, 14.—16. 11. 1957.

KOSS, L. G., and G. R. DURFEE: Diagnostic cytology and its histopathologic bases. London: Pitman Med. Publ. Co. Ltd. 1961.
— M. R. MELAMED, and W. W. DANIEL: In situ epidermoid carcinoma of the cervix and vagina following radiotherapy for cervical cancer. Cancer (Philad.) **14**, 353—360 (1961).
— F. W. STEWART, F. W. FOOTE, M. J. JORDAN, G. M. BADER, and E. DAY: Some histological aspects of behavior of epidermoid carcinoma in situ and related lesions of the uterine cervix. A long-term prospective study. Cancer (Philad.) **16**, 1160—1211 (1963).
—, and W. H. WOLINSKA: Trichomonas vaginalis cervicitis and its relationship to cervical cancer. A histocytological study. Cancer (Philad.) **12**, 1171—1193 (1959).
KOTTMEIER, H. L.: Carcinoma of the cervix. A study of its initial stages. Acta obstet. gynec. scand. **38**, 522—543 (1959).
— Évolution et traitement des épithéliomas. Rev. franç. Gynéc. **56**, 821—825 (1961).
— K. KARLSTEDT, L. SANTESSON, and G. MOBERGER: Histopathological problems concerning the early diagnosis of carcinoma of the cervix. Ciba Found. Study Group Nr **3**, p. 20—27. London: J. and A. Churchill Ltd. 1959.
— E. VASQUEZ-FERRO, A. WACEK, J. W. JENNY, and H. WENNER-MANGEN: Inspection technics for carcinoma in situ. Symposium. Schiller test on carcinoma in situ. Acta cytol. (Philad.) **5**, 415—421 (1961).
KRAKE, K. H.: Zur Früherkennung des Kollumkarzinoms in der täglichen Praxis. Zbl. Gynäk. **82**, 1481—1487 (1960).
KRIEGER, J. S., and L. J. MCCORMACK: The individualization of therapy for cervical carcinoma in situ. Surg. Gynec. Obstet. **109**, 328—332 (1959).
KRIMMENAU, R.: Zur Differentialdiagnose gesteigert atypisches Epithel und Epidermisierung auf Zervixpolypen. Zbl. Gynäk. **80**, 1138—1145 (1958).
— Beitrag zur Technik der „Konisation" an der Portio uteri. Geburtsh. u. Frauenheilk. **18**, 1471—1477 (1958).
KRONE, H. A.: Die Bedeutung der Konisation für die Früherfassung des Portiokarzinoms. 2. Öst./Schweiz./Bayr. Gynäkologentagg, Lindau, 30. 9.—3. 10. 1959. Ref. Geburtsh. u. Frauenheilk. **20**, 291 (1960).
— Zum Problem des präinvasiven Gebärmutterkarzinoms. Diagnose und Therapie des „gesteigert atypischen Plattenepithels" der Cervix uteri und ihre Ergebnisse. Dtsch. med. Wschr. **87**, 340—347 (1962).
KRÜCKEMEYER, K.: Gedanken zur Problematik des sog. Oberflächen-Karzinoms der Portio uteri. Dtsch. med. J. **14**, 465—467 (1961).
KRÜGER, E. H.: Über die Topographie kolposkopischer Befunde und histologischer Epithelveränderungen an der Portio uteri. Zbl. Gynäk. **79**, 789—796 (1957).
— Zur Diagnose und Therapie des „sog. Oberflächenkarzinom". Zbl. Gynäk. **79**, 1421—1430 (1957).
— Möglichkeiten und Grenzen der Kolpophotographie. Geburtsh. u. Frauenheilk. **17**, 529—536 (1957).
— Über das Gefäßbild beim beginnenden Karzinom. Zbl. Gynäk. **79**, 1669—1677 (1957).
— Zur Frage der Gewebsentnahme bei suspekter Portio zur Klärung der klinischen Verdachtsdiagnose. Geburtsh. u. Frauenheilk. **18**, 271—277 (1958).
LAMBERT, B., and J. D. WOODRUFF: Spinal cell atypia of the cervix. Cancer (Philad.) **16**, 1141—1150 (1963).
LANCEREAUX (1856): Zit. nach G. N. PAPANICOLAOU. Acta Un. int. Cancr. (Brux.) **14**, 249—254 (1958).
LANG, W. R.: The comparison between cytology and colposcopy in the detection of early cancer. Acta Un. int. Cancr. (Brux.) **14**, 340—343 (1958).
— Colposcopy, neglected method of cervical evaluation. J. Amer. med. Ass. **166**, 893—897 (1958).
— The cervical portio from menarche on: A colposcopic study. Ann. N.Y. Acad. Sci. **97**, 653—661 (1962).
—, and A. E. RAKOFF: Colposcopy and cytology. Comparative values in the diagnosis of cervical atypism and malignancy. Obstet. and Gynec. **8**, 312—317 (1956).
— — and G. TATARIAN: Cytologic and histologic correlation of colposcopic findings. Surg. Gynec. Obstet. **104**, 717—721 (1957).

LANGE, P.: Clinical and histological studies on cervical carcinoma. Precancerosis, early metastases and tubular structures in the lymph nodes. Acta path. microbiol. scand. **50**, Suppl. **143**, 9—162 (1960).

LANGREDER, W.: Kritisches zur vaginalen zytologischen Diagnostik. Zbl. Gynäk. **76**, 633 (1954).

— Neue Methoden der Krebsfrüherfassung. Geburtsh. u. Frauenheilk. **18**, 517—522 (1958).

— Das Zytophor, ein Instrument zur Massenuntersuchung auf weiblichen Genitalkrebs. Krebsforsch. u. Krebsbekämpf. **41**, 304—308 (1959).

LAPID, L. S., and M. A. GOLDBERGER: Exfoliative dyskaryotic cells associated with atypical cervical lesions. Amer. J. Obstet. Gynec. **61**, 1324—1328 (1951).

LATOUR, J. P. A.: Results in the management of preclinical carcinoma of the cervix. Amer. J. Obstet. Gynec. **81**, 511—514 (1961).

— L. B. BROWN, and L. A. TURNBULL: Preclinical carcinoma of the cervix. Amer. J. Obstet. Gynec. **74**, 354—360 (1957).

LAX, H.: Das Oberflächenkarzinom. (Eine Stellungnahme zu HINSELMANNs 32 Thesen und MESTWERDTs Atlas der Kolposkopie.) Z. Geburtsh. Gynäk. **138**, 105—153, 186—189 (1953).

LEE, L. E., Jr., P. J. MELNICK, and H. M. WALSH: Carcinoma in situ of the uterine cervix. Surg. Gynec. Obstet. **102**, 677—682 (1956).

LEEB, H., u. R. ULM: Das präklinische Carcinoma colli uteri. Diagnostik und Therapie. Gynaecologia (Basel) **149**, 81—89 (1960).

LEONHARDT, A.: Histologische Untersuchungsergebnisse an der obligatorisch amputierten Portio uteri bei kolposkopisch atypischem Epithel. Zbl. Gynäk. **81**, 736—744 (1959).

LEVRIER, M., et R. CATOR: Cytodiagnostic des cancers génitaux féminins. C. R. Soc. franç. Gynéc. **30**, 259—265 (1960).

LIMBURG, H.: Die Frühdiagnose des Uteruscarcinoms, 3. Aufl. Stuttgart: Georg Thieme 1956.

— Vergleich zwischen Zytologie und Colposkopie in der Entdeckung von Frühkarzinomen. Acta Un. int. Cancr. (Brux.) **14**, 321—325 (1958).

LINDENSCHMIDT, W., and P. STOLL: Occurrence of dyskaryotic cells in trichomonas infestation. Acta cytol. (Chic.) **2** (1), 11 (1958).

LISSE, K.: Die Behandlung des „Oberflächen-Carcinom" an der Universitäts-Frauenklinik Berlin (Charité). Arch. Geschwulstforsch. **22**, 106—120 (1963).

LISTON, W. G., and W. A. LISTON: A study of trichomonas vaginitis in hospital practice in Edinburgh. J. Obstet. Gynaec. Brit. Emp. **46**, 474—502 (1939).

LITTMANN, H., u. W. WALZ: Kolpophotographie. Photogr. u. Forsch. **6**, 144—149 (1955).

LÖNNE, F.: Die Kolposkopie im Rahmen der „wirksamen gesetzmäßigen Krebsbekämpfung". Zbl. Gynäk. **62**, 51—52 (1938).

— Früherfassung des weiblichen Genitalcarcinoms durch Aufklärungspropaganda und Vorsichtsuntersuchungen. Arch. Gynäk. **173**, 67—80 (1942).

LOMBARD, H. L., and E. A. POTTER: Epidemiological aspects of cancer of the cervix. Cancer (Philad.) **3**, 960—968 (1950).

LÜCKE, A., u. E. KLEBS: Beitrag zur Ovariotomie und zur Kenntnis der Abdominalgeschwülste. Virchows Arch. path. Anat. **41**, 1—14 (1867).

LUKSCH, F., and T. SEBEK: A comparison of the results of cytological and colposcopic investigation of carcinoma of the cervix. Čs. Gynek. **22** (36), 119—123 (1957).

MACKENZIE, L. L.: The cytology of early squamous-cell carcinoma of the cervix. Amer. J. Obstet. Gynec. **69**, 629—642 (1955).

MACMILLAN, H. J. C.: Uterine carcinoma. Verification of cytologic findings by giant histologic sections. Obstet. and Gynec. **15**, 163—174 (1960).

MADEJ, J.: Die Anwendung der Milchsäurelösung als Kontrastmittel in der erweiterten Kolposkopie. Geburtsh. u. Frauenheilk. **22**, 1427—1432 (1962).

MAJEWSKI, A.: Wege und Ziele in der Früherkennung des Gebärmutterhalskrebses. Jena: Gustav Fischer 1956.

— Die Noradrenalinprobe als neues Hilfsmittel der Kolposkopie. Geburtsh. u. Frauenheilk. **20**, 983—988 (1960).

—, u. A. PLATEN: Kolposkopische Befunde beim Carcinoma in situ und Mikrocarcinom am Collum uteri. Arch. Gynäk. **196**, 629—633 (1962).

MAMZACK, R.: Über die Frühdiagnose und Früherfassung der Kollum-Karzinomfälle in der gynäkologischen Sprechstunde. Prophylaxe **1**, 421—423 (1955).

MANDLEBAUM, F. S. (1900): Zit. nach G. N. PAPANICOLAOU. Acta Un. int. Cancr. (Brux.) **14**, 249—254 (1958).
— The diagnosis of malignant tumors by paraffin sections of centrifuged exudates. J. Lab. clin. Med. **2**, 580 (1917).
MANGLANO, J. I.: Der Glykogennachweis in Carcinomata in situ, „beginnenden" und fortgeschrittenen Plattenepithelcarcinomen des Collum uteri. Arch. Gynäk. **194**, 586—593 (1961).
MARSAN, C., M. LECOQ et A. SICARD: La signification des frottis cytologiques de la classe III. Presse méd. **68**, 2291—2294 (1960).
MARTI, T.: Bieten die Schillersche Reaktion und die Kolposkopie eine hundertfache Sicherheit bei der Frühdiagnose eines Plattenepithelkrebses an der Portio? Zbl. Gynäk. **63**, 1460—1462 (1939).
MARTIN, R., u. K. HARRICHHAUSEN: Die Möglichkeiten der Vorsorgeuntersuchungen in der gynäkologischen Sprechstunde. Münch. med. Wschr. **103**, 1835—1837 (1961).
MARTINS, A. F., u. I. DREICON: Therapie des Oberflächencarcinoms. An. bras. Ginec. **49**, 363—368 (1960).
MASCALL, N.: Some reflections on the trichomonas vaginalis. Brit. J. vener. Dis. **30**, 156—162 (1954).
MASIN, M., and F. MASIN: Cresyl violet staining in exfoliative gynecologic cytology. Obstet. and Gynec. **15**, 702—710 (1960).
MASTERSON, J. G.: An analysis of untreated intra-epithelial carcinoma of the cervix. Proc. 3rd Nat. Canc. Conf., **1956**, p. 671—673.
MATUSCHKA, M. v.: Unsere histologische Technik zur Aufarbeitung von Konisationen, ganzen Uteri und Uteri mit anhängenden Parametrien. Geburtsh. u. Frauenheilk. **22**, 498—505 (1962).
McDONALD, J. R., and A. C. BRODERS: Malignant cells in serous effusions. Arch. Path. **27**, 53—60 (1939).
McKAY, D. G., B. TERJANIAN, D. POSCHYACHINDA, P. A. YOUNGE, and A. T. HERTIG: Clinical pathologic significance of anaplasia (atypical hyperplasia) of the cervix uteri. Obstet. and Gynec. **13**, 2—21 (1959).
McLAREN, H. C.: The treatment of carcinoma in situ. Acta Un. int. Cancr. **16**, 385—388 (1960).
—, and M. E. ATTWOOD: Methods of diagnosing cervical carcinoma-in-situ. Brit. med. J. **1961 II**, 1111—1113.
MENKEN, F.: Früherfassung des Collumcarcinoms durch Photokolposkopie. Photogr. u. Wiss. **2**, 15—18 (1954).
— Photocolposcopie et stéréophotocolposcopie pour l'enregistrement des modifications superficielles du col de l'utérus. Gynéc. prat. **6**, 195—200 (1955).
MESTWERDT, G.: Elektive Therapie des Mikrokarzinoms am Collum uteri? Zbl. Gynäk. **73**, 558—567 (1951).
— Über das Schicksal der Matrixbezirke an der Portio. Zbl. Gynäk. **73**, 1072—1073 (1951).
— Atlas der Kolposkopie, 2. Aufl. Jena: Gustav Fischer 1953.
— Über „Präkanzerosen" am Collum uteri. Strahlentherapie **103**, 214—223 (1957).
— Vergleich zwischen Zytologie und Colposkopie in der Entdeckung von Frühkarzinomen. Acta Un. int. Cancr. (Brux.) **14**, 343—346 (1958).
—, u. A. MÖNCKEBERG: Über die Beziehungen zwischen Karzinomentwicklung und dem kolposkopisch gefundenen atypischen Epithel an der Portio. Geburtsh. u. Frauenheilk. **7/8**, 156—172 (1948).
—, u. H. WESPI: Atlas der Kolposkopie, 3. Aufl. Stuttgart: Gustav Fischer 1961.
MEYBERG, J.: Der cytologische Ausstrich als brauchbare Methode für die Diagnostik und Lokalisation der Entzündung von Vagina, Portio und Cervix. Arch. Gynäk. **192**, 221—228 (1960).
— Die Konisation der Cervix uteri bei 120 Frauen. Geburtsh. u. Frauenheilk. **22**, 243—250 (1962).
MEYER, R.: Über Epidermoidalisierung (Ersatz des Schleimepithels durch Plattenepithel an der Portio vaginalis uteri nach Erosion an Cervixpolypen und in der Cervicalschleimhaut). Ein Beitrag zur Frage der Stückchendiagnose und des präcancerösen Stadiums. Zbl. Gynäk. **47**, 946—960 (1923).

MEYER, R.: The histological diagnosis of early cervical carcinoma. Surg. Gynec. Obstet. **73**, 129—139 (1941).
MICHALKIEWICZ, W., L. A. PRZYBORA, S. SIMM, and M. WOLNA: Recurrence and therapeutic problems in cervical dysplasia and in situ cancer. Cancer (Philad.) **16**, 1212—1221 (1963).
MICHALZIK, K.: Portio-Karzinom. Frühdiagnose. Morphologie. Genese. München u. Berlin: Urban & Schwarzenberg 1959.
MIKULICZ-RADECKI, F. v.: Können Vorsichtsuntersuchungen und Krebsberatungsstellen die Früherfassung der Genitalcarcinome fördern? Arch. Gynäk. **189**, 336—343 (1957).
— Über die Verbesserung der Heilungsresultate beim Carcinoma colli uteri im Laufe der letzten 43 Jahre. Strahlentherapie **111**, 1—7 (1960).
MILLER, E. M., and E. v. HAAM: A comparison of the vaginal aspiration and cervical scraping technics in the screening process for uterine cancer. Acta cytol. (Philad.) **5**, 214—216 (1961).
MILLIGAN, M., L. A. CARROW, and V. EGGERS: A source of false positives in cytologic interpretation. Amer. J. Obstet. Gynec. **78**, 599—603 (1959).
MOORE, J. G., D. G. MORTON, J. W. APPLEGATE, and W. HINDLE: Management of early carcinoma. Amer. J. Obstet. Gynec. **81**, 1175—1182 (1961).
MORARI, M., u. R. STRAMETZ: Ergebnisse der Zytodiagnostik und Kolposkopie bei der Früherfassung von Kollumkarzinomen. Krebsarzt **8**, 185—198 (1953).
MORICARD, R.: Problèmes statistiques des erreurs apportées par les frottis vaginaux dans le diagnostic précoce du cancer du col. Gynéc. et Obstét. **54**, 294—331 (1955).
—, et R. CARTIER: Transformation d'épithélioma pavimenteux intra-épithéliaux du col utérin en épithélioma invasifs. Étude de six observations. Gynéc. et Obstét. **56**, 333—352 (1957).
MURRAY, E. G.: Studien über Veränderungen des Zellinhaltes der Vagina. Arch. Gynäk. **165**, 635—710 (1938).
MUSSEY, E.: Carcinoma in situ of the uterine cervix. Symposium. Proc. Mayo Clin. **35**, 513—518 (1960).
—, and E. H. SOULE: Carcinoma in situ of the cervix. A clinical review of 842 cases. Amer. J. Obstet. Gynec. **77**, 957—972 (1959).
NAVRATIL, E.: Frühdiagnose des Uteruscarcinoms. (Erstellung von Statistiken. Genauigkeit der Zytodiagnostik.) In: SEITZ-AMREICH, Biologie und Pathologie des Weibes, Bd. 4, S. 717—725. München u. Berlin: Urban & Schwarzenberg 1955.
— Vergleich zwischen Zytologie und Colposkopie in der Entdeckung von Frühkarzinomen. Acta Un. int. Cancr. (Brux.) **14**, 346—349 (1958).
— Zytodiagnostisches gynäkologisches Zentrum. Krebsarzt **14**, 478—484 (1959).
— F. BAJARDI u. E. BURGHARDT: Weitere Ergebnisse der Krebsfährtensuche an der Universitäts-Frauenklinik Graz. Wien. klin. Wschr. **71**, 781—783 (1959).
— E. BURGHARDT u. F. BAJARDI: Ergebnisse der Erfassung präklinischer Karzinome an der Universitäts-Frauenklinik Graz. Krebsarzt **11**, 193—196 (1956).
— — —, and W. NASH: Simultaneous colposcopy and cytology used in screening for carcinoma of the cervix. Amer. J. Obstet. Gynec. **75**, 1292—1297 (1958).
NEVERMANN: Die Hamburger Krebsberatungsstellen. Zbl. Gynäk. **77**, 1153—1154 (1955).
NEVINNY-STICKEL, H.: Probeexzision oder Konisation? Med. Mschr. **14**, 448—451 (1960).
NIEBURGS, H. E.: A comparative study of different techniques for the diagnosis of cervical carcinoma. Amer. J. Obstet. Gynec. **72**, 511—515 (1956).
—, and E. R. PUND: Specific malignant cells exfoliated from preinvasive cancer of the cervix uteri. Amer. J. Obstet. Gynec. **58**, 532—536 (1949).
— — Detection of cancer of the cervix uteri. Evaluation of comparative exfoliative cytology diagnosis: A study of 10,000 cases. J. Amer. med. Ass. **142**, 221—225 (1950).
— H. REISMAN, and B. PACHECO: Interpretation of cellular changes preceding invasive uterine cervix carcinoma. Cancer (Philad.) **16**, 480—501 (1963).
— I. STERGUS, E. M. STEPHENSON, and B. L. HARBIN: Mass screening of the total female population of a county for cervical carcinoma. J. Amer. med. Ass. **164**, 1546—1551 (1957).
NOGALES, F.: Carcinoma „in situ". Acta ginec. (Madr.) **4**, 425—436 (1953).
NOLD, B.: Über die atypische Umwandlungszone der Portio. Das kolposkopische Bild. Med. Bild **3**, 142—144 (1960).
NOVAK, E.: Gynecological and obstetrical pathology. With clinical and endocrine relations. Philadelphia: W. B. Saunders Co. 1947.

NOVAK, J.: Zur Diagnose und Behandlung des intraepithelialen Gebärmutterkarzinoms. Wien. klin. Wschr. **69**, 985—988 (1957).

NYBERG, R., B. TÖRNBERG, and B. WESTIN: Colposcopy and SCHILLER's iodine test as an aid in the diagnosis of malignant and premalignant lesions of the squamous epithelium of the cervix uteri. Acta obstet. gynec. scand. **39**, 540—556 (1960).

NYKLÍČEK, O.: Cell dyskaryosis in the vaginal cytology. Neoplasma (Bratisl.) **7**, 187—192 (1960).

OBER, K. G.: Cervix uteri und Lebensalter. Die Bedeutung der Formwandlungen der Zervix für die Krebsdiagnostik und die Frage der sogenannten Portioerosion. Dtsch. med. Wschr. **83**, 1661—1670, 1671, 1672 (1958).

—, u. H. P. BÖTZELEN: Technik, Vor- und Nachteile der Konisation der Cervix uteri. Geburtsh. u. Frauenheilk. **19**, 1051—1060 (1959).

—, u. E. BONTKE: Sitz und Ausdehnung der Carcinomata in situ und der beginnenden Krebse der Cervix. Arch. Gynäk. **192**, 55—68 (1959).

— C. KAUFMANN u. H. HAMPERL: Carcinoma in situ, beginnendes Karzinom und klinischer Krebs der Cervix uteri. Geburtsh. u. Frauenheilk. **21**, 259—297 (1961).

— P. SCHNEPPENHEIM, H. HAMPERL u. C. KAUFMANN: Die Epithelgrenzen im Bereich des Isthmus uteri. Arch. Gynäk. **190**, 346—383 (1958).

OBER, W. B., and L. REINER: Cancer of the cervix in Jewish women. Schweiz. Z. allg. Path. **18**, 774—780 (1955).

OKAGAKI, T., V. LERCH, P. A. YOUNGE, D. G. MCKAY, and A. Y. KEVORKIAN: Diagnosis of anaplasia and carcinoma in situ by differential cell counts. Acta cytol. (Philad.) **6**, 343—347 (1962).

OKI, T.: On the relation of glycogen and carcinoma of cervix of uterus. Jap. med. World **7**, 108—113 (1927).

OLSON, A. W., and E. E. NICHOLS: Leukoplakia of the cervix — the mosaic and papillary pattern. Amer. J. Obstet. Gynec. **82**, 895—902 (1961).

OSBAND, R., and W. NICHOLSON JONES: Carcinoma in situ in pregnancy. Amer. J. Obstet. Gynec. **83**, 599—606 (1962).

PALMER, R.: Méthode d'examens des épithéliomas cervicaux sans signes fonctionnels. Colposcopie et technique de prélèvement biopsique (conduite tenue à l'hôpital Broca pour le dépistage et le diagnostic du cancer intra-épithélial). Rev. franç. Gynéc. **56**, 745—746 (1961).

PAPANICOLAOU, G. N.: New cancer diagnosis. Proc. Third Race Betterment Conf. **1928**, p. 528.

— The sexual cycle in the human female as revealed by vaginal smears. Amer. J. Anat. **52**, 519—637 (1933).

— A new procedure for staining vaginal smears. Science **95**, 438—439 (1942).

— Cytologic diagnosis of uterine cancer by examination of vaginal and uterine secretions. Amer. J. clin. Path. **19**, 301—308 (1949).

— A survey of the actualities and potentialities of exfoliative cytology in cancer diagnosis. Ann. intern. Med. **31**, 661—674 (1949).

— Observations on the origin of histiocytes in secretions of the female genital tract. Anat. Rec. **112**, 69 (1952).

— Observations on the origin and specific function of the histiocytes in the female genital tract. Fertil. and Steril. **4**, 472—478 (1953).

— Cytological evaluation of smears prepared by the tampon method for the detection of carcinoma of the uterine cervix. Cancer (Philad.) **7**, 1185—1190 (1954).

— Atlas of exfoliative cytology. Cambridge (Mass.): Harvard University Press 1954.

— Exfoliative cytologic patterns in carcinoma in situ correlated with histopathologic findings Proc. 3rd Nat. Canc. Conf. **1956/57**, p. 652—658.

— Historical development of cytology as a tool in clinical medicine and in cancer research. Acta Un. int. Cancr. (Brux.) **14**, 249—254 (1958).

—, and E. L. BRIDGES: Simple method for protecting fresh smears from drying and deterioration during mailing. J. Amer. med. Ass. **164**, 1330—1331 (1957).

—, and H. F. TRAUT: Diagnosis of uterine cancer by the vaginal smear. New York: The Commonwealth Fund 1943.

— —, and A. A. MARCHETTI: The epithelia of woman's reproductive organs. New York: The Commonwealth Fund 1948.

PARKER, R. T., W. K. CUYLER, L. A. KAUFMANN, B. CARTER, W. L. THOMAS, R. N. CREADICK, V. H. TURNER, C. H. PEETE Jr., and W. B. CHERNY: Intraepithelial (stage 0) cancer of the cervix. A 13 year cumulative study of 485 patients. Amer. J. Obstet. Gynec. **80**, 693—710 (1960).

PEALE, A. R.: Pathologic aspects of carcinoma in situ of the cervix. Obstet. and Gynec. **13**, 657—664 (1959).

PEMBERTON, F. A., and G. VAN S. SMITH: The early diagnosis and prevention of carcinoma of the cervix. A clinical pathologic study of borderline cases treated at the free hospital for women. Amer. J. Obstet. Gynec. **17**, 165—176 (1929).

PETERSEN, O.: Precancerous changes of the cervical epithelium in relation to manifest cervical carcinoma. Clinical and histological aspects. Acta radiol. (Stockh.) **127**, 9—168 (1955).

— Diskussionsbemerkung zu C. KAUFMANN u. K. G. OBER, The morphological changes of the cervix uteri with age, and their significance in the early diagnosis of carcinoma. Ciba Found. Study Group No. 3, p. 80—81. London: J. and A. Churchill Ltd. 1959.

— Les épithéliomas intra-épithéliaux en dehors de la gestation. Conséquences thérapeutiques. Transformation des épithéliomas intra-épithéliaux en épithéliomas invasifs. Rev. franç. Gynéc. **56**, 815—820 (1961).

PETRACCA, A.: Accorgimenti di tecnica per la diagnosi precoce del cancro dell'utero con l'analisi di 5428 strisci vaginali. Minerva ginec. **14**, 343—344 (1962).

PHILIPP, E.: Neue Gesichtspunkte für die Erkennung und Behandlung des Gebärmutterkrebses. (Cytodiagnostik, Krebsberatungsstelle, Oberflächencarcinom u.a.) Schlesw.-Holst. Ärztebl. 8, 41—48 (1955).

— Vorschläge für die Einrichtung cytodiagnostischer Untersuchungsstellen. Med. Klin. **52**, 2190—2193 (1957).

PIPBERGER, H. V., u. E. D. FREIS: Automatische Analyse kardiologischer Analog-Daten mittels elektronischer Rechenmaschinen. Med. Dok. **4**, 58—61 (1960).

POMERANCE, W., H. J. GREENE, H. E. NIEBURGS, and A. OPPENHEIM: Patient acceptance and comparative value of three different methods of obtaining vaginal smears for the detection of carcinoma of the cervix. Amer. J. Obstet. Gynec. **77**, 183—187 (1959).

POUCHET, F. A.: Théorie positive de l'ovulation spontanée et de la fécondation des mammiféres et de l'espèce humaine, borée sur l'observation de toute la série animale. Paris: J. B. Baillière 1847.

PRONAI, K.: Zur Lehre von der Histogenese und dem Wachstum des Uteruscarcinoms. Arch. Gynäk. **89**, 596—607 (1909).

PRZYBORA, L. A., and A. PLUTOWA: Histological topography of carcinoma in situ of the cervix uteri. Cancer (Philad.) **12**, 263—277 (1959).

PUND, E. R., J. B. NETTLES, J. D. CALDWELL, and H. E. NIEBURGS: Preinvasive and invasive carcinoma of the cervix uteri. Amer. J. Obstet. Gynec. **55**, 831—837 (1948).

PUNDEL, J. P.: Acquisitions récentes en cytologie vaginale hormonale. Paris: Masson & Cie. 1957.

—, et F. SCHWACHTGEN: Le dépistage précoce du cancer du col utérin par les méthodes modernes. Étude critique des diverses techniques à l'attention du praticien. Gynéc. prat. **7**, 7—24 (1956).

— — Le terrain hormonal des infections vaginales à trichomonas. Gynaecologia (Basel) **144**, 44—50 (1957).

QUENSEL, U. (1919): Zit. nach G. N. PAPANICOLAOU: Acta Un. int. Cancr. (Brux.) **14**, 249—254 (1958).

QUENSEL, U.: Zur Frage der Zytodiagnostik der Ergüsse seröser Höhlen. Methodologische und pathologisch-anatomische Bemerkungen. Acta med. scand. (Stockh.) **68**, 427—457 (1928).

— Zytologische Untersuchungen von Ergüssen der Brust- und Bauchhöhlen mit besonderer Berücksichtigung der karzinomatösen Exsudate. Acta med. scand. (Stockh.) **68**, 458—501 (1928).

QUINKE, H.: Ueber fetthaltige Transsudate. Hydrops chylosus und Hydrops adiposus. Dtsch. Arch. klin. Med. **16**, 121—139 (1875).

RANDERATH, E., u. G. HIERONYMI: Zur Frage des sog. Oberflächenkarzinoms der Portio uteri. Münch. med. Wschr. **98**, 1269—1274 (1956).

REAGAN, J. W.: A cytologic study of incipient carcinoma. Amer. J. clin. Path. **22**, 231—236 (1952).
—, and S. F. PATTEN Jr.: Dysplasia: a basic reaction to injury in the uterine cervix. Ann. N.Y. Acad. Sci. **97**, 662—682 (1962).
RECKEN, D.: Beobachtungen bei Nachuntersuchungen des atypischen Epithels der Portio. Geburtsh. u. Frauenheilk. **15**, 683—692 (1955).
REICHEN, G.: A propos du diagnostic précoce du cancer du col de l'utérus. Rev. franç. Gynéc. **47**, 201—205 (1952).
RIBA, L. W.: Resistant trichomoniasis in the female. Amer. J. Obstet. Gynec. **73**, 174—179 (1957).
RISSMANN, E., G. KERN u. H. ZU EULENBURG: Erfahrungen mit der Flächenlochkarte im Rahmen der gynäkologischen Krebsfrühdiagnostik. Arch. Gynäk. **199**, 540—548 (1964).
RIVA, H. L., J. D. HEFNER, and D. M. KAWASAKI: Carcinoma in situ of the cervix. A review of 156 cases. Obstet. and Gynec. **17**, 525—530 (1961).
ROGOVENKO, S. S.: Conoid diathermoexcision of the cervix uteri in precancerous diseases. Vop. Onkol. **7**, 68—74 (1961).
ROTH, O. A.: Das Vaginalsekret. In: H. J. STREICHER u. S. SANDKÜHLER, Klinische Zytologie. Stuttgart: Georg Thieme 1953.
RUBIN, I. C.: The pathological diagnosis of incipient carcinoma of the uterus. Amer. J. Obstet. Gynec. **62**, 668—676 (1910).
RUNGE, H., u. P. STOLL: Das Problem des sogenannten Oberflächenkarzinoms der Portio. Dtsch. med. Wschr. **80**, 1069—1072, 1120—1124 (1955).
—, u. H. ZEITZ: Zur Frage der Genese des Collumcarcinoms. Acta Un. int. Cancr. **15**, 398—402 (1959).
SANDERS, W. R. (1864): Urinuntersuchung bei Blasen-Ca. Zit. nach G. N. PAPANICOLAOU. Acta Un. int. Cancr. (Brux.) **14**, 249—254 (1958).
SCAPIER, J., E. DAY, and G. R. DURFEE: Intraepithelial carcinoma of the cervix; a cytohistological and clinical study. Cancer (Philad.) **5**, 315—323 (1952).
SCHAUENSTEIN, W.: Histologische Untersuchungen über atypische Plattenepithelien an der Portio und an der Innenfläche der Cervix uteri. Arch. Gynäk. **85**, 576—616 (1908).
SCHEFFEY, L. C., K. A. BOLTEN, and W. R. LANG: Colposcopy. Aid in diagnosis of cervical cancer. Obstet. and Gynec. **5**, 294—306 (1955).
—, and W. R. LANG: Prevention of cancer of the cervix and management of carcinoma in situ Congr. internat. de Gynécol. et d'Obstétr. Genève **1954**, p. 182—185.
— W. R. LANG, and G. TATARIAN: An experimental program with colposcopy. Amer. J. Obstet. Gynec. **70**, 876—888 (1955).
SCHILLER, W.: Untersuchungen zur Entstehung der Geschwülste. I. Teil: Collumcarcinom des Uterus. Virchows Arch. path. Anat. **263**, 279—367 (1927).
— Untersuchungen zur Entstehung der Geschwülste. II. Teil: Uterusmyom. Virchows Arch. path. Anat. **263**, 368—395 (1927).
— Über die Frühstadien des Portiocarcinoms und ihre Diagnose. Arch. Gynäk. **133**, 211—283 (1928).
— Zur histologischen Frühdiagnose des Portiocarcinoms. Zbl. Gynäk. **52**, 1562—1567 (1928).
— Zur klinischen Frühdiagnose des Portiocarcinoms. Zbl. Gynäk. **52**, 1886—1892 (1928).
— Jodpinselung und Abschabung des Portioepithels. Zbl. Gynäk. **53**, 1056—1064 (1929).
— Die Frühdiagnose des Carcinoms der weiblichen Geschlechtsorgane. Wien. klin. Wschr. **1931 II**, 1533—1536.
— Bedeutung der Kolposkopie, Probeabschabung und Probeexcision für die Diagnose des Gebärmutterhalskrebses. Wien. klin. **1932 II**, 176—177.
— Early diagnosis of carcinoma of the cervix. Surg. Gynec. Obstet. **56**, 210—222 (1933).
— Zur Frühdiagnose des Karzinoms der Portio uteri. Mschr. Krebsbekämpf. **2**, 7—14 (1934).
— Early diagnosis of carcinoma of the portio uteri. Amer. J. Surg. **26**, 269—280 (1934).
— Prosoplastische Veränderungen des Portioepithels und ihre Beziehungen zum sogenannten Vaginalcyclus und zur Carcinombildung. Arch. Gynäk. **155**, 415—442 (1934).
— The diagnosis of carcinoma of the cervix in a very early stage. Lancet **1936 I**, 1228—1232.
— Pathology of the cervix. Amer. J. Obstet. Gynec. **34**, 430—438 (1937).

SCHILLER, W.: Leukoplakia, leukokeratosis, and carcinoma of the cervix. Amer. J. Obstet. Gynec. **35**, 17—38 (1938).
— Clinical behavior of early carcinoma of the cervix. Surg. Gynec. Obstet. **66**, 129—139 (1938).
— Bemerkungen zu „Das Oberflächenkarzinom". Arch. Gynäk. **185**, 640 (1955).
SCHLEIDEN (1838): Zit. nach G. N. PAPANICOLAOU: Acta Un. int. Cancr. (Brux.) **14**, 249—254 (1958).
SCHMIDT-ELMENDORFF, H. R.: Prophylaxe des Zervixkarzinoms. Zbl. Gynäk. **76**, 2215—2222 (1954).
SCHMITT, A.: Eine Gradeinteilung für die funktionelle Zytodiagnostik in der Gynäkologie. Geburtsh. u. Frauenheilk. **13**, 593—603 (1953).
— Kolposkopische Befunde und ihre photographische Wiedergabe. Ciba-Symposium **3**, 109—113 (1955).
— Die Kolpophotographie im Colorbild. Photogr. u. Wiss. **5**, 21—23 (1956).
— The value of colposcopy in the diagnosis of cancer of the cervix. Proc. 3rd Nat. Canc. Conf. **1956/57**, p. 619.
— Colposcopy detection of atypical and cancerous lesions of the cervix. Obstet. and Gynec. **13**, 665—671 (1959).
SCHNEPPENHEIM, P., H. HAMPERL, C. KAUFMANN u. K. G. OBER: Die Beziehungen des Schleimepithels zum Plattenepithel an der Cervix uteri im Lebenslauf der Frau. Arch. Gynäk. **190**, 303—345 (1958).
SCHOTTLÄNDER, J.: Zur Histologie und Histogenese des Uteruskarzinoms mit besonderer Berücksichtigung metaplastischer Vorgänge. Zbl. Gynäk. **31**, 750—751 (1907).
—, u. F. KERMAUNER: Zur Kenntnis des Uteruskarzinoms. Berlin. S. Karger 1912.
SCHROEDER, C.: Krebsvorsorge und praktischer Arzt. Dtsch. med. Wschr. **78**, 1758—1760 (1953).
SCHRÖDER, R.: Lehrbuch der Gynäkologie, 5. Aufl. Leipzig: Georg Thieme 1959.
SCHUBERT, G.: Praktische und theoretische Gesichtspunkte bei den Frühstadien weiblicher Krebserkrankungen. Med. Klin. **49**, 14—22 (1954).
—, u. H. J. SCHMERMUND: Moderne Gesichtspunkte bei der Behandlung des Oberflächenkarzinoms am Collum uteri. Arch. Geschwulstforsch. **6**, 333—347 (1954).
SCHÜLLER, E.: Cytologie des weiblichen Genitalkarzinoms. (Wien. Beitr. z. Geburtsh. u, Gynäkol.) Wien u. Bonn: Wilhelm Maudrich 1955.
— Diskussionsbemerkung zu: The occurrence of dyscaryotic cells in carcinoma in situ. Acta cytol. (Chic.) **1** (1), 45—46 (1957).
— Carcinoma colli uteri incipiens. Arch. Gynäk. **190**, 520—548 (1958).
— The epithelia of the uterine endocervix. Acta cytol. (Chic.) **3**, 333—337 (1960).
SCHÜMMELFEDER, N.: Die Fluorochromierung tierischer Zellen mit Acridinorange. Naturwissenschaften **35**, 346 (1948).
— Über Beziehungen zwischen Stoffwechselaktivität und Acridinorangespeicherung von Zellen. Naturwissenschaften **36**, 58 (1949).
— Die Fluorochromierung des lebenden, überlebenden und toten Protoplasmas mit dem basischen Farbstoff Acridinorange und ihre Beziehung zur Stoffwechselaktivität der Zelle. Virchows Arch. path. Anat. **318**, 119—154 (1950).
— Zur histochemischen Bedeutung der Fluorescenzmetachromasie des Acridinorange. Acta histochem. (Jena), Suppl. **1**, 148—151 (1958). (I).
— Cytochemische Befunde. In: HENNING u. WITTE, Internat. Symposium über Klinische Cytodiagnostik. Stuttgart: Georg Thieme 1958 (II).
— Die Akridinorange-Fluorochromierung in der zytologischen Krebsdiagnostik. Ther. Ber. (Bayer) **34**, 195—200 (1962).
— E. BONTKE u. G. KERN: Zur Frage der fluoreszenzmikroskopischen Cytodiagnostik. Zbl. allg. Path. path. Anat. **102**, 318—319 (1960).
— K. J. EBSCHNER u. E. KROGH: Die Grundlage der differenten Fluorochromierung von Ribo- und Desoxyribonukleinsäure mit Acridinorange. Naturwissenschaften **44**, 467—468 (1957).
— G. KERN u. E. KERN-BONTKE: Die Acridinorange-Fluorochromierung in der gynäkologischen Zytodiagnostik bösartiger Tumoren. Mitteilungsdienst GBK 2. 482—502 (1962).

SCHÜMMELFEDER, N., E. KROGH u. K. J. EBSCHNER: Färbungsanalysen zur Acridinorange-Fluorochromierung. Vergleichende histochemische und fluoreszenzmikroskopische Untersuchungen am Kleinhirn der Maus mit Acridinorange- und Gallocyanin-Chromalaun-Färbungen. Histochemie **1**, 1—28 (1958).

SCHULMAN, H., and D. CAVANAGH: Intraepithelial carcinoma of the cervix. The predictability of residual carcinoma in the uterus from microscopic study of the margins of the cone biopsy specimen. Cancer (Philad. **14**, 795—800 (1961).

SCHWANN (1839): Zit. nach G. N. PAPANICOLAOU. Acta Un. int. Cancr. (Brux.) **14**, 249—254 (1958).

SCOTT, J. W., W. B. WELCH, and T. F. BLAKE: Bloodless technique of cold knife conization (ring biopsy). Amer. J. Obstet. Gynec. **79**, 62—66 (1960).

SCOTT, R. B., and L. A. BALLARD: Problems of cervical biopsy. Ann. N. Y. Acad. Sci. **97**, 767—781 (1962).

—, and J. W. REAGAN: Diagnostic cervical biopsy technique for the study of early cancer. Value of the cold-knife conization procedure. J. Amer. med. Ass. **160**, 343—347 (1956).

SEECOF u. BOETSCH (1924): Zit. nach G. N. PAPANICOLAOU. Acta Un. int. Cancr. (Brux.) **14**, 249—254 (1958).

SHORR, E.: A new technic for staining vaginal smears: II. Science **91**, 579—580 (1940).

— A new technic for staining vaginal smears: III. a single differential stain. Science **94**, 545—546 (1941).

SIEGEL, P.: Weitere cytologische Untersuchungsergebnisse bei Uteruscarcinomen an der Univ.-Frauenklinik Hamburg-Eppendorf. Med. Klin. **50**, 243—244 (1955).

SIEGLER, E. E.: Are spindle-shaped squamoid cells suggestive of a distinct type of carcinoma or of a distinct degree of cellular maturity? Acta cytol. (Chic.) **2**, 272—277 (1958).

SIMM, S.: The cytology of the metaplastic changes of the cervical erosion. Gynaecologia (Basel) **147**, 80—91 (1959).

SLATE, T. A., J. W. MERRITT, and C. R. KENNEDY: Trichomoniasis and its relation to cervical atypia and epidermoid carcinoma of the cervix. West. J. Surg. **68**, 298—303 (1960).

SMOLKA, H.: Die Anwendbarkeit der gynäkologischen Zytodiagnostik in Klinik und Praxis. Geburtsh. u. Frauenheilk. **18**, 88—100 (1958).

— Cervicale Zellelemente im Vaginalinhalt und ihre differentialdiagnostische Bedeutung in der cytologischen Abstrichbeurteilung. Arch. Gynäk. **195**, 53—59 (1961).

—, u. B. BERIĆ: Die Beeinflussung des Portioabstriches durch Kolposkopie-Reagenzien. Zbl. Gynäk. **80**, 1113—1114 (1958).

—, u. H. J. SOOST: Grundriß und Atlas der gynäkologischen Cytodiagnostik. Stuttgart: Georg Thieme 1956.

SOKOLOVSKY, R. M., A. B. DERAGNE, and Z. I. MALISHEVA: Morphological diagnosis of carcinoma in situ of uterine cervix. Vop. Onkol. **7**, 43—54 (1961).

SONG, Y. S., H. FANGER, and T. H. MURPHY: Significance of performing dual smear examinations in a mass screening survey for uterine cancer. Amer. J. Obstet. Gynec. **78**,1309—1311 (1959).

SOOST, H. J.: Vermeidbare technische Fehler bei der Herstellung zytologischer Präparate. Zbl. Gynäk. **80**, 622—627 (1958).

— Die Bedeutung des Ortes der Entnahme für die zytologische Krebsfährtensuche. Krebsarzt **13**, 408—420 (1958).

— Zur Frühdiagnose des Collumcarcinoms in der Praxis. Dtsch. med. Wschr. **85**, 517—518, 521—522 (1960).

— Zytodiagnostik als Teamwork zwischen Praxis und Labor. Mkurse ärztl. Fortbild. **10**, 225—226 (1960).

— Was leistet die gynäkologische Cytodiagnostik in der Krebsfährtensuche und in welchem Umfang kann der in der Praxis tätige Arzt sich ihrer bedienen? Hrsg. von der Arbeitsgemeinschaft Krebserkennung und Krebsbekämpfung in Bayern.

—, u. R. NEVIN: Die Tamponentnahme in der gynäkologischen Krebsfährtensuche. Medizinische **38**, 1754—1756 (1959).

—, u. R. PICHLMAYER: Vergleichende Untersuchungen über Fixierungsmöglichkeiten und den Versand zytologischer Präparate. Münch. med. Wschr. **101**, 1368—1370 (1959).

SOULE, E. H., and D. C. DAHLIN: Cytodetection of preclinical carcinoma of the cervix: 12 years' experience with initial screening and repeat cervical smears. Symposium. Proc. Mayo Clin. **35**, 508—513 (1960).

STAFL, A., A. LINHARTOVA u. V. DOHNAL: Das kolposkopische Bild der Felderung und seine Pathogenese. Arch. Gynäk. **199**, 223—242 (1963).

STEMMER, W.: Die Färbetechnik in der Vaginalzytologie. Ars med. (Basel) **43**, 318—320 (1953).

STERN, E.: Rate, stage and patient age in cervical cancer. An analysis of age specific discovery rates for atypical hyperplasia, in situ cancer and invasive cancer in a well population. Cancer (Philad.) **12**, 933—937 (1959).

STOECKEL, W.: Die Kolposkopie, die Diagnose und die Therapie des Portiokarzinoms. Diskussionsbemerkungen zu dem Vortrag von TREITE in der Sitzg der Berl. Gynäk. Ges. vom 15. Mai 1942. Zbl. Gynäk. **66**, 1590—1596 (1942).

STOLL, P.: Über die statistische Erfassung kolposkopischer und zytologischer Befunde in der Gynäkologie. Zbl. Gynäk. **82**, 642—646 (1960).

— Das Scheidensekret. Morphologie, Cytologie, Cyclus. Arch. Gynäk. **195**, 21—30 (1961).

— H. G. BACH u. L. RIEHM: Zytologische Karzinom-Suche in der gynäkologischen Poliklinik. Erfahrungen der Universitäts-Frauenklinik Heidelberg in den Jahren 1951—1955. Dtsch. med. Wschr. **80**, 1178—1182 (1955).

— E. MARTIN u. E. GAULRAPP: Abnorme und atypische Plattenepithelzellen im Vaginalsekret. Geburtsh. u. Frauenheilk. **14**, 509—518 (1954).

—, u. H. MUTH: Die Bedeutung des Vaginalsmear in der Differentialdiagnose gutartiger gynäkologischer Erkrankungen. Geburtsh. u. Frauenheilk. **12**, 424—435 (1952).

—, u. H. POLLMANN: Erfahrungen mit Albothyl in der gynäkologischen Praxis. Beitrag zur kolposkopischen und zytologischen Kontrolle der Behandlung von Fluor und Portioerosion. Münch. med. Wschr. **99**, 1719—1726 (1957).

—, u. L. RIEHM: Über die statistische Erfassung histologischer Befunde in der Gynäkologie. Zbl. Gynäk. **76**, 452—459 (1954).

— — u. H. G. BACH: Der „verdächtige" Ausstrich in der gynäkologischen Zytologie. Gynaecologia (Basel) **139**, 39—50 (1955).

STOPPELLI, I.: Il microscopio a fluorescenza come mezzo di ricerca in ostetricia e ginecologia. I. Possibilità di indagini nel depistage e nella diagnosi citologica dell'epitelioma del collo dell'utero. Monit. ostet.-ginec., N.S. **31**, 736—749 (1960).

STÜPER, P.: Kritik an den Erfolgsstatistiken über die Früherfassung der Kollumkarzinome durch die Zytodiagnostik. Geburtsh. u. Frauenheilk. **15**, 606—610 (1955).

SUSSMAN, W.: Detection of gynecologic cancer by fluorescence microscopy. A simple, rapid method suitable for mass screening. Amer. J. Obstet. Gynec. **82**, 1273—1276 (1961).

Symposium: Früherkennung des Collumcarcinoms. Leistungen und Grenzen der Kolposkopie, Cytologie und Histologie. Berlin-Göttingen-Heidelberg: Springer 1957.

— Advantages and disadvantages of various techniques of obtaining material for routine cytological examinations. Review of techniques of vaginal smears. Acta cytol. (Chic.) **4**, 221—235 (1960).

— Material obtained by cervical scraping only. Acta cytol. (Chic.) **4**, 242—245 (1960).

— Material obtained by two techniques: (a) Vaginal smears and (b) cervical smears. Acta cytol. (Chic.) **4**, 246—251 (1960).

— Material obtained by three techniques: (a) Vaginal smears, (b) cervical smears and (c) endocervical smears. Acta cytol. (Chic.) **4**, 252—256 (1960).

TAKEUCHI, A., and D. G. MCKAY: The area of the cervix involved by carcinoma in situ and anaplasia (atypical hyperplasia). Obstet. and Gynec. **15**, 134—145 (1960).

TAYLOR, C. W.: Histomorphology of carcinoma in situ. Acta cytol. (Philad.) **5**, 285—286 (1961).

TERRIS, M.: Epidemiology of cervical cancer. Ann. N.Y. Acad. Sci. **97**, 808—813 (1962).

TERZANO, G.: Diskussionsbemerkung zu: Occurrence of dyscaryotic cells in invasive cervical carcinoma. Acta cytol. (Chic.) **1** (1), 48 (1957).

THEISS, B.: Symptomatologie der Frühstadien des Collumcarcinoms. Diss. Köln 1963.

THORNTON, W. N., Jr., and D. E. SMITH: The relationship of the squamocolumnar junction and the endocervical glands to the site of origin of carcinoma of the cervix. Amer. J. Obstet. Gynec. **78**, 1060—1073 (1959).

TIETZE, K.: Über eine Tamponausstrichmethode in der zytologischen Diagnostik. Geburtsh. u. Frauenheilk. **18**, 746—753 (1958).

TÖRNBERG, B., B. WESTIN, and A. NORLANDER: Fluorescence microscopy and acridin-orange staining in the cytological diagnosis of atypical changes in cervical epithelium. Acta obstet. gynec. scand. **39**, 517—527 (1960).

TOWNSEND, L., and N. A. BEISCHER: The treatment of carcinoma-in-situ of the uterine cervix. Med. J. Aust. **47**, (II), 408—410 (1960).

TREITE, P.: Die Frühdiagnose des Plattenepithel-Karzinoms am Collum uteri. Stuttgart: Ferdinand Enke 1944.

TRIFON, H. M.: Detection and localization of preclinical carcinoma of the cervix by contact smears. Surg. Gynec. Obstet. **106**, 495—501 (1958).

ULM, R.: Organisation und Problematik des zytodiagnostischen Zentrums in Wien. Krebsarzt **14**, 489—503 (1959).

— R. BACHER, H. JANISCH, E. KOFLER u. H. KREMER: Ergebnisse des Zytodiagnostisch-Gynäkologischen Zentrums in Wien 1958—1961. Krebsarzt (Wien) **18**, 94—102 (1963).

UMIKER, W., L. PICKLE, and B. WAITE: Fluorescence microscopy in exfoliative cytology. An evaluation of its application to cancer screening. Brit. J. Cancer **13**, 398—402 (1959).

VÁSQUEZ-FERRO, E. C.: La biopsia selectiva del cuello uterino. Sem. méd. (B. Aires) **115**, 741—748, 768 (1959).

VÖGE, A.: Kolposkopisch faßbare Portioveränderungen, ausgewertet mit dem Elektronenrechner IBM 650. Geburtsh. u. Frauenheilk. **20**, 698—702 (1960).

WACHTEL, E.: Experimental cancer of the uterus in C_3H strain mice. J. Obstet. Gynaec. Brit. Cwlth **68**, 101—105 (1961).

WADDELL, K. E., J. S. WELCH, and D. G. DECKER: Positive cytologic findings in preclinical squamous cell epithelioma of the uterine cervix: surgical management. Symposium. Surg. Clin. N. Amer. **41**, 1025—1031 (1961).

WAGNER, D.: Die Bedeutung der Supravitalfärbung nach STEMMER für die Zytodiagnostik in der gynäkologischen Praxis. Geburtsh. u. Frauenheilk. **20**, 194 (1960).

— Über die atypische Umwandlungszone der Portio. Der zytologische Befund. Med. Bild **3**, 145—147 (1960).

— Die Erfassung des rezidivierenden Oberflächenkarzinoms am Collum uteri nach konservativer Therapie. Geburtsh. u. Frauenheilk. **21**, 944—961 (1961).

—, u. O. FETTIG: Zytologische und histologische Untersuchungen zur atypischen Umwandlungszone. Geburtsh. u. Frauenheilk. **21**, 156—169 (1961).

— H. P. KALMUS u. H. STEGMANN: Die Bedeutung der Nativfärbung für die Zytodiagnostik in der gynäkologischen Praxis. Geburtsh. u. Frauenheilk. **21**, 138—143 (1961).

—, u. H. STEGMANN: Ein neues Verfahren der Registrierung und statistischen Auswertung eines klinischen Krankengutes. Zbl. Gynäk. **81**, 378—385 (1959).

WALSCHE (1843): Zit. nach G. N. PAPANICOLAOU. Acta Un. int. Cancr. (Brux.) **14**, 249—254 (1958).

WALZ, W.: Früherfassung des Portiokarzinoms mit Hilfe der Kolposkopie, Zytologie und Kolpomikroskopie. Geburtsh. u. Frauenheilk. **15**, 949 (1955).

— Über die Früherfassung des Portiokarzinoms. Ergebnisse aus einem Zeitraum von 5 Jahren. Geburtsh. u. Frauenheilk. **18**, 243—256 (1958).

WANDALL (1944): Zit. nach G. N. PAPANICOLAOU. Acta Un. int. Cancr. (Brux.) **14**, 249—254 (1958).

WASCHKE, G.: Zur Leistungsfähigkeit der Vaginalabstrich-Diagnose und der Kolposkopie bei der Früherfassung des Portiokarzinoms. Zbl. Gynäk. **73**, 81—85 (1951).

— Über die Verwendbarkeit der Kolposkopie und der Cytodiagnostik bei Reihenuntersuchungen in gynäkologischen Geschwulstberatungsstellen. Zbl. Gynäk. **74**, 435—438 (1952).

— Ergebnisse gynäkologischer Krebsvorsorgeuntersuchungen bei 10000 Frauen. Ärztl. Wschr. **9**, 398—399 (1954).

— Die Bedeutung des Sichtlochkartenverfahrens für die Einrichtung und Auswertung von Krebsstatistiken an Frauenkliniken. Zbl. Gynäk. **81**, 748—755 (1959).

WATTEVILLE, H. DE, W. GEISENDORF et L. DANON: Le diagnostik précoce du cancer du col et son traitement au stade non invasif. Bull. Féd. Soc. Gynéc. Obstét. franç. **4**, Suppl. 1, 38—79 (1952).

WAY, S.: The Diagnosis of Early Carcinoma of the Cervix. London: J. and A. Churchill Lt
1963.

WEBER, M.: Bericht über die Tätigkeit der gynäkologischen Konsiliarstellen in Nordrhei
Westfalen in den Jahren 1952—1957. Geburtsh. u. Frauenheilk. **19**, 119—134 (1959).

— Krebsbekämpfung in Nordrhein-Westfalen durch Vorsichtsuntersuchung in den Kreb
beratungsstellen 1952—1960. Mitteilungsdienst GBK **2**, 235—247 (1961).

WEILL, G., et S. DELAGE: Moyens actuels de dépistage du cancer, du col utérin en pratiqu
courante. Strasbourg méd., N.S. **10**, 419—422 (1959).

WEINER, I., L. BURKE, and M. A. GOLDBERGER: Carcinoma of the cervix in jewish wome
Amer. J. Obstet. Gynec. **61**, 418—422 (1951).

WESPI, H. J.: Erfahrungen mit der systematischen Kolposkopie an der Züricher Fraue
klinik. Zbl. Gynäk. **32**, 1762—1776 (1938).

— Entstehung und Früherfassung des Portiokarzinoms. Basel: Benno Schwabe & Co. 194

— Kolpophotographie. Gynaecologia (Basel) **131**, 65—73 (1951).

— Altersverteilung und Latenzzeit bei Portiokarzinom. Gynaecologia (Basel) **133**, 169—17
(1952).

— Colposcopy in the diagnosis of cervical pathology. J. Obstet. Gynaec. (Ludhiana) **15**
171—186 (1954).

— Vergleich zwischen Zytologie und Colposkopie in der Entdeckung von Frühkarzinomen
Acta Un. int. Cancr. (Brux.) **14**, 350—352 (1958).

— Die Kolpophotographie. Oncologia (Basel) **11**, 66—71 (1958).

— Rationelle Früherfassung des weiblichen Genitalkarzinoms. Gynaecologia (Basel) **147**
356—371 (1959).

—, u. W. LOTMAR: Fortschritte der Kolpophotographie und ihre Bedeutung. Gynaecologi
(Basel) **137**, 281—306 (1954).

—, u. H. SAUTER: Der Einfluß von Alter und Geburtenzahl auf die Entstehung des Genital-
carcinoms. Z. Krebsforsch. **53**, 347—357 (1943).

WHEELER, C. B., Jr.: Carcinoma of the cervix with early stromal invasion. Amer. J. Obstet.
Gynec. **72**, 119—124 (1956).

WIDAL, (1890): Zit. nach G. N. PAPANICOLAOU. Acta Un. int. Cancr. (Brux.) **14**, 249—25
(1958).

WIED, G. L.: Differentialdiagnostische Betrachtungen über den cytologischen Vaginalabstrich.
Dtsch. Gesundh.-Wes. **5**, 1444—1450 (1950).

— Eine Untersuchung über die Zweckmäßigkeit gefärbter oder vitaler Präparate für die
Zytodiagnostik. Geburtsh. u. Frauenheilk. **11**, 897—909 (1951).

— Importance of the site from which vaginal cytologic smears are taken. Amer. J. clin. Path.
25, 742—750 (1955).

— The potentialities of the smear technique for the differentiation of noninvasive and invasive
cervical carcinoma. Amer. J. Obstet. Gynec. **71**, 793—805 (1956).

— The interpretation of inflammatory reactions in the vagina, cervix and endocervix by
means of cytologic smears. Amer. J. clin. Path. **28**, 233—242 (1957).

—, and G. F. BAHR: Vaginal, cervical and endocervical cytologic smears on a single slide.
Obstet. and Gynec. **14**, 362—367 (1959).

—, u. W. CHRISTIANSEN: Die Zytolyse von Epithelien des Vaginalsekretes. Geburtsh. u.
Frauenheilk. **13**, 986—995 (1953).

— — Bedeutung und Einfluß der Bakterienflora im zytologischen Vaginalausstrich. Zbl.
Bakt., 1. Abt. Med. Hyg. Bakt. Virusforschg. u. Parasitol. **160**, 413—424 (1953/54).

—, u. A. M. DARGAN: Die cytologische Differenzierung verschiedener Ausbreitungsgrade des
Collumcarcinoms. Arch. Gynäk. **189**, 358—363 (1957).

—, y J. R. DEL SOL: Es posible diferenciar el carcinoma invasor del cérvix uterino del carci-
noma "in situ" empleando la citologia exfoliativa? Acta ginec. (Madr.) **9**, 49—63 (1958).

— G. LEGORRETA, D. MOHR, and A. RAUZY: Cytology of invasive cervical carcinoma and
carcinoma in situ. Ann. N.Y. Acad. Sci. **97**, 759—766 (1962).

WIHMAN, G.: A contribution to the knowledge of the cellular content in exudates and transu-
dates. Acta med. scand. **130**, Suppl. 205, 1—124 (1948).

WILDNER, G. P.: Krebskrankenerfassung und Krebskrankenstatistik. Krebsforsch. u. Krebs-
bekämpf. **41**, 253—279 (1959).

WILLIAMS, J.: Cancer of the uterus. Harveian Lectures for 1886. London: K. H. Lewis 1888.
WINTER, G.: Die Früherfassung des Krebses in der Zukunft. Arch Gynäk. **173**, 80—85 (1942).
WINTER, G. F.: Neue klinische Erfahrungen beim Oberflächenkarzinom. Geburtsh. u. Frauenheilk. **18**, 484—487 (1958).
WURCH, T. A., et J. P. ISAAC: Nouvelle technique de coloration histologique différentielle en trois temps pour le diagnostic des cancers des voies génitales de la femme par la méthode cytologique. Rev. franç. Gynéc. **46**, 319—325 (1951).
WYNDER, E. L.: Circumcision as a preventive factor against cancer of the cervix. Proc. 3rd Nat. Canc. Conf. **1956/57**, p. 603—607.
— Die Beschneidung in der Prophylaxe des Kollumkarzinoms. Dtsch. med. Wschr. **82**, 1333—1336 (1957).
— J. CORNFIELD, P. D. SCHROFF, and K. R. DORAISWAMI: A study of environmental factors in carcinoma of the cervix. Amer. J. Obstet. Gynec. **68**, 1016—1052 (1954).
—, and S. D. LICKLIDER: The question of circumcision. Cancer (Philad.) **13**, 442—445 (1960).
— N. MANTEL, and S. D. LICKLIDER: Statistical considerations on circumcision and cervical cancer. Amer. J. Obstet. Gynec. **79**, 1026—1030 (1960).
WYSS, H. J.: Zusammenhang zwischen kolposkopischem und histologischem Befund in der Schillerschen Abschabung. Arch. Gynäk. **194**, 365—394 (1961).
YOUNGE, P. A.: Preinvasive carcinoma of the cervix. Arch. Path. **27**, 804—805 (1939).
— A gynecologist's evaluation of methods of early cancer diagnosis. In: F. HOMBURGER and W. H. FISHMAN, The Laboratory Diagnosis of Cancer of the Cervix. New York: S. Karger 1956.
— Cancer of the uterine cervix. A preventable disease. Obstet. and Gynec. **10**, 469—481 (1957).
— Problems concerning the diagnosis and treatment of carcinoma in situ of the uterine cervix. Amer. J. Roentgenol. **79**, 479—483 (1958).
— A. T. HERTIG, and D. ARMSTRONG: A study of 135 cases of carcinoma in situ of the cervix at the Free Hospital for Women. Amer. J. Obstet. Gynec. **58**, 867—892 (1949).
—, and A. Y. KEVORKIAN: Carcinoma in situ of the cervix. The problems of detection and evaluation in regard of the therapy. Ciba Found. Study Gr. No 3, 83—103. London: J. and A. Churchill Ltd. 1959.
ZACHERL, H.: Schwierigkeiten der histologischen Diagnose der Anfangsstadien des Collumcarcinoms. Arch. Gynäk. **189**, 346—355 (1957).
—, u. E. SCHÜLLER: Diagnostische und therapeutische Probleme beim beginnenden Kollumkarzinom. Wien. med. Wschr. **107**, 32—35 (1957).
ZADEK, I.: Die Zytologie der Exsudate und Transsudate. In: HIRSCHFELD u. HITTMAIR, Handbuch der allgemeinen Hämatologie, Bd. 1, S. 1373—1418. Berlin u. Wien: Urban & Schwarzenberg 1933.
ZECHNER, F.: Die Krebskrankenstatistik in Österreich. Krebsarzt **15**, 244—250 (1960).
ZEMANSKY, A. P.: Examination of fluids for tumor cells. Analysis of 113 cases checked against subsequent examination of tissue. Amer. J. med. Sci. **175**, 489—504 (1928).
ZIMMER, S.: Erfahrungen mit der Zytodiagnostik bei der Karzinomfährtensuche in der Praxis. Dtsch. Gesundh.-Wes. **1957**, 1466—1468.
— Zur Methodik der Früherkennung des Kollumkarzinoms in der Sprechstunde des praktischen Arztes. Z. ärztl. Fortbild. **51**, 94—96 (1957).
— Über die Anwendung krebsprophylaktischer Untersuchungsmethoden in der Praxis. Forsch. Fortschr. dtsch. Wiss. **33**, 193—197 (1959).
— Schwierigkeiten und Erfolge bei der Anwendung krebsprophylaktischer Untersuchungsmethoden in der Praxis. Z. ärztl. Fortbild. **53**, 321—323 (1959).
ZINSER, H. K.: Was wird aus den Matrixbezirken an der Portio? Zbl. Gynäk. **71**, 1164—1173 (1949).
— Die vitalzytologische Karzinomdiagnose. Z. Geburtsh. Gynäk. **133**, 74—106 (1950).
— Vergleichende Untersuchungen mit der Kolposkopie und Cytologie. Arch. Gynäk. **180**, 55—58 (1951).
— Zur Anwendung spezieller Färbemethoden in der Zytodiagnostik. Z. Geburtsh. Gynäk. **140**, 299—313 (1954).
— Die Zytodiagnostik in der Gynäkologie, 2. Aufl. Jena: Gustav Fischer 1957.

ZINSER, H. K.: The unfixed dyscaryotic cells under the phase contrast microscope. Acta cytol. (Chic.) **1** (1), 36—37 (1957).
— Vergleich zwischen Zytologie und Colposkopie in der Entdeckung von Frühkarzinomen. Acta Un. int. Cancr. (Brux.) **14**, 353—354 (1958).
— Gynäkologische Karzinomfrühdiagnostik. Strahlentherapie **107**, 635—643 (1958).
— Organisatorische Fragen der cytologischen Krebsfrühdiagnostik. Mitteilungsdienst GBK **3**, 1—9 (1959).
— Organisation der Zytologie, Anwendung und Ausbildung. Krebsforsch. u. Krebsbekämpf. **41**, 283—293 ((1959).
— Das zytodiagnostische gynäkologische Zentrum. Krebsarzt **14**, 484—489 (1959).
— Studien an der gefäßinjizierten Zervix. Geburtsh. u. Frauenheilk. **20**, 651—657 (1960).
— Ergebnisse und Erfahrungen cytologischer Zentren der Gesellschaft zur Bekämpfung der Krebskrankheiten in Nordrhein-Westfalen 1957—1961. Mitteilungsdienst GBK **2**, 247—254 (1961).
— Erfahrungen und Ergebnisse zytologischer Zentren. (Ein Fünfjahresbericht.) Zbl. Gynäk. **84**, 905—917 (1962).
—, u. H. DIEGRITZ: Fortschritte und Grenzen der Frühdiagnostik des Kollum-Karzinoms. Geburtsh. u. Frauenheilk. **12**, 782—804 (1952).
—, u. G. KERN: Kritische Betrachtungen zur Karzinomfrühdiagnostik. Geburtsh. u. Frauenheilk. **18**, 105—118 (1958).
— H. MEISSNER u. H. P. BÖTZELEN: Diagnostische und therapeutische Betrachtungen an 403 Frühfällen. Geburtsh. u. Frauenheilk. **23**, 321—342 (1963).
—, K. H. ROSENBAUER: Untersuchungen über die Angioarchitektonik der normalen und pathologisch veränderten Cervix uteri. Arch. Gynäk. **194**, 73—112 (1960).
— — Untersuchungen an der gefäßinjizierten Cervix uteri. Geburtsh. u. Frauenheilk. **20**, 657—660 (1960).

Subject Index

The page numbers in *italics* indicate principal references.

GPSR Compliance
The European Union's (EU) General Product Safety Regulation (GPSR) is a set of rules that requires consumer products to be safe and our obligations to ensure this.

If you have any concerns about our products, you can contact us on

ProductSafety@springernature.com

In case Publisher is established outside the EU, the EU authorized representative is:

Springer Nature Customer Service Center GmbH
Europaplatz 3
69115 Heidelberg, Germany

www.ingramcontent.com/pod-product-compliance
Ingram Content Group UK Ltd.
Pitfield, Milton Keynes, MK11 3LW, UK
UKHW021303051126
16364UKWH00004B/5
9783662251508